Risk Communication in Public Health Emergencies

"Dr. Melville offers a timely and very thought-provoking book. Reflecting on the COVID-19 pandemic, it is easy to acknowledge the important role of crisis and emergency risk communication. The book is well written, and the case studies portray easily relatable examples for most professionals responsible for communications or who are positioned on the periphery of the communications functions. The skills to be gained in these pages will strengthen our collective ability to respond efficiently, effectively, and cohesively to health security challenges during the next pandemic or during the next disaster in your area of responsibility."

Stephen Murphy, PhD, MPH, MBA, Program Director – MS in Health Security, and Director of the Region 6 Center for Health Security and Response Readiness at Tulane University C. S. Weatherhead School of Public Health and Tropical Medicine

Risk Communication in Public Health Emergencies

Practical Guidance Rooted in Theory

Kathleen G. V. Melville
Tulane University Celia Scott Weatherhead School of Public Health and Tropical Medicine

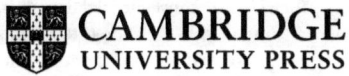

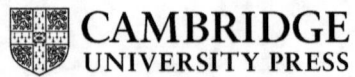

Shaftesbury Road, Cambridge CB2 8EA, United Kingdom

One Liberty Plaza, 20th Floor, New York, NY 10006, USA

477 Williamstown Road, Port Melbourne, VIC 3207, Australia

314–321, 3rd Floor, Plot 3, Splendor Forum, Jasola District Centre, New Delhi – 110025, India

103 Penang Road, #05-06/07, Visioncrest Commercial, Singapore 238467

Cambridge University Press is part of Cambridge University Press & Assessment, a department of the University of Cambridge.

We share the University's mission to contribute to society through the pursuit of education, learning and research at the highest international levels of excellence.

www.cambridge.org
Information on this title: www.cambridge.org/9781009449038

DOI: 10.1017/9781009449069

© Kathleen G. V. Melville 2025

This publication is in copyright. Subject to statutory exception and to the provisions of relevant collective licensing agreements, no reproduction of any part may take place without the written permission of Cambridge University Press & Assessment.

When citing this work, please include a reference to the DOI 10.1017/9781009449069

First published 2025

A catalogue record for this publication is available from the British Library

A Cataloging-in-Publication data record for this book is available from the Library of Congress

ISBN 978-1-009-44903-8 Paperback

Cambridge University Press & Assessment has no responsibility for the persistence or accuracy of URLs for external or third-party internet websites referred to in this publication and does not guarantee that any content on such websites is, or will remain, accurate or appropriate.

....

Every effort has been made in preparing this book to provide accurate and up-to-date information that is in accord with accepted standards and practice at the time of publication. Although case histories are drawn from actual cases, every effort has been made to disguise the identities of the individuals involved. Nevertheless, the authors, editors, and publishers can make no warranties that the information contained herein is totally free from error, not least because clinical standards are constantly changing through research and regulation. The authors, editors, and publishers therefore disclaim all liability for direct or consequential damages resulting from the use of material contained in this book. Readers are strongly advised to pay careful attention to information provided by the manufacturer of any drugs or equipment that they plan to use.

Contents

List of Case Study Contributors vi

1 Why You Need to Care about Emergency Risk Communication 1

Part I Precrisis Planning

2 Precrisis Planning Is Necessary for Public Information and Emergency Communications: Leveraging What You've Got 25

3 Identifying Who Needs to Know What and When: It's Not a Surprise What Your Audiences Need to Know 51

4 Addressing the Information Needs of the Public and Medical Community during a Public Health Emergency 76

5 How to Get the Message Out: Understanding All of Your Communication Channels and When to Use Them 107

Part II Communicating during a Health Emergency

6 Initial Messages during a Health Emergency: Addressing Uncertainty and Creating Trust with the Public 139

7 Maintenance Messages during a Health Emergency: How to Protect the Public's Health and Debunking Misinformation 164

8 Communicating during Long Public Health Emergencies: Creating Health Communication Campaigns 201

Part III Communicating and Planning after a Health Emergency

9 Pivoting from Crisis Management to Recovery: Communicating the End of a Health Emergency 225

10 Evaluating Emergency Risk Communication and Engaging in Public Education for the Next Emergency 257

Part IV Crisis Leadership

11 Effective Communication during a Health Emergency: The Role of the Spokesperson and Working with the Media 281

12 Crisis Leadership: Staying Steady on Unsteady Ground 305

Index 327

List of Case Study Contributors

Paige A. Gray, MPH
Case Study of Public Health Crisis: Outbreak of *Legionella* in Central Ohio Hospital (2019)

Laura Herrmann, MPH
Derailment of Norfolk South Train in East Palestine, Ohio: An Analysis of Crisis & Emergency Risk Communication

Jaime Jimenez, MPH
Case Study: The Water Crisis in Jackson, Mississippi

Maxwell M. Leonhardt, MD, MPH
Disaster Communications in Dallas, Texas: Using CERC Principles to Analyze CDC Communications When the Ebola Epidemic Came to the United States

Madison Dulas, MSW, MS-DRL, LGSW
Intersection of the California Camp Fire and CERC Principles

Mae M. Brooks, MPH
Analysis of CERC Framework during the Flint Water Crisis

Emma Caroli de la Rosa MPH
2022 Mpox Outbreak in Louisiana

Jessica Worthington, MPH
An Analysis of the Georgia Department of Public Health's Response to COVID-19

Julie Mayo Lamberte, MSPH
The EVALI Public Health Emergency and the Response by the Georgia Department of Public Health

Lynn A. Walkiewicz, PhD, MSW
Maine Messaging during the time of COVID-19: The Leadership Style of Dr. Nirav Shah

Kishla Askins, MPH
Analyzing Prime Minister of New Zealand Jacinda Ardern's COVID-19 Communication Using the CERC framework

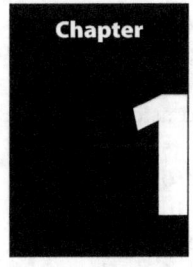

Chapter 1

Why You Need to Care about Emergency Risk Communication

Chapter Objectives
- Identify how to use this book to support emergency communication planning, implementation, and evaluation.
- Describe different public health communication terms.
- Name the six Crisis and Emergency Risk Communication (CERC) principles.
- Explain the CERC framework and phase-based messaging framework.
- Summarize how risk perception impacts emergency risk communication.
- Explain the importance of strong relationships between leaders and communication officers.

Between December 2019 and May 2023, the world was ravaged by a virus that caused as much destruction as Achilles during the Trojan War. The COVID-19 pandemic impacted individuals worldwide, regardless of their geographic location, religious or political beliefs, occupation, or social standing. People's experience was directly impacted by lockdown measures, physical distancing, masks, vaccine recommendations, or illnesses of self or friends or family members, as well as by how their local and national elected officials and public health leaders managed and communicated about the pandemic. As people went into lockdown, they went online and found a flood of information both true and false about the pandemic. The constant deluge of online information, the new and evolving outbreak, and the worldwide impact created a complex health emergency.

Public health agencies worldwide faced a global pandemic. Despite decades of tabletop discussions, functional exercises, and even real-life health emergencies like H1N1 and Ebola to help us prepare and respond to a global pandemic, the US public health system experienced early setbacks that impacted its attempts to contain the outbreak: faulty tests created by the Centers for Disease Control and Prevention (CDC), mixed messaging on the use of masks due to personal protective equipment shortages, the inadequate Strategic National Stockpile, and the lack of a suitable national testing strategy. As the outbreak evolved, the public health system faced issues regarding vaccine effectiveness, vaccine hesitancy, pandemic fatigue, and a politicization of public health recommendations. The complexity of the outbreak further exacerbated communication challenges, resulting in conflicting messages from US government leaders at the federal and state levels. The public was often left wondering what the most accurate information was, who the most credible leader to trust was, and, ultimately, what the best action to take to avoid severe illness was.

As public health leaders, medical doctors, health care providers, emergency management officials, government officials, and graduate students, it is imperative to understand what emergency risk communication is and how to leverage such a powerful tool before, during, and after health emergencies. In the United States, during the COVID-19 emergency response, pandemic playbooks and emergency risk communication strategies developed over decades by previous administrations were tossed aside by White House officials.[1,2,3] Instead of coordinating pandemic response efforts at the federal level to ensure access to needed medical resources and supplies across the United States, the White House viewed the unfolding health emergency without adequate appreciation for the seriousness and scale of the risk. Further, instead of leveraging emergency risk communication principles, the President continued to deny the health threat, and his communication strategy was to overly reassure the public and avoid addressing the uncertainty of the situation through statements like, "The Coronavirus is very much under control in the USA."[2] While career public health professionals and medical doctors like Dr. Nancy Messonnier, Dr. Anthony Fauci, and Dr. Deborah Birks tried to engage in transparent communication about the health risks and potential disruption to life posed by COVID-19, their messages to the public were often walked back by the White House, creating confusion and dispelling the trust of the American public.[2]

Used appropriately and in tandem with dedicated emergency response plans, emergency risk communication can get the right information to the right people at the right time to prevent severe health impacts.[4] Previously, emergency risk communication was a tool used by some medical doctors and public information officers (PIOs) within health departments, but today, with the emergence of new health emergencies around the world, the ability to understand and use emergency risk communication should no longer be reserved for those at the top of these organizations; rather, it needs to be a basic core capacity that anyone working in public health, health care, or emergency response can understand and utilize in their jobs. Much like putting on a seat belt when getting into a car, emergency risk communication needs to be the first thing we consider in emergency planning and response, not an afterthought for fixing something that has already gone wrong.

COVID-19 revealed severe cracks in the public health system,[5] including:

- The need for more comprehensive regional and national disease registries, especially for infectious diseases
- The need to develop efficient mechanisms and detection tools to more rapidly and accurately identify cases of COVID-19 and other infectious diseases
- The need for laboratories to scale up testing
- The need to streamline future responses and educate stakeholders on the measures and actions to take during a health emergency
- The need for worker education and development to address misinformation
- The need for better private–public partnerships to address supply chain issues for personal protective equipment
- The need for additional workforce development and training in the public and private sectors to ensure that the various stakeholders are capable of responding to outbreaks as is pertinent to their skills and positions.

The reduction of federal appropriations to support public health preparedness in the United States creates a predictable situation: Gutted health departments will be unable to prepare for or respond to the next inevitable health emergency. The 2021 Public Health

Workforce Interests and Needs Survey discovered that many are leaving the public health workforce, and the pandemic is often cited as a cause:

> Nearly one-third of state and local public health employees (32%) said they are considering leaving their organization in the next year – 5% to retire and 27% for another reason. Among those who said they're considering leaving, 39% said the pandemic has made them more likely to leave. Looking out further, 44% said they are considering leaving within the next five years.[6]

With a burned-out and fed-up workforce coupled with the reduction of public health authorities across the United States, one could think that the future of public health is dismal. But when considering crises and emergencies, out of destruction and loss come opportunity and renewal.[7,8]

The opportunity is here for health departments, health care systems, emergency management, and graduate students in these fields to learn what went wrong in COVID-19, what can be learned from these mistakes, and what can be done to ensure similar mistakes do not occur in the future. Through after-action reviews, government agencies can look at the cracks in their own institutions to understand what relationships need to be built and how to continue to uphold their mission to protect the health and safety of citizens.

How to Use This Book

This book focuses on crisis and emergency risk communication (CERC) to educate and inform current and future public health leaders, health care providers, emergency management officials, government officials, and graduate students on how to plan, create, disseminate, and evaluate emergency risk communication during health emergencies. The CDC's CERC framework is highlighted to demonstrate its application of emergency risk communication strategies and activities to health emergencies.[4,9] Case studies written by public health students from Tulane University analyze health emergencies like COVID-19, Mpox, and the Norfolk Southern train derailment using the CERC framework to understand how to communicate accurate and actionable health information. Additional theories like risk perception, the health belief model, agenda setting, mindfulness, and transformational leadership and their relevance to emergency risk communication are included. To deepen the reader's exploration and learning of emergency risk communication through practical application, mini case studies, examples, and discussion questions are provided.

This book is made up of four parts: precrisis planning, communicating during a health emergency, communicating and evaluating after a health emergency, and crisis leadership.

- Part I: Precrisis Planning builds the foundation for emergency communications by outlining critical steps in the communication planning process, identifying key audiences, and addressing the unique information needs of the medical community during a health emergency.
- Part II: Communicating during a Health Emergency provides specific practices and guidelines for constructing messages during the various phases of an emergency response.
- Part III: Communicating and Evaluating after a Health Emergency outlines how to pivot from emergency messaging to messages of renewal. It also offers key tips on learning lessons from the emergency response.

- Part IV: Crisis Leadership provides key tips and best practices on being a spokesperson. It is Media Relations 101. This part also provides practical guidance on how to be an effective leader during a health emergency.

Health Emergencies and Public Health Preparedness

Health emergencies can be defined as emergent situations with health consequences that overwhelm routine health department capacities and capabilities.[10] For health departments to be ready to respond to health emergencies, engaging in public health emergency preparedness (PHEP) activities is crucial. PHEP activities include establishing an infrastructure to support emergency operations (i.e., emergency operations centers, Incident Command Structures) and identifying key personnel to assist in this.[10] The ability of health departments to leverage and integrate public health preparedness with existing systems and public health practices allows for emergency response activities to be quickly scaled up during health emergency responses.[10]

Health emergencies often impact not only community residents but also businesses and nongovernmental organizations. Developing and maintaining relationships within the community and engaging with these stakeholders prior to a health emergency are key preparedness activities. Key preparedness activities fall under three main categories: preplanned and coordinated rapid response capability; expert and fully staffed workforce; and accountability and quality improvement.

- Preplanned and coordinated rapid response capability includes understanding hazards and vulnerabilities within the community (i.e., community health assessments and populations at risk); knowledge of legal authority and liability barriers for the health agency; roles and responsibilities; Incident Command Systems; public engagement; epidemiological functions; laboratory functions; countermeasures and mitigation strategies; mass health care; public information and communication; and robust supply chains.[10]
- Expert and fully staffed workforce means having a skilled workforce that can perform well during a health emergency and leaders who can manage the health emergency, engage with stakeholders, and effectively communicate response operations and mitigation strategies.[10]
- Accountability and quality improvement include testing operational capabilities, performance management, and financial tracking.[10]

Another key feature of public health preparedness is understanding the legal authority that public health departments have during a declared health emergency. State laws dictate the amount of legal power that health officials have during a formally declared emergency to enact measures to protect the health and safety of a community:

> Once a public health emergency is declared, designated officials can harness powers that are typically unavailable without legislative approval, by issuing emergency orders. These expansive powers may include deploying military personnel, commandeering property, restricting freedom of movement, halting business operations, and suspending civil rights and liberties.[11]

See Chapter 3 for more on public health powers.

Public Health Communication Terminology

"Communication" is often considered an umbrella term, something casually used with an assumption that its definition is the same to everyone. Often, however, it turns out that people are not on the same page, resulting in project delays and even financial losses. These same assumptions are also made regarding health communication, risk communication, crisis communication, and emergency risk communication. The terms "crisis" and "emergency" are often overused, and if one listens to the news media, everything is now a crisis. To help create a common understanding of terms, this first chapter will outline common terms used in public health preparedness and response. Let's define these terms to understand how they will be used throughout this book.

Health Communication

It is important to understand health communication, as it is fundamental to the work of public health and for programs designed to change behavior. Health communication is "the study and use of communication strategies to inform and influence individual and community decisions that enhance health."[12] Health communicators use a wide range of methods to design communication programs relating to media literacy, media advocacy, public relations, advertising, education entertainment, individual and group instruction, and partnership development.[12] Some of these methods will also be used in emergency risk communication activities, so it is helpful for emergency risk communicators to understand how public health programs use these methods and maintain partnerships during nonemergency times.

Health communication from the perspective of a health department involves communicating information at the population or community level, not at the individual level. Within health departments, there is often a team or program called the "health promotion" or "health education" team. This type of health promotion or health education is what is generally referred to by public health staffers as routine, day-to-day public health communication. Health departments want to inform, influence, and motivate groups of people to take action to improve or maintain their health.[13] Health promotion activities focus on adolescent health, sexual health, breastfeeding, school health, physical activity, and immunizations.[14]

An example of a federal health promotion program is the Move Your Way campaign developed by the US Department of Health and Human Services (HHS).[15] The campaign is focused on getting citizens to live healthier lives by increasing their physical activity. By focusing on the entire nation, the campaign is designed to inform, influence, and motivate a group of people to act together: a key component of health promotion activities.

On an individual level, an example of health communication is speaking with your health care provider – a doctor, nurse, nurse practitioner, naturopath, acupuncturist, therapist – about your current health status or health concerns. This basic, interpersonal, one-to-one communication is focused solely on the individual and the individual's health. In terms of study samples, the sample size in this case is one. This type of individual communication between patient and health care provider is also important during health emergencies. Research continues to show that health care providers are a trusted source of information during emergencies.[16]

Risk Communication

Another key term used by public health practitioners, health care providers, and emergency management officials is "risk communication." Generally, the definition for "risk communication" is the same across multiple agencies and industries: communication messages that alert people to some type of hazard or threat to life or property. For public health practitioners, risk communication focuses on the risks and benefits of a given action to protect one's health.[17]

Let's examine risk communication related to the benefits and risks of getting the vaccine for measles, mumps, rubella, and varicella (MMRV), a vaccine for children and young adults attending college. In the United States, CDC recommends all children get two doses of MMRV vaccine, starting with the first dose at 12–15 months of age and with the second dose at 4–6 years of age. Additionally, students who will attend post-high school educational institutions and who are likely to live in close quarters with others, such as in dormitories or shared housing, need to get additional doses of MMRV vaccine. The benefit of getting the MMRV vaccine is immunity protection against measles, mumps, rubella, and varicella.

The risks associated with getting a vaccine, or even with taking certain medications, are side effects. For the MMRV vaccine, the side effects include a sore arm from the shot, fever, and a mild rash. In some cases, the MMRV vaccine can cause swelling of the neck or checks or a temporary low platelet count (the cells that help with blood clotting). In rare cases, as with most vaccines, a person can experience a severe allergic reaction also known as anaphylaxis. This type of allergic reaction can occur in people who have a life-threatening reaction to components that make up the vaccine, such as gelatin or the antibiotic neomycin.

In this example of risk communication, the individual ultimately needs to decide whether they want to take the action recommended by their health care provider. The individual weighs the risks and the benefits and determines whether the benefits outweigh the risks. This type of decision-making is characterized by a theory called "significant choice" and is based on a person making a rational decision. The significant choice framework comes from the work of Thomas Nilsen and is defined as a choice made based on the best information available when the decision must be made.[18]

The implication here for health communicators regarding risk communication is that there is a power differential between the person sharing the risk information and the person receiving the risk information. Those receiving the information are in a submissive and vulnerable position. This is why it is so critical for communicators to understand the power and influence that is wielded when engaging in risk communication. The stakes become even higher in emergency risk communications. In this situation, for individuals to make the best decision – to make their significant choice – they are relying on those sharing the risk information to be fully truthful, honest, and transparent with the information that is being provided.

Let's take risk communication a step further and explore how risk communication can be used as a form of risk management. The US National Research Council defines risk communication as a two-way flow of information – including fact and opinion – with the goal of facilitating better risk management decisions.[19] Here's an example of risk communication that includes a two-way exchange of information to lead to better risk management.

Mini-Case Study: Triangle Lake, Oregon

Individuals living in rural Oregon near Triangle Lake began raising concerns about pesticides being used in industrial forest management practices in Oregon's coastal mountains. In 2010, residents of the area were approached by a researcher from Emory University who conducted an initial investigation by collecting urine samples from the community members. The results of that study – which indicated elevated levels of pesticides but not high enough for a public health concern – were shared with the Oregon Department of Forestry.[20] Oregon Health Authority (OHA) was contacted to perform a community health assessment to see whether pesticides were present in the area and whether there were any potential health effects from the pesticide use. OHA launched an investigation, and various samples were collected for analysis, including urine, water, soil, and foods.[20,21] The investigation eventually ruled out pesticide exposure through drinking water, soil, and homegrown food, leaving the culprit to be air exposure.[22] The OHA report revealed that residents had been exposed to the chemicals atrazine and 2,4-D.[21,23,24]

This example shows how risk communication was used as risk management that created a dialogue between the community, private companies, and the government to inform risk management decisions. Engaging in risk communication as a dialogue removes the power differential and provides an opportunity for communities to engage in emergency responses. See Chapter 10 for more on engaging the public through community-based participatory research.

Crisis Communication

"Crisis communication" is another common term used in both private and public sectors. In the public relations industry, crisis communication is most often related to responding to a situation with the goal of maintaining the reputation of the business. This perspective is known as "reputation management" – ensuring that the image of the business or organization does not deteriorate to such a degree that it negatively impacts product sales, stock prices, and other financial assets.

A crisis is defined as an unexpected event or series of events that creates a perceived threat, has an element of surprise, and has high levels of uncertainty.[7] There are three key aspects of an organizational crisis: heightened media attention, shortened response time, and uncertainty.

These characteristics of heightened media attention, shortened response time, and an uncertain situation can be seen in an anthrax attack that occurred in the United States in 2001: The anthrax attack drew widespread media attention, the nature of the threat to humans required the government to act fast to contain and mitigate health harm, and given the nature of the situation – a terrorist attack – the situation was very uncertain. A year after the attack, I served as an intern in Washington, DC, for then US Senator Tom Daschle. Senator Daschle was one of the people targeted during the attack. Staff members would share the story of what happened on the day of the attack, the hazmat procedures that were put in place, and how staff dealt with being exposed to such a lethal substance. Luckily no one on Senator Daschle's staff died, but some of the postal workers exposed to the anthrax through the mail service did die due to their exposures.

For emergency risk communicators the anthrax attack showed the need for message consistency, timeliness, and accuracy. Because the situation – a bioterrorism attack – was a novel situation for CDC to respond to, there was limited science on how to mitigate the health threat. Plus, CDC's pressroom only had a few people working there, with no clear crisis communication plans or policies in place. As a result, CDC had over 80 spokespeople communicating during the response. Having 80 spokespeople speaking to the press is not an ideal situation during a crisis.[25] As a result, CDC took the time to learn from the anthrax response and thus began the development of the CERC term and theoretical framework.[17]

Crisis and Emergency Risk Communication: CERC Framework and Phase-Based Messaging

CERC consists of messages that include the urgency of crisis communication and the need to communicate risks and benefits to stakeholders in the public.[4,17] CERC is the communication model and framework CDC created in 2002.[17] The first edition of CERC was initially created as a manual to support federal relations between agencies and the press. The 2014 CERC manual includes 12 modules focused on explanations of crisis communication and the psychology of a crisis, message development, crisis communication plans, spokesperson guidelines, working with the media, public health law, and human resource considerations. It also includes references to the National Incident Management System (NIMS) and the use of Joint Information Centers to coordinate health information between agencies involved in an emergency response.

"CERC can be described as a standardized methodology for the communication function of government agencies responding to public health emergencies."[17] The CERC framework has been used to analyzed to numerous health emergencies including pandemic influenza, hospital emergencies, severe winter storms, H1N1, and food recalls.[17] Since CERC has been a foundational mainstay in the field of public health, case studies using the CERC framework will be shared throughout this book. These case studies were created by students at Tulane University's Celia Scott Weatherhead School of Public Health and Tropical Medicine who participated in the Disaster and Emergency Communications class taught by the author.

CERC Principles

The CERC framework focuses on six principles as the tenets for effective CERC: Be First, Be Right, Be Credible, Express Empathy, Promote Action, and Show Respect (see Figure 1.1). The framework also includes explanations of how to create messages for different phases of the crisis communication life cycle (i.e., precrisis, initial, maintenance, recovery, and evaluation).[4,9,26] In short, the CERC framework provides an outline of the what and how of CERC.

> Be First: Crises are time-sensitive. Communicating information quickly is always important. For members of the public, the first source of information often becomes the preferred source. If your agency is legally required to respond to the emergency, being the first agency to release information is important for legitimizing the response operations and mitigating the health threat to the community.[4,9,26]
>
> Be Right: Accuracy establishes credibility. Information can include what is known, what is not known, and what is being done to fill in the gaps. Accuracy of information supports organizational credibility. For an organization to be right in the early stages of an emergency, addressing uncertainty is critical. See Chapter 6 for specifics on addressing uncertainty.[4,9,26]

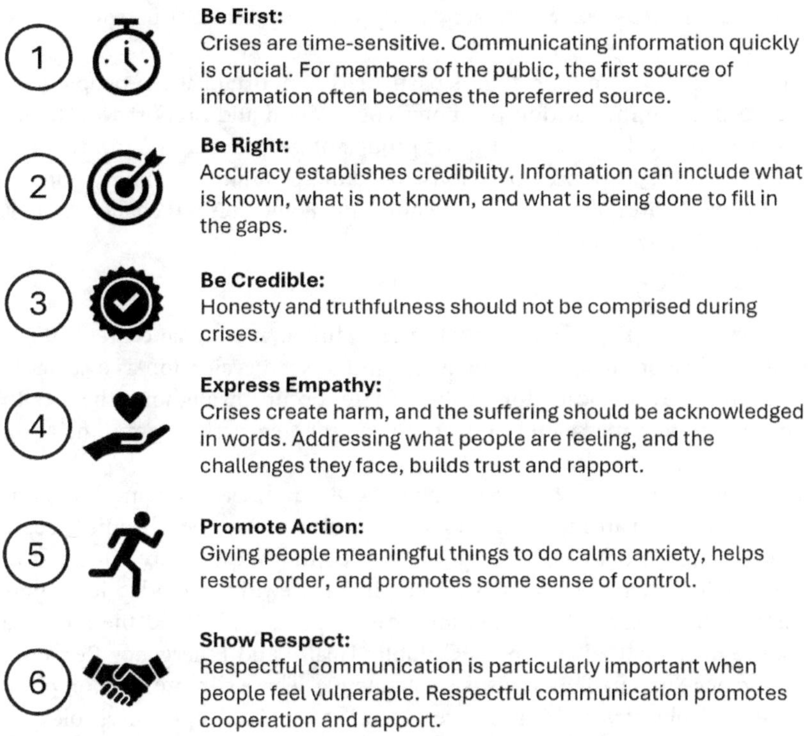

Be First:
Crises are time-sensitive. Communicating information quickly is crucial. For members of the public, the first source of information often becomes the preferred source.

Be Right:
Accuracy establishes credibility. Information can include what is known, what is not known, and what is being done to fill in the gaps.

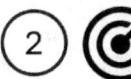
Be Credible:
Honesty and truthfulness should not be comprised during crises.

Express Empathy:
Crises create harm, and the suffering should be acknowledged in words. Addressing what people are feeling, and the challenges they face, builds trust and rapport.

Promote Action:
Giving people meaningful things to do calms anxiety, helps restore order, and promotes some sense of control.

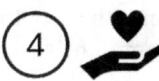
Show Respect:
Respectful communication is particularly important when people feel vulnerable. Respectful communication promotes cooperation and rapport.

Figure 1.1 The Crisis and Emergency Risk Communication (CERC) framework principles
This figure describes the six principles of the CERC framework that are the tenets for effective crisis and emergency risk communication. The CERC principles were identified by the US Centers for Disease Control and Prevention in 2002.
Source: United States Centers for Disease Control and Prevention (CDC). The use of this material does not imply endorsement by CDC, Agency for Toxic Substances and Disease Registry, United States Department of Health and Human Services, or the United States Government of the author. This material is available on the CDC website free of charge: www.cdc.gov/zika/about/needtoknow.html

Be Credible: Honesty and truthfulness should not be compromised during crises. Being open, honest, and transparent about what the agency knows and what the agency is doing is necessary during emergency operations. This also supports organizational credibility and establishes trust between the agency and the community affected by the emergency.[4,9,26]

Express Empathy: Crises create harm, and this suffering should be acknowledged in words. Addressing what people are feeling and the challenges they face builds trust and rapport. Crises cause disruption, fear, and anxiety; health emergencies impact one's well-being. Health is a currency that is hard to replace once it is gone. Expressing empathy acknowledges the disruption, fear, and loss that have occurred. When a spokesperson authentically expresses empathy, they can change impersonal perceptions of the organization in a connected and personal way that transforms the organization from an "it" to "we." Expressing empathy can build trust and rapport with those affected by the emergency.[4,9,26]

Promote Action: Giving people meaningful things to do calms anxiety, helps restore order, and promotes a restored sense of control. Providing people in an emergency with meaningful action steps reduces anxiety and promotes a sense of personal control.[4,9,26]

Show Respect: Respectful communication is particularly important when people feel vulnerable. Respectful communication promotes cooperation and rapport with those affected by the emergency, but also with those groups of people and organizations who are assisting with the response operations. Working in multidisciplinary and multijurisdictional responses often leads to organizational and cultural challenges that can slow or even stall activities.[4,9,26]

CERC Phases

There are five phases in the CERC framework: precrisis, initial, maintenance, resolution, and evaluation phase. The original CERC manual distinguished evaluation as a separate phase; subsequent updates advocate for evaluation to occur throughout the health emergency to inform public messaging and optimize emergency risk communication activities.[4,9,26]

During the precrisis phase, those routine public health and health promotion communication activities relating to immunizations, physical activity, and chronic disease prevention are occurring. In addition, emergency risk communicators are engaging in public health preparedness activities such as developing, reviewing, and adapting emergency risk communication plans. These communication plans go beyond the required emergency response plans that adhere to CDC Public Health and Emergency Response funding and Emergency Support Functions (see Chapter 2). These communication plans include communication objectives, key audiences, identified spokespeople, thresholds for communication activities, links to currently available public information such as websites or FAQs, and even sample messaging.

Another key preparedness activity for emergency risk communications during the precrisis phase is to reach out to other communicators, partner agencies, and stakeholder groups to maintain relationships. It's often very helpful to talk through proposed messaging to create and strengthen message consistency across partner agencies and stakeholder groups.

The next phase of the emergency is the initial phase. This phase begins when some catalyst has occurred to start the health emergency. For example, in a foodborne illness or infectious disease outbreak, the numbers of cases drastically increase. In some cases, it may be a death of a community member that signals the start of the health emergency. Once the initial phase begins, there are immediate emergency risk communication concerns to address. The CERC principles can help with developing and delivering key messages during the initial phase of the emergency. During the initial phase, being first, right, credible, and empathic, showing respect, and promoting action are necessary to build organizational credibility and take organizational responsibility for the health emergency.

With social media, agencies, organizations, and businesses often are no longer the first ones to release emergency information. Often agencies, organizations, and businesses are alerted *by* social media about a health emergency. However, during the initial phase of a health emergency, it is critical for the government agency that is legally accountable and responsible per state statue and Emergency Support Functions to release credible, accurate, and honest information as soon as possible. As we know from the definition of a crisis, there will be heightened media attention, a shorted response time, and a lot of uncertainty. All these components are exacerbated early on in a crisis.

The initial phase is usually short and lasts from 24 to 48 hours. Generally, after this amount of time, more information has been obtained and test results have been validated. In health emergencies, samples and test results provide key clues about their cause. Even while health agencies wait for the scientific test results to come in, key crisis information must be shared with the public about what has happened, what the agency knows at this time, what the agency does not know, and what the agency is doing to find more information and respond to the health emergency. Providing this type of information addresses the uncertainty of the crisis. Stating what the agency knows and what the agency does not know currently supports truthfulness, openness, and honesty. This will bolster the credibility of the organization overall. Hiding or intentionally not releasing information has never worked out for any agency or business in the short or long term.

The next phase of the emergency is the maintenance phase. Typically, health agencies spend a lot of time in this phase. This phase can last from a week to years, as was seen during the COVID-19 pandemic. During the maintenance phase, as more information is becoming available about the cause of the health emergency, more detailed risk information by population group can be shared. For example, pregnant women, children, and those with underlying health conditions tends to be the most vulnerable during health emergencies. By communicating their specific health risks, these groups can make informed decisions on how to protect their health. However, there might be additional groups that are affected by the health emergency. During the maintenance phase, tailored messages can be created for each population group that is affected by the health emergency, indicating the risk level for each group. Additionally, there may be pharmaceutical interventions that are available. During the maintenance phase, communicating about interventions is a vital component to mitigating the health threat.

Once the health threat has been mitigated, the health emergency moves into the resolution phase. This phase is also called the "recovery phase" by emergency management officials. At this point, the health agency begins to pivot away from emergency communication and moves into educational messaging. During the recovery phase, messages of renewal or returning to a new normal may be published. Depending on the severity of the emergency, memorials may be held or physical monuments constructed to remember those affected by the emergency. During the recovery phase, there are often policy changes that may occur both internally within the agency and externally as elected officials write new legislation related to the health emergency.

The final phase of the health emergency is the evaluation phase. Seasoned health practitioners and emergency managers know that evaluations can occur during the emergency response and after. Interim progress reviews, hotwashes, and after-action reviews provide an opportunity to investigate what worked, what didn't work, and what can be improved for the next response. Inevitably these types of evaluations focus heavily on emergency response operations and little on the actual communication during the event. Veteran risk communicators know that evaluating emergency risk communication activities takes a dedicated vision and intention to do so. There is a benefit to reviewing communication-specific activities, policies, and procedures.

Let's take a brief look at how CDC public health communicators applied phase-based messaging during Hurricane Katrina. Public health communicators excelled at pre-event health information dissemination and delivered messages in advance to mitigate issues due to short-term power outages during and after the storm.[27] However, the length of the emergency response, coupled with severe flooding and a second hurricane, complicated emergency risk communication activities. Different types of information were needed at different times in each of these emergency situations. For example, health information was needed on how people could protect themselves from storm debris and storm winds. Later, guidance was needed on preventing drowning, carbon monoxide poisoning, electrical hazards, and driving in floodwater. As emergency shelters opened, health information was needed on personal hygiene, infection control, storing food safely, stress reduction, and management of chronic disease.

After the health emergency, CDC public health communicators reviewed communication messages, policies, and procedures to learn what worked and what did not. Through the Hurricane Katrina response, CDC learned that phase-based messaging was key to meeting information demands throughout a health emergency. Plus, depending on the type of health emergency – flooding, wildfires, infectious diseases, foodborne illnesses – strategic communication planning could drive the development of health messages for each phase of the specific health emergency. This would create a basic communication plan for different types of health emergencies and establish specificity regarding the types of messaging needed at different times throughout an emergency.

The Role of Risk Perception in Emergency Risk Communication

As emergency risk communicators plan for and respond to health emergencies using the CERC framework and other theories, it is imperative for communicators to understand the public's risk perception. Risk perception derives from the probability and severity of a threat mixed with emotions, knowledge, attitudes, and beliefs. How people perceive risks is informed by how much knowledge they have about a particular risk, how they feel about the risk, and whether the risk was chosen or imposed upon them.[28-31] A key challenge emergency risk communicators face when communicating about a health risk is the visibility of the risk. For example, when someone is ill, there are symptoms such as a fever, a runny nose, or a cough. However, during the COVID-19 pandemic, emergency risk communicators struggled to give the public direction on how to avoid a risk they couldn't see. In contrast to communicating about almost invisible health risks, emergency management and forestry PIOs can easily communicate about weather- and land-related risks such as tornadoes, floods, earthquakes, severe winter weather, and wildfires because people can see them and usually have some understanding of these threats. The unfortunate benefit of having gone through COVID-19 is that people across the globe now have direct experience of engaging with contact tracing, isolation and quarantine, mask wearing, and vaccination campaigns. Emergency risk communicators can leverage this prior experience of COVID-19 to support future emergency risk communication messaging.

To understand the complexities of emergency risk communication, one needs to take a step back and consider why this area is so complex and inherently challenging to communicate. Research on emergency risk communication comes from multiple disciplines, including psychology, economics, business, public relations, public health, and disaster sociology. Crises and emergencies can cause disruption at individual, community, societal, and even global levels. Regardless of the scope and scale of the emergency, the communication needs are complicated due to the following variables:

- Emergency type
- Cause
- Risk to health and property
- Geographic location
- Socioeconomic status of those affected by the emergency
- Number of stakeholders impacted by the emergency
- Business and political interests

These multiple factors prompted researchers in the late 1970s to investigate why communicating risks to the public was so complicated. In a landmark research paper, Paul Slovic offered clear insights into how people view risk and why people view risks differently.[28] In this quantitative study, Slovic had technical experts and members of the public judge different hazards. For hazards that fall under the category of dread risk (i.e., things that are uncontrollable, catastrophic, fatal, and have an inequitable distribution), the public want to see these types of risks reduced and want strict regulations in place to reduce these risks. In contrast, experts viewed these dread risks very differently and were more likely to accept the riskiness of the hazard compared to members of the public. Slovic began to realize there is a psychological component of why people think about and understand risks differently: Risk perception involves a subjective assessment of the risk.[32]

A part of this subjective assessment of the risk is based upon one's instinctual desire for survival coupled with previous knowledge and experience, attitudes, and beliefs. As a result, during unknown situations that are out of one's control and are imposed upon people without their choice, fear can play a major role in perceiving risk. When things are uncertain, the human brain works hard to make sense of the situation and through the "affect heuristic" and judges the situation as simply good or bad.[29] "Risk as feelings refers to our fast, instinctive and intuitive reactions to danger. Risk as analysis brings logic, reason and scientific deliberation to bear on hazard management."[29]

One's initial judgments about a risk ultimately impact what decisions one makes about that risk. If a person perceives there is a benefit in taking an action or decision – such as getting a vaccine during a health emergency – the perceived risk of harm from the medical intervention is likely to decrease. "This result implies that people base their judgements of an activity or a technology not only on what they think about it but also on how they feel about it. If their feelings toward an activity are favorable, they are moved toward judging the risks as low and the benefits as high; if their feelings toward it are unfavorable, they tend to judge the opposite – high risk and low benefit."[29]

The challenge for emergency risk communicators is making the risk tangible at the personal or individual level but also communicating the risk at the community level. Ultimately, emergency risk communication is about population health, impacting hundreds of thousands of people during a health emergency. However, individual risk perception is all about the individual, and as the numbers grow larger in emergency risk communication messages, individuals may begin to lose interest. Such numbers are simply too big for a person to relate to or comprehend. This process is called "psychosocial numbing," and it is exemplified in the following quote by Albert Szent-Gyorgi: "I am deeply moved if I see one man suffering and would risk my life for him. Then I talk impersonally about the possible pulverization of our big cities with a hundred million dead. I am unable to multiply one man's suffering by a hundred million."[29]

Threat and dread are frequent emotional reactions to perceived threats and form a part of outrage – the negative emotional reaction by the public regarding an emergency.[33] Components of outrage are based on how the public judges the impact and causes of an emergency through factors such as trust, control, voluntariness, dread, and familiarity.[33] By understanding how the public is perceiving the risks and impacts of an emergency, emergency risk communicators can develop messages that consider the public's outrage. By combining the 12 factors of outrage with phase-based emergency messaging, communicators can develop messages that are attuned to the public and stakeholders affected by an emergency. Table 1.1 is based upon the outrage factors as defined by Peter Sandman and includes updated descriptions and examples.[33]

Table 1.1 Outrage factors with descriptions and examples

Outrage factor	Description and examples
Voluntary vs. coerced	A person chooses the risk vs an organization imposes the risk upon a person or community. Coerced threats are more likely to create outrage.
Natural vs. industrial	An act of God, natural disaster, or naturally occurring pandemic vs a lab leak or nuclear power reactor malfunction. Industrial or human-made threats are more likely to create outrage.
Familiar vs. exotic	A familiar act like driving a car can be perceived as less risky: The more we do it, the more familiar something is. In contrast, self-driving cars are more exotic – the technology is new and less familiar to us. Exotic threats are more likely to create outrage.
Not memorable vs. memorable	The use of symbolization and media images can make a situation more memorable, such as the images of the Deepwater Horizon oil rig explosion and footage of oil gushing from the well that were constantly shown on TV. Odors related to a chemical emergency such as that of the 2023 Southern Norfolk train derailment can create a memorable event. The more personal the experience, the more memorable it will be, and the more outrage it will generate.
Not dreaded vs. dreaded	Dreaded threats create a perceived lack of control over catastrophic consequences and highly fatal events that result in an individual feeling fear. When people don't dread something, they are likely to experience less outrage.
Chronic vs. catastrophic	Chronic risks become absorbed into society and become familiar, such as health risks from cancer, heart disease, or smoking. Catastrophic risks – events those that are less likely to happen such as contracting Ebola in the United States – can cause more outrage than chronic, ongoing hazards.
Knowable vs. unknowable	Knowable risks provide certainty, as there is available science and data about the hazards. In contrast, unknowable risks such novel viruses or issues with new vaccines create uncertainty and can cause more outrage.

Table 1.1 (cont.)

Outrage factor	Description and examples
Individually controlled vs. controlled by others	Like the outrage factor of voluntary vs coerced, if an individual can control the hazards, they are less likely to experience outrage. In contrast, if the hazard is controlled by others, the public is likely to experience more outrage. For example, the Flint water crisis was under the control of the government, not individuals.
Fair vs. unfair	The unequitable distribution of risks and hazards can create outrage. About 40% of Flint, Michigan's population lives below the poverty line and the impacts of lead poisoning on children have lifelong consequences. Many view the Flint water crisis as an unfair distribution of risk to the community.
Morally irrelevant vs. morally relevant	When hazards transgress society's morals – the accepted customs of conduct among the community – outrage can occur. The issue of vaccine mandates can stimulate outrage among the public.
Trustworthy sources vs. untrustworthy sources	Receiving health information from trusted sources such as medical doctors can reduce outrage. However, if the public feels betrayed by those trusted sources of information, enormous outrage could occur.
Responsive process vs. unresponsive process	When organizations engage in honest, transparent, respectful, accurate, and empathetic communication during emergency responses, there is less likely to be outrage. When organizations are secretive, withholding, lack respect, or lie, outrage will occur.

In addition to considering the public's outrage, a final challenge facing emergency risk communicators is navigating the politicization of public health and its impact on risk perception. In the United States, emergency risk communicators must strike a balance of messaging that protects the public's health while respecting the constitutional rights of its citizens. While this has always been an issue, the COVID-19 pandemic has sparked fierce debate about how much authority public health agencies should have during an emergency and about deferring to parental authority regarding childhood vaccinations instead of relying upon evidence-based science of communicable disease prevention.

The Partnership of Organizational Leadership and Communication Officers

For emergency risk communication activities to work effectively, organizational leadership needs to identify risk communication as a priority function for the health agency during routine public health activities and emergencies. By establishing the importance of risk communication for the agency, organizational leadership signals to the rest of the agency that risk communication is not an afterthought when conducting public health work but a necessary and integral part to communicating and working with the public, stakeholders, and other government agencies.

It would be ideal for organizational leadership to have a strong working relationship with the communication officers within the agency. Communication officers or PIOs play a critical role in the development and dissemination of messages and the management of Joint Information Centers during health emergencies.[34] The messages that are created by PIOs and subject matter experts are communicated through the health department's leadership team via press releases, media briefings, and stakeholder meetings. Health department leadership – especially those designated as spokespeople – has a key role to play in personalizing the emergency response activities, gaining support from the public and stakeholders for emergency response operations, and as the face of the emergency.

While most communications occur during the emergency response, having the support of agency leadership during precrisis and postcrisis stages to support message testing, communications training, and evaluation of communication activities is imperative to the effectiveness of emergency risk communication messaging. Ensure that organizational structures and procedures are established to facilitate effective emergency risk communication, such as: clearly defined clearance and review processes; identified and trained spokespeople; current social media policies; preidentified vendors to rapidly receive funding to support the development of communication campaigns; and executed memorandums of understanding for nonagency communication experts and PIOs to support emergency response activities as surge staff.

Case Study of Public Health Crisis: Outbreak of *Legionella* in Central Ohio Hospital (2019)
Paige A. Gray, MPH

Overview of Crisis/Situation
Legionnaires' disease (LD) is a severe type of pneumonia caused by bacteria of the genus *Legionella*.[35] LD is caused by inhalation exposure to the droplets of the bacteria, and the bacteria thrive in environments such as large water systems that have not been properly maintained.[36] Most healthy individuals exposed do not end up getting LD, but certain individuals are at increased risk for developing LD. These include those aged 50 years and older, those with chronic lung disease, such as chronic obstructive pulmonary disease (COPD), those with weakened immune systems, or those who are on medication that weakens the immune system.[35] As is clear, it is of significant concern when LD outbreaks do occur, especially in settings where those most at risk might be present, such as hospital settings.[35] We will now examine an outbreak of LD that occurred in Ohio in 2019.

In 2019, an Ohio hospital system known as Mount Carmel opened another location, Mount Carmel Grove City, on April 28, 2019. The private, 210-bed hospital was defined as being "large-scale [and] comprehensive" by the news channels.[38] It would offer a comprehensive cancer center, complex neuroscience services, and a newborn intensive care unit, bringing a full-scale health system to the south of Columbus. Just a month after the grand opening, Mount Carmel Grove City announced it was undergoing a "possible" LD outbreak after its sixth reported case. In total, 16 patients would be diagnosed with LD during the outbreak at this new and state-of-the-art facility, resulting in one death. Mitigation efforts included water restrictions for patients, staff, and visitors, as well as the installment of water filters and disinfection of the water supply through hyperchlorination.[39,40,41]

The timeline of key events was as follows[37]:
- Three positive cases were confirmed at Mount Carmel Grove City (earliest reported on May 15, 2019).
- The first LD case was diagnosed at the facility between April 29 and May 7.
- Cases were confirmed via urine antigen testing.
- Five later cases were reported between May 8 and May 20.
- The onset of LD cases occurred from May 12 to May 29.
- The hospital reported to the Ohio Department of Health (ODH) cases of confirmed LD as of May 16.
- Water samples were taken from May 23 through June 1.
- Samples for water testing were taken from the second and fourth to seventh floors and emergency department, confirming *Legionella* through polymerase chain reaction testing in the emergency department and on the seventh floor.
- A fourth case was determined as a result.
- The first declaration to the public of this as an outbreak of LD occurred on May 31, at a then-current total of six confirmed LD cases.
- May 31: ODH releases a "rare adjudication order" to the hospital to take immediate action or not accept any new patients.
- May 31: Water restrictions were put in place.
- June 1: ODH Director, Amy Acton, discusses the outbreak with the public via a news conference.[42]
- Disinfection operations were set up for the entire water system by June 2.
- Hyperchlorination was expected to be completed by June 2.
- June 2: A patient who contracted LD during the outbreak died.
- June 6: Temporary water filters were installed by the hospital as a barrier to the transmission of the bacteria.
- June 6: ODH lifts water restrictions on floors at the hospital.[44]
- June 11: A 16th case of LD was confirmed (noting that incubation of the disease can take up to 14 days) and permanent supplemental disinfection system was installed.
- June 13: Leadership from the hospital announced the cause of the outbreak and the corrective actions.
- June 24: A press release from the hospital was published regarding total confirmed cases and demographic data, along with a source of the outbreak, and that corrective action was taken.
- July 9: A fifth lawsuit was filed against the hospital due to illness related to LD, citing hospital negligence.

Overview and Analysis of CERC Principles and Phase-Based Messaging

According to CDC, there are six CERC principles that lead to effective emergency and risk communications. These principles ensure that resources in a crisis are properly managed, communication is delivered effectively, and decisions are made swiftly and accurately with regard to the data available.[45] These principles enable preplanning functions in crisis and disaster scenarios in which trained spokespeople can adapt to various situations and so be prepared during every phase of the situation. These six CERC principles as defined in CDC'S CERC 2014 manual are as follows:

1. Be First: Communication of information quickly and being the first source of information to the public are key.
2. Be Right: There must be information in the message about what is known, what is not known, and what is being done to fill in the gaps of knowledge.

3. Be Credible: This encompasses honesty as the best policy during the crisis; do not compromise your honesty.
4. Express Empathy: Acknowledge and address what the community is feeling in times of crisis and disaster. Ensure that messages address what people are feeling and the challenges they may be facing.
5. Promote Action: Give the community activities to do to limit the crisis and restore order, and outline clear paths toward resolving the crisis or disaster.
6. Show Respect: Communication should be respectful and promote cooperation. Phase-based messaging works in line with the CERC principles to ensure that specific types of information are communicated outward during a crisis. Communication efforts and various priorities are shifted throughout the phases of a crisis, and communicators who work with the public need to respond accordingly.[45]

The five phases of the CERC rhythm are precrisis, initial, maintenance, resolution, and evaluation. Messaging during a crisis starts in the initial phase, where rapid communication to those affected groups should be evident.[45] Additionally, messages should explain the risks of the threat, what the agency is doing to control the spread and identify the source of the outbreak, and promote action in terms of what people can do to protect themselves. In the maintenance phase, more information should be coming out about the crisis and what the agency is doing. Keeping the public informed of the facts and mitigating any misinformation should be priorities. The resolution phase should focus on recovery from the crisis and the promotion of public policy changes that may have emerged due to the crisis.[45] As the crisis dissipates, evaluations on how the situation was managed start to develop and the evaluation phase begins. Utilization of CERC phase-based messaging in line with the CERC principles minimizes negative public responses and maintains public trust in the health care agency.

During the 2019 outbreak of LD at Mount Carmel Grove City, some of the CERC principles were evident in Mount Carmel's communications to the public, but some of its messaging was severely lacking. In the following subsections we will analyze some of the messages put out during the LD outbreak at Mount Carmel Grove City and highlight the various phases during which each message was published. Please note that the CERC principle Be Right was absent from the communication response and so is not included in this analysis.

Be First
When it comes to the principle of "being first," in this situation Mount Carmel Grove City did not react in as timely a manner as it should have, nor did it act as the initiator of informing the public. In one of its first messages, the hospital released a general statement to the public informing the community that the hospital was working with the health department and CDC to confirm the source of the outbreak and informing the public that the hospital was confident that all operations could be maintained without disruption:

> Working with local health officials, we've determined at least seven confirmed cases of Legionnaires' Disease in individuals who recently received treatment at Mount Carmel Grove City. We are partnering with Franklin County Public Health (FCPH) and the Ohio Department of Health (ODH), in conjunction with the CDC, to identify the source of bacteria.
>
> We are running additional tests on water sources throughout the hospital, and our entire water supply is undergoing supplemental disinfection. We're confident that we can safely maintain the full services of the hospital while we study this situation.

For most people, the risk of developing Legionnaires' Disease is low; however, individuals with chronic, underlying medical conditions are at increased risk. If you have been hospitalized and developed a cough, muscle aches, headaches, fever chills, or shortness of breath, please contact your primary care physician.

As always, the safety of our patients is our top priority. We will continue testing the water over the next few weeks in coordination with FCPH, ODH, and CDC.

As we learn more, we will provide updates to our patients and community.[46]

This statement was informative but lacked a few aspects of an initial CERC phase-based message, including information regarding a timeline of events and who to contact for more information. Regarding the principle of "being first," it was only after the declaration was made by the ODH on May 3 of an outbreak and of immediate action being taken that the hospital made its statement.[47,48] The rare adjudication order that the ODH Director, Amy Acton, issued was to ensure that Mount Carmel Grove City took the necessary steps to protect public health.[49]

Additionally, the spokesperson for the parent company of the hospital, Trinity Health, noted "the health system followed the guidelines in place for investigating individual cases . . . it's not uncommon to see sporadic cases that have nothing to do with being in a health-care facility."[46] CDC guidance states that LD outbreaks can be associated with travel, health care, and potable water systems, and declaring an outbreak requires there to have been "two or more cases associated with the same possible source during a 12-month period."[36] This goes against the Trinity Health spokesperson's statement as: (1) We know that individuals with LD were admitted to the hospital for a separate illness and were later diagnosed with LD and (2) the individuals who contracted the illness were admitted and stayed in the hospital at around the same time. The hospital was slow to communicate the LD risk to the public, and its eventual public message indicated that "it followed the guidelines in place," which could be perceived as a lack of transparency about *what* they knew and *when* they knew about the source of the outbreak.

Be Credible
Mount Carmel Health System is part of a network of hospitals spanning central Ohio. In 2019, the health care system had multiple full-service hospitals open. It was also undergoing investigation regarding accusations of a doctor's malpractice and murder through deliberate fentanyl overdosing of patients at two of its locations. With the opening of Mount Carmel Grove City, and with it already being under such scrutiny, we can assume that Mount Carmel Health System knew its credibility was being examined by the public,[50] which led to a lack of openness and transparency in its dealing with the LD outbreak. During the maintenance phase of the outbreak, the media was starting to notice this. *The Columbus Dispatch*, a local news outlet, noted in an article about the outbreak: "The building of the new hospital in Grove City was not without controversy from the beginning."[51] This article then discussed the closing of one Mount Carmel hospital in an area of Columbus where it was much needed, and it also highlighted the story of Dr. Husel, the doctor accused of the murder of 14 patients over multiple years. During his trial, Dr. Husel was acquitted of those 14 patient deaths.[51]

Mount Carmel's lack of public discussion of the outbreak generated distrust among the public, indicating that its credibility was severely lacking. Most of Mount Carmel's actions in dealing with the outbreak came about only after it was told to do so by the ODH. The public noticed this, and those currently in the hospital's care were outraged.[48]

Express Empathy

During the maintenance phase of the crisis, while the full investigation of the water system was underway, Mount Carmel Health System was having its spokesperson relay messages to the public. Dr. Streck, the Chief Clinical Operations Officer of Mount Carmel Health System, released a statement confirming the death of one of the patients who had contracted LD, and he went on to advise on what to do if one contracts LD. In his statement, he not only contradicted himself but also sounded like he was reading from a script: "We are deeply saddened to confirm that one of the patients who was diagnosed with Legionnaires' disease passed away today . . .. We can say it's too early to determine the final cause of death."[52] In his statement, he acknowledges the patient's death but does not acknowledge LD as a contributing factor. This could be seen as very misleading by the public as he was trying to prevent blame for the patient's death being attached to the hospital. However, a statement was made from the ODH Director, Amy Acton, on the patient's death that same evening. ODH noted it as a "*Legionella*-related death of a Mount Carmel Grove City patient," and it went on to state that "we share a concern for all impacted by this outbreak."[35]

Show Respect

During the maintenance phase of this health emergency, multiple statements made by Mount Carmel Grove City failed to show respect not just to the public and patients, but also to the business partners the hospital was supposed to be working with during the outbreak. One example of this is the delay in the hospital undertaking action. According to the timeline of events, the first cases were reported to FCPH as of May 16, 2019, but water restrictions were not implemented and the public was not notified until May 31.[41] A delay in action indicates a failure to show respect to the community. Secondly, as mentioned earlier, the blame game played by Mount Carmel's parent company, Trinity Health, regarding ODH's delayed outbreak response action indicated a lack of respect and cooperation. Trinity Health noted that it did not announce the outbreak until it was confirmed that the cases were all related to its own hospital system when in fact the numbers had already passed the CDC threshold of greater than two reportable cases.[36]

Promote Action

A resolution message from a hospital allows it to give the public more information regarding the questions that many in a community might have: What has been done? Why did this occur? Who was at fault? When the President of Mount Carmel Health System, Sean McKibben, addressed the community, he noted that better disinfection and increased environmental testing could have prevented this situation. Actions noted were the installation of a supplemental disinfection system and 24/7 monitoring controls, as well as an updated protocol to flush the water system in every patient room daily.[41] Additionally, McKibben wanted Mount Carmel to be a change leader in industry and for it to be a part of the new task force that ODH had created for *Legionella* to address the issues surrounding policy changes and regulations regarding *Legionella* in health care settings. Mount Carmel produced a thorough message to the community once the outbreak had concluded, stating that it had resolved the crisis and was committed to change.

Implications for Practitioners and Organizations Based on an Analysis of CERC Principles

Communication in a crisis, such as an outbreak in a hospital, is critical to minimizing negative health outcomes for the public. This takes us back to the CERC principle of "the right message at the right time from the right person can save lives."[45] Three key takeaways are noted from this crisis as lessons to be learned; these will be discussed in the following subsections.

Response Timeliness
A quicker response from the hospital system once LD was suspected should have occurred. Two weeks passed before action was taken to protect patients or an announcement was made to the public. The hospital was indeed testing the water supply, but it did not implement any other actions until the outbreak was declared. At that point, there were six confirmed cases, and a linkage had already been established to the hospital. When asked to explain the reason for this delay, the hospital blamed ODH and waited for confirmation of the outbreak.

Adopt a Proactive Strategy
Having an established policy in place for dealing with an outbreak leads to proactivity in dealing with possible future outbreaks. Mount Carmel Grove City, being part of a larger health system, should have had an established policy and practice in place for dealing with an outbreak of LD that aligned with best practices and guidelines following CDC recommendations. Instead, the hospital was forced to be reactive, changing its practices and altering its protocols after the outbreak had occurred to better equip itself to prevent potential future outbreaks. Instead, the hospital should have been more proactive, especially as this was a new hospital that was supposedly state-of-the-art.

Transparency Is Crucial
The last implication of this crisis is that transparency with the public is crucial. The messages given to the public should be concise, transparent, and forthright. In this crisis, little information was given during the outbreak from the hospital system itself through any of the available channels. Its website and social media were silent. This could be due to the fact that it was already battling negative media attention stemming from a separate incident involving a doctor accused of malpractice and murder and so it was trying to keep this outbreak as quiet as possible, but this lack of transparency did more damage. Mount Carmel Grove City should have addressed the situation publicly in its media strategy and informed the public promptly. The lack of transparency from the hospital led to its credibility being questioned.

Conclusion
Mount Carmel Grove City had big plans for this new facility opening, but due to an oversight in its planning process the hospital is now tainted by its failure to follow appropriate processes and oversight measures, which led to an outbreak of LD within a month of its opening. The hospital should develop effective crisis communication plans, especially on how to respond to outbreaks and mitigate risks, which will benefit it in the long term.

End-of-Chapter Reflection Questions

1. What emergency responses have you participated in? How was the communication different compared to day-to-day public health communication?
2. Compare and contrast where in your agency you see health communication, risk communication, and emergency risk communication occurring. Does your agency currently use emergency risk communication principles during health emergencies? Evaluate what works well and what needs improvement.

3 What emergency responses have been successful for your agency? Which responses have not been as successful? How would the use of phase-based messaging help in planning, sharing, and evaluating emergency risk messaging?

4 Think about your own personal risk perceptions. How do they impact your actions in your personal life? How are your personal risk perceptions reflected in your professional work?

5 Identify at least two ways you want to improve emergency risk communication at your agency. Consider who else needs to be involved, what resources are needed, how much time is needed, how you will evaluate whether these improvements are successful, and how these improvements will be maintained over time.

References

1 Parker CF, Stern EK. The Trump Administration and the COVID-19 Crisis: Exploring the Warning-Response Problems and Missed Opportunities of a Public Health Emergency. *Public Adm* 2022;10.1111/padm.12843.

2 Abutaleb Y, Paletta D. *Nightmare Scenario: Inside the Trump Administration's Response to the Pandemic That Changed History.* New York, HarperCollins Publisher, 2021.

3 Slavitt A. *Preventable.* New York, St. Martin's Publishing Group, 2021.

4 CDC. *Crisis and Emergency Risk Communication October 2002.* Atlanta, GA, CDC, 2002.

5 Tulenko K, Vervoort D. Cracks in the System: The Effects of the Coronavirus Pandemic on Public Health Systems. *Am Rev Public Adm* 2020;**50**(6–7):455–66.

6 de Beaumont. Findings 2024. 2021. https://debeaumont.org/phwins/2021-findings/ (Accessed May 1, 2024).

7 Seeger M, Sellnow T, Ulmer R. *Communication and Organizational Crisis.* London, Bloomsbury Academic, 2003.

8 Ulmer R, Sellnow T, Seeger M. *Effective Crisis Communication: Moving from Crisis to Opportunity.* New York, Sage Publications, 2010.

9 CDC. *Crisis and Emergency Risk Communication October 2018.* Atlanta, GA, CDC, 2018.

10 Nelson C, Lurie N, Wasserman J, Zakowski S. Conceptualizing and Defining Public Health Emergency Preparedness. *Am J Pub Health* 2007;**97**:s9–s11.

11 Haffajee R, Paremt WE, Mello MM. What Is a Public Health "Emergency"? *New Eng J Med* 2014;**371**(11):986–88.

12 National Cancer Institute. Making Health Communication Programs Work. *Health and Human Services.* n.d. www.cancer.gov/publications/health-communication (Accessed March 13, 2024).

13 CDC. Healthy People 2023. 2020. www.cdc.gov/nchs/healthy_people/hp2030/hp2030.htm (Accessed May 1, 2024).

14 Parrott R. Emphasizing "Communication" in Health Communication. *J Commun* 2006;**54**(4):751–87.

15 HHS. *Move Your Way Community Resources.* Washington, DC: US Department of Health and Human Resources, 2023.

16 Suran M, Bucher K. False Health Claims Abound, but Physicians Are Still the Most Trusted Source for Health Information. *JAMA* 2024;**331**(19):1612–13.

17 Seeger M, Reynolds B, Day AM. Crisis and Emergency Risk Communication: Past, Present, and Future. In: Finn F, Winni J, editors. *Crisis Communication.* Berlin, De Gruyter Mouton, 2020; 401–18.

18 Nilsen TR. *Ethics of Speech Communication* (1st edition). New York, Bobbs-Merrill, 1966.

19 NRC. *Improving Risk Communication*. Washington, DC: National Academies Press, 1989.

20 Templeton A. 6 Things You Should Know About the Triangle Lake Pesticide Investigation. *OPB*. 2012. www.opb.org/news/article/6-things-you-should-know-about-the-triangle-lake-p/ (Accessed May 1, 2024).

21 Oregon Health Authority. Highway 36 Exposure Investigation. 2014. www.oregon.gov/oha/ph/healthyenvironments/trackingassessment/environmentalhealthassessment/hwy36/pages/index.aspx (Accessed May 1, 2024).

22 Learn S. Triangle Lake residents press for moratorium on aerial spraying in private forests near schools, homes. *The Oregonian*. 2013. www.oregonlive.com/environment/2013/05/residents_near_triangle_lake_p.html (Accessed May 1, 2024).

23 Mortensen C. Concerns Arise Over Pesticide Spray Near School. *Eugene Weekly*. 2015. https://eugeneweekly.com/2015/09/17/concerns-arise-over-pesticide-spray-near-school/ (Accessed May 1, 2024).

24 Oregon Health Authority. Exposure Investigation Portland, Oregon. 2014. www.oregon.gov/oha/ph/healthyenvironments/trackingassessment/environmentalhealthassessment/hwy36/pages/index.aspx (Accessesd May 1, 2024).

25 Barrett MS. Spokespersons and Message Control: How the CDC Lost Credibility during the Anthrax Crisis. *Qual Res Rep Commun* 2005;**6**(1):59–68.

26 CDC. *Crisis and Emergency Risk Communication October 2014*. Atlanta, GA, CDC, 2014.

27 Vanderford ML, Nastoff T, Telfer JL, Bonzo SE. Emergency Communication Challenges in Response to Hurricane Katrina: Lessons from the Centers for Disease Control and Prevention. *J Appl Commun Res* 2007;**35**(1):9–25.

28 Slovic P. Perception of Risk. *Science* 1987;**236**(4799):280–85.

29 Slovic P. *The Feeling of Risk: New Perspectives on Risk Perception*. London, Earthscan; 2010.

30 Ropeik D. The Perception Gap: Recognizing and Managing the Risks That Arise When We Get Risk Wrong. *Food Chem Toxicol* 2012;**50**(5):1222–25.

31 Malecki KMC, Keating JA, Safdar N. Crisis Communication and Public Perception of COVID-19 Risk in the Era of Social Media. *Clin Infect Dis* 2021;**72**(4):697–702.

32 Glik DC. Risk Communication for Public Health Emergencies. *Annu Rev Public Health* 2007;**28**:33–54.

33 Sandman PM. Responding to Community Outrage: Strategies for Effective Risk Communication. 2012. www.psandman.com/media/RespondingtoCommunityOutrage.pdf (Accessed May 1, 2024).

34 FEMA. *National Incident Management System Basic Guidance for Public Information Officers*. Washington, DC, US Federal Emergency Management Agency (FEMA), 2020.

35 CDC. About Legionnaires Disease and Pontiac Fever. 2019. www.cdc.gov/legionella/about/index.html (Accessed April 14, 2022).

36 CDC. Legionnaires Disease Outbreaks | Legionella. www.cdc.gov/legionella/outbreaks.html (Accessed March 18, 2022).

37 OSHA. Legionellosis (Legionnaires' Disease and Pontiac Fever) – Overview. www.osha.gov/legionnaires-disease (Accessed April 14, 2022).

38 Croft S. Mount Carmel opens new hospital in Grove City. *10tv.com*. 2019. www.10tv.com/article/news/local/mount-carmel-opens-new-hospital-grove-city-2019-may/530-f754621f-61f9-4f05-8921-e4cba8378436#:~:text=Mount%20Carmel%20Grove%20City%20opens%20April%2028.&text=Large%2Dscale%20comprehensive%20health%20care,beds%20with%20 all%20private%20rooms (Accessed March 13, 2022).

39. Breedlove A. Legionnaires' Disease at Mt. Carmel Grove City Hospital (6/24/19). *Franklin County Public Health*. 2019. https://myfcph.org/legionella/ (Accessed March 26, 2022).

40. 10tv Web Staff. 16 confirmed cases of legionnaires' related to outbreak at Mount Carmel Grove City. *10tv.com*. 2019. www.10tv.com/article/news/local/16-confirmed-cases-legionnaires-related-outbreak-mount-carmel-grove-city-2019-jun/530-daf06ea2-cfeb-4012-912b-b908f49fe318 (Accessed March 13, 2022).

41. Haeberle B. Mount Carmel Grove City failed to disinfect water lines that attributed to Legionnaires' outbreak. *10tv.com*. 2019. www.10tv.com/article/news/investigations/10-investigates/mount-carmel-grove-city-failed-disinfect-water-lines-attributed-legionnaires-outbreak-2019/530-d90b53c7-f9bc-4a63-8312-c2030a755cfa (Accessed March 13, 2022).

42. Ohio Dept. of Health Director Dr. Amy Acton. *The Columbus Dispatch*. 2019. www.youtube.com/watch?v=Wrbb-wmYJHE (Accessed April 22, 2024).

43. Henry M. Patient dies in outbreak at hospital. *The Columbus Dispatch*. 2019. www.dispatch.com/story/lifestyle/health-fitness/2019/06/03/patient-dies-in-outbreak-at/4940613007/ (Accessed March 13, 2022).

44. Statement from Director of Health on Lifting Water Restrictions on Floors at Mount Carmel Grove City. *Ohio Department of Health*. 2019. https://odh.ohio.gov/media-center/odh-news-%20releases/statement-director-health-lifting-water-restrictions-mount-carmel-grove-city (Accessed March 13, 2022).

45. Centers for Disease Control and Prevention. CERC Manual | Crisis & Emergency Risk Communication (CERC). 2020. https://emergency.cdc.gov/cerc/manual/index.asp (Accessed March 13, 2022).

46. Media Statement on behalf of Ed Lamb, president & CEO, Mount Carmel Health System. *Mount Carmel Health*. 2019. www.mountcarmelhealth.com/assets/hidden/documents/mchs-media-statement-june-5.pdf. (Accessed March 13, 2022).

47. Rouan R. Grove City hospital has disease outbreak. *The Columbus Dispatch*. n.d. www.dispatch.com/story/lifestyle/health-fitness/2019/06/01/grove-city-hospital-has-disease/5006727007/ (Accessed March 13, 2022).

48. Legionnaires' Disease at Mt. Carmel Grove City Hospital. *Franklin County Public Health*. 2019. https://myfcph.org/legionella/#:~:text=Franklin%20County%20Public%20Health%20is,was%20the%20potable%20water%20system (Accessed November 4, 2024).

49. Director of Health Issues Adjudication Order to Protect Public Health. *Ohio Department of Health*. 2019. https://odh.ohio.gov/media-center/odh-news-releases/director-health-issues-adjudication-order-to-protect-public-health (Accessed March 13, 2022).

50. del Valle JC. Jury deliberates again today in murder case of doctor accused of overprescribing fentanyl to the dying. *CNN*. 2022 www.cnn.com/2022/04/12/us/william-husel-ohio-doctor-closing-arguments-mistrial-motion/index.html (Accessed April 15, 2022).

51. Zachariah H. Hospital probing how disease originated. *The Columbus Dispatch*. 2019. www.dispatch.com/story/lifestyle/health-fitness/2019/06/01/hospital-probing-how-disease-originated/4999996007/ (Accessed March 18, 2022).

52. Media Statement from Dr. Richard Streck, Chief Clinical Operations Officer, Mount Carmel Health System. *Mount Carmel Health*. 2019. www.mountcarmelhealth.com/assets/documents/mchs_media-statement_june-2.pdf (Accessed April 1, 2022).

53. Statement from Director of Health on Patient's Death at Mount Carmel Grove City. *Ohio Department of Health*. 2019. https://odh.ohio.gov/media-center/odh-news-releases/statement-director-%20of-health-patients-death-mount-carmel-grove-city (Accessed March 18, 2022).

Part I Precrisis Planning

Chapter 2

Precrisis Planning Is Necessary for Public Information and Emergency Communications
Leveraging What You've Got

Chapter Objectives
- Describe how to conduct a communication audit.
- Summarize how the Public Health Emergency Preparedness capabilities are related to emergency risk communication planning.
- Present the roles and responsibilities of key crisis communication team members.
- Describe the function of a Joint Information Center.
- Explain how partnerships play a role in emergency risk communication.
- Present the steps involved in conducting message testing.

Overview of Planning for Public Health Emergencies and Leveraging Current Crisis Communication Plans

Since the early 2000s, thousands of public health officials and practitioners have been trained in emergency risk messaging principles, and creating an emergency risk communication plan is part of that training.[1] Health departments that receive federal public health preparedness funding through the Centers for Disease Control and Prevention (CDC) cooperative agreement must develop a crisis communication plan to demonstrate emergency risk communication functionality.[2] As outlined in the Public Health Emergency Preparedness (PHEP) capabilities, assessing the current state of a health agency's ability to respond to and communicate about a health emergency is part of the emergency preparedness and response capabilities planning model.[3]

Assessing the current state of the health department's ability to respond to a health emergency includes analyzing resource elements, which include planning documents, human resources (i.e., skilled workers), and physical resources such as office space, computers, and other items needed to respond to an emergency. For emergency risk communicators, this means reviewing and updating communication plans to identify missing or outdated information, unclear processes and procedures, and updates to who serves as a spokesperson or the identification of additional subject matter experts. Reviewing crisis and emergency risk communication (CERC) plans, toolkits, standard operating procedures, and who serves as key subject matter experts is a crucial preparedness activity. Engaging in these preparedness activities will also help strengthen relationships within the agency and support cross-team and cross-program coordination.

A communication audit entails reviewing existing materials within your organization and identifying where to make improvements. Organizations often conduct communication audits to ensure their materials are in line with their brand, identity, and communication policies, but audits can also assess what information materials are available to a given program or, in some cases, to a revised outdated program.[4] Communication audits review relevant policies related to reviewing and clearing documents for public consumption, identified spokespeople, and media and social media usage for official business. For emergency risk communication, communication audits are usually conducted before or after an emergency response.

When a communication audit is conducted before an emergency, it will focus on how much information (e.g., communication materials) is available on a given topic such as influenza, *E. coli*, measles, hepatitis C, or other health threats that could arise in the community. The audit will also assess when the information was created and whether the materials need to be revised and updated. When communication audits happen after an emergency, they are usually part of an after-action review (AAR) to improve organizational processes during an emergency. See Chapter 10 for more on evaluation and AARs.

Conducting a Communication Audit

To conduct a communication audit during the precrisis phase, follow these five steps:

1. Identify priority health threats for the community that the health agency serves. These health threats could include the flu season, common foodborne illness outbreaks (e.g., salmonella), or smoke from wildfires. Check with leadership if you are unsure on how to prioritize health threats.
2. Create an inventory of the communication materials available to communicate about the health threat. These communication materials can include communication toolkits, talking points, social media messages, press release templates or previously used press releases, webpage copy, and fact sheets. Using a spreadsheet is a good way to keep track of what materials are available by health threat. It is also a good idea to include when the item was created and last reviewed.
3. Identify what is missing or what is outdated. Make a plan to create and/or edit communication materials and make sure to work in coordination with subject matter experts and leadership. Consider coordinating with community members to gather their feedback on the materials as part of a message testing process.
4. Once the communication materials have been created and edited, hold a briefing meeting to update key communication staff, program staff, and leadership about what materials have been created, where the materials are, and how they will be used during an emergency. You can also work with your preparedness program to identify how the new materials could be tested, such as during a tabletop discussion or functional exercise.
5. Make a note to check and review these materials both annually and following an emergency in which they were employed.

If new messages need to be created, consider testing those messages to ensure they will resonate with and reach target audiences. See later in this chapter for more on message testing.

Communication Plans, Planning, and Toolkits

Since 2001, CDC has funded state and local health departments through the PHEP cooperative agreement program, which provides critical funds for health departments to create and sustain information and communication systems, conduct routine surveillance efforts for infectious diseases, provide community education and risk communication, organize exercises, and identify ways to address vulnerable populations.[5]

CDC outlines 15 public health and emergency preparedness and response capabilities[2]:

1 Community Preparedness
2 Community Recovery
3 Emergency Operations Coordination
4 Emergency Public Information and Warning
5 Fatality Management
6 Information Sharing
7 Mass Care
8 Medical Countermeasure Dispensing and Administration
9 Medical Material Management and Distribution
10 Medical Surge
11 Nonpharmaceutical Interventions
12 Public Health Laboratory Testing
13 Public Health Surveillance and Epidemiological Investigation
14 Responder Health and Safety
15 Volunteer Management

Emergency risk communication and messaging can be found in all of these preparedness capabilities. When your organization is in the precrisis, preparedness stage, it is key that emergency risk communicators understand emergency response operations. This fundamental understanding is so important because, for each key operation area, communicators need to develop messaging that explains what their organization is doing and what the public can do to protect their health. Nonpharmaceutical interventions will be developed by subject matter experts and implemented by health department staff, but emergency risk communicators will need to share and educate the public about nonpharmaceutical interventions through public messaging. Additionally, within the PHEP capability guidance, there are key areas where some functions overlap with emergency risk communication. For example, Capability 2: Community Recovery coordinates with Capability 4: Emergency Public Information and Warning to develop messages and identify audiences impacted by the emergency.

For emergency risk communicators, it is important to understand Capability 4: Emergency Public Information and Warning. This capability outlines key functions and tasks that must take place to facilitate effective emergency communication in a health emergency. These functions include:

1 Activate the emergency public health information system.
2 Determine the need for a Joint Information Center/System.
3 Establish and participate in information system operations.
4 Establish avenues for public interaction and information exchange.
5 Issue public information, alerts, warnings, and notifications.

The key is for these PHEP functions to align with an emergency risk communication plan that strategically guides communication during a health emergency. For emergency risk communicators, the key is to crosswalk the Capability 4: Emergency Public

Information and Warning with the CERC's recommended components of a crisis communication plan.

The 2014 CERC manual outlines required components of the crisis communication plan[6,7]:

- Signed endorsements from senior leadership.
- Designate responsibilities for the public information team.
- Information verification and clearance procedures.
- Establish agreements on release authorities (who releases what and when).
- Media contact lists.
- Plan to coordinate public health response teams.
- Designate spokespeople.
- Notification procedures for public information and preparedness and response teams.
- Contact lists for emergency response partners.
- Have agreements and procedures to join Emergency Operations Center and/or Joint Information Center/System (JIC).
- Develop procedures to secure needed resources.
- Outline information dissemination efforts.
- Lists of stakeholders, including who they are, where they are located, and how to reach them.

Crisis communication plans need to include the materials identified during a communication audit that can be used during a health emergency. The following sections crosswalk the PHEP capabilities with sections of a CERC plan to provide practical guidance on how to revise and update existing communication plans.

Function 1: Activate the Emergency Public Health Information System

This function ensures that the crisis communication team and spokespeople are alerted to the health emergency and can provide information to the public.

The core tasks of the function are:

- Identify key personnel (including spokespeople, subject matter experts, public information officers) to implement and disseminate emergency risk communication.
- Identify the location of a physical or virtual Joint Information Center or Joint Information System.
- Outline how key personnel will be notified about the emergency.
- Identify the roles and responsibilities of those who are responsible for emergency risk communication.
- Ensure key personnel are trained.
- Clarify roles between and among partner agencies regarding public information activities.

What Does This Look Like in a CERC Plan?

Within a crisis communication plan, clearly outline who will act as spokespeople and for what emergency response they will be used. Also clarify when particular spokespeople will be used depending on the magnitude and severity of the emergency response. For example, for some foodborne illness outbreaks, having an epidemiologist serve as a spokesperson is appropriate as they will be the expert on the outbreak investigation. However, if the outbreak involves multiple counties or a high-profile organization, having a health officer or health department as spokesperson is more appropriate.

Next, include members of the crisis communication team and identify what roles and responsibilities they will hold. In this, it is critical to identify individuals with specific skillsets related to writing, communication, media monitoring and analysis, media relations, and website and social media management. If you have a small agency, you may need to identify staff from programs outside of the preparedness program. For example, if the preparedness program only staffs three individuals, leveraging staff from the immunization program or nursing division will be necessary during a health emergency. If staff do not have the necessary skills or need to receive training, ensure that the preparedness program facilitates the necessary training and tracks which individuals have received training.

Developing Sustainable Crisis Communication Teams

In addition to outlining policies and procedures, CERC plans designate who will carry out emergency risk communication activities. Two key tenets of public health preparedness include scaling operations to meet emergency response demands and having a skilled workforce that is able to perform during health emergencies. A health department that leverages and integrates public health preparedness with existing systems and public health practices will be able to quickly scale up their emergency response activities during an active response.[8]

An expert and fully staffed workforce includes having skilled team members who can perform during a health emergency and leaders who can manage the health emergency, engage with stakeholders, and effectively communicate response operations and mitigation strategies. To develop a sustainable crisis communication team, first look internally at current staff labor categories and skillsets and then determine if, and when, external support is needed. Table 2.1 outlines the key roles needed for a crisis communication team.

Communication plans can add other positions depending on the scope and scale of the health emergency. Additionally, if a Joint Information Center is established, there may be more roles to consider, such as a Joint Information Center manager, who oversees the administration of the JIC and may coordinate public email inquiries regarding the emergency response.

Function 2: Determine the Need for a Joint Information Center/System

This function focuses on coordinating public information, both internally within the health agency and externally with other jurisdictions and agencies. A point of distinction is needed here: A JIC can be created either as a structure internal only to public health (i.e., a public health JIC) or public health can participate in a JIC created by an emergency management agency (i.e., emergency management JIC).

The core tasks of this function are:
- Coordinate with emergency management to determine the need for a public health JIC and coordinate with emergency management.

Table 2.1 Crisis communication team member roles and responsibilities

Role	Responsibility
Spokespeople	Designated to speak to the media on behalf of the agency during a health emergency. Spokespeople personalize and humanize the agency during health emergencies.
Subject matter experts	Experts on a particular health topic area who provide technical and scientific information and review content for public health messaging. Can include health officers, epidemiologists, infectious disease doctors, and immunization specialists.
Media relations	Coordinate with the media and spokespeople for interviews and press briefings.
Website managers	Oversee and manage content on the health department website. Coordinate when to disseminate information with public information officers.
Social media managers	Oversee and manage social media channels. Monitor channels for comments and sentiment analysis. Coordinate when to disseminate information with public information officers.
Public information officers	Manage emergency communications and coordinate with personnel from media relations, website management, social media management, call centers, and JIC to ensure coordinated and consistent messages. Establish communications strategy. Coordinate media monitoring.
Hotline/call center coordinators	Oversee and manage emergency hotlines/call centers. Share public inquiry data as input for the development of communications strategy.
Translators	Translate information into multiple languages.
Interpreters	Sign language interpreters assist during media briefings.
508 compliance coordinators	Ensure people with disabilities can equitably access relevant documents and information.

- If a public health JIC is not activated, identify who will participate in an emergency management JIC.
- Coordinate the delivery of public information from the JIC through four common functions: information gathering, information dissemination, operations support, and liaison roles.

What Does This Look Like in a CERC Plan?

JICs are a part of the National Incident Management System (NIMS), and they were developed to coordinate communication activities across multiple agencies during emergency management disaster responses.[9] In a traditional JIC, a physical location is set up for public information officers from different agencies to develop messages based on their agency's role in the response, and the incident commander approves the message before it is released. The virtual form of this coordinating center is called a Joint Information System. This book will refer to both a Joint Information Center and a Joint Information System as a JIC.

CDC and local public health departments often operationalize JICs to organize internal communication functions and coordinate with other health departments. This is called a public health JIC.[3] The public health JIC functions as the main media distribution point during health emergencies and ensures the distribution of consistent and accurate information.[10,11]

The following functions of a JIC were used as part of the CDC 2005 severe acute respiratory syndrome (SARS) emergency response[10]:

- Issue local public health announcements and updated information on the outbreak and response efforts.
- Disseminate information about the health emergency, its management, and the possible need for travel restrictions, isolation, and quarantine measures.
- Establish a "news desk operation" to coordinate and manage media relations activities.
- Provide a location for state, local, and federal communication and emergency response personnel to meet and work side by side on developing key messages, handling media inquiries, and writing media advisories and briefing documents.
- Respond to frequently asked questions by developing fact sheets, talking points (key messages), and question-and-answer documents.
- Coordinate requests for spokespeople and subject matter experts.
- Issue media credentials to the press.
- Address other local/regional information requests related to the outbreak that require distribution to the media and the general public.
- Develop, coordinate, and manage local websites as required.

Public health JICs are often established to coordinate internal and external emergency risk communication activities. For example, health departments work on outbreaks on a regular basis, with many of them never reaching a declared health emergency status. In these situations, activating an external JIC is not necessary because the outbreak situation does not overwhelm current resources and current resources can handle the public health incident. Instead, the health agency may bring together an internal JIC to coordinate communication across multiple internal programs. However, when outbreaks are larger and require more communications support, creating a JIC will scale up communication activities and the number of people working on communication activities. Remember, emergencies start at the local level. During communication planning and review, it is good practice to develop a threshold or trigger chart that outlines that when certain conditions are reached, a JIC will be activated. Procedures for activating and maintaining the structure of a JIC if one is activated will be outlined in a later section of this chapter.

How Best to Engage with Partner Agencies

A key factor to establishing a public health JIC is including partner agencies. Health departments respond to outbreaks and other smaller health threats on a regular basis, but sometimes they need additional support when local systems are overwhelmed. It is imperative for health department staff to know and understand what local resources are available to handle health emergencies and what trigger events or thresholds will initiate a formal emergency response declaration and multidisciplinary and multijurisdictional responses.

When a formal health emergency is declared, local and state health departments can request additional resources. Depending on the situation, other government agencies may also be involved. Consider the following quote: "When you want to go fast, go alone. When you want to go farther, go together." This quote is relevant to large-scale emergencies because multiple government agencies will be involved in the response, all of which will have key tasks and responsibilities to carry out. However, even in large-scale emergency responses, one agency is designated the lead; this lead role is determined by the type of emergency (i.e., natural disaster, terrorism, health, etc.).

Designating who does what is often established through formal training, tabletop exercises, full-scale exercises, and, of course, real-world experience. These are key activities that happen during the precrisis phase of a health emergency. Developing a regular frequency for meetings, tabletops, and function exercises will help build relationships and maintain trust between and among agencies. For emergency risk communicators, establishing communications-specific tabletop exercises and meeting discussions with other communicators, public information officers, and identified spokespeople will create a strong working relationship with internal public health staff and with communicators external to the agency.

When a relationship is established with another agency, it is imperative to maintain and nurture that relationship over time. Knowing the responsibilities of other agencies and identifying key staff in other agencies – such as the public information officer for the transportation department or the forestry department – could help make an emergency response more efficient. Having these preidentified relationships in place before an emergency occurs makes agency collaboration during a response easier, more effective, and more efficient.[12] Trying to develop relationships and build trust with new response partners during a health emergency can be challenging.[13]

Further, when public health agencies participate in an emergency that is led and managed by emergency management – whether at the local, state, or federal level – within the JIC the health agency serves as the subject matter expert for health and medical issues and questions. For example, under Emergency Support Function 8 (ESF 8), public health and medical services annex,[14,15] when emergency management is leading an emergency response, the public health function is supporting delivery of medical countermeasures, equipment and supplies, and technical assistance. Further, under ESF 8, the public health function is to communicate emergency risk information, including proactive actions the public can take to protect their health.

Function 3: Establish and Participate in Information System Operations

This function focuses on how to engage with CERC activities through monitoring the media, conducting media briefings, and addressing rumors:
- Participate in public information sharing.
- Control rumors.

- Provide a single point of dissemination of information for public health and health care issues.

What Does This Look Like in a CERC Plan?

Within the CERC plan, it is critical to outline such matters as issuing press releases, establishing an incident-specific emergency website, holding media briefings, and establishing call centers. Understanding how the agency will address rumors is important. See Chapter 7 information on addressing rumors.

For health emergency responses, it is critical to streamline communication so that the public, stakeholders, and media inquiries are identified, documented, and responded to in an efficient manner. One way to streamline emergency communication is to funnel emergency inquiries to specific emergency response phone numbers and emails. These emergency-specific communication channels are often used when a JIC is established.

Function 4: Establish Avenues for Public Interaction and Information Exchange

Provide ways for the public to contact the health agency during an emergency, such as:
- Establish systems for handling public and media inquiries.
- Post incident-related information on health agency websites.
- Use social media platforms and text messaging.
- Identify, protect, and ensure information exchange occurs with hard-to-reach and socially vulnerable populations.

What Does This Look Like in a CERC Plan?

Within the CERC plan, it is critical to outline how and when certain types of media relations activities are used, such as issuing press releases, establishing an incident-specific emergency website, holding media briefings, and establishing call centers. Leverage the agency's digital channels to share and disseminate information, including the agency website, social media channels, GovDelivery newsletters, and text messaging. See Chapter 5 for more information on communication channels. Coordinating with the public health and preparedness program can help identify the locations of hard-to-reach and socially vulnerable populations. See Chapter 3 for more information on identifying audiences.

Function 5: Issue Public Information, Alerts, Warnings, and Notifications

Use CERC principles to disseminate critical health and safety information to the media, the public, and other stakeholders.

The core tasks include:
- Comply with jurisdictional legal guidelines when communicating information.
- Disseminate information to the public using message maps (including those who are deaf or hard of hearing or have visual impairments, limited English proficiency, diverse cultural backgrounds, cognitive limitations, or those who do not use traditional media).
- Disseminate information to responder organizations.

What Does This Look Like in a CERC Plan?

This function of the crisis communication plan leverages communication messages such as talking points, webpage copy, social media messages, fact sheets, and webpages about the virus, among others, all of which can be used during an emergency. It is also imperative that communication materials be available in multiple formats. Although not a state requirement, 508 compliance is a federal law that requires US federal agencies to provide accessible information to people with disabilities when using electronic and information technology.[16]

Finally, the crisis communications plan needs to outline procedures regarding information distribution to stakeholders, the public, and the media. For example, identify what communication channels will be used to send press releases to the media. If a specific media email list is established, identify how that will be used during a health emergency and who has the ability to send such releases. If a GovDelivery email newsletter is established, outline how that will access the system and send the message.

Key Tip: Emergency Communication Clearance Processes, Release Schedules, and Updating Published Materials

As outlined earlier, a crisis communication plan will include communication clearance processes and procedures, including a release schedule and processes for updating published materials. The *communication clearance process* is a critical step for agency leadership and subject matter experts to review and approve emergency messaging before it is officially released to the public, media, partner agencies, and stakeholders. This final review ensures the emergency messaging is scientifically accurate and does not violate agency policies. The *release schedule* is managed by the communications team and outlines how often information will be released. For example, during the initial phase of an emergency, information may be updated every 24 hours. As the emergency moves into the maintenance phase, information may be updated weekly. As the emergency moves into the recovery phase, information may be updated monthly. A *process for updating published materials* ensures that the emergency information available on the agency's website and social media channels is accurate and up to date. When updating published materials, it is helpful to designate a subject matter expert to review agency web pages in order to ensure the posted information remains accurate. It is also imperative to outline how often the review of published materials will take place (e.g., daily, weekly, monthly). Finally, designate a web or communications team member to make the actual updates.

When developing a communication clearance process, consider the following:

- Who needs to review the document? Consider agency leadership, subject matter experts, and the policy team. Give each reviewer specific instructions on what to look for when reviewing. For example, have subject matter experts look at the accuracy of the content and have a communications specialist focus on proofreading and grammar issues. It is a best practice to have the policy team review the documents to ensure emergency messages do not impact current agency policies.
- How will the review process take place? For example, will you send the materials by email or create a specific SharePoint site to facilitate the review process?

- Who is the final approver? Often the highest-ranking official of the agency gives final approval regarding a message. If the Incident Command System has been activated, the Incident Commander may be the final approver.
- How much time is needed to review? It is a best practice to provide reviewers with clear deadlines and timelines for review. For example, if the information needs to be sent to the media in 2 hours, tell the reviewers they only have 1 hour for review, which provides the communications team with 1 hour to address edits and package the materials for release.

Mini-Case Study: Douglas Complex Fire

On July 26, 2013, lightning and thunderstorms moved into Douglas County in central Oregon, and a lightning strike ignite multiple wildfires, which were collectively referred to as the "Douglas Complex Fire."[17] The Douglas Complex Fire was made up of three separate fires – the Milo branch fire, the Rabbit Mountain/Union Creek fire, and the Dad's Creek/Panther Butte fire – impacting land and communities.[18] The Oregon Office of the State Fire Marshall and the Oregon Department of Forestry coordinated fire operations and evacuations. While the fire threatened land and property, the smoke from the wildfire began impacting the community's health. Air quality readings from the Oregon Department of Environmental Quality indicated "unhealthy" and "hazardous" levels in some areas of the state.[18,19]

The local health departments began working with the Oregon Department of Forestry, which was the lead agency managing the emergency response efforts. The fire's scope and severity overwhelmed local resources, and additional state and federal resources were requested.

When the state health department got involved, they used the CERC toolkit for wildfires to guide public messaging. The toolkit had been developed earlier that year and included samples of phase-based messaging: messages designed for the precrisis, initial, maintenance, and recovery phases of a health emergency. For the initial and maintenance phases, the toolkit was color-coded with a red band at the top of the page so that people could flip right to the predeveloped crisis messages they could send out.

During the emergency response, emergency risk communicators discovered that the predeveloped messaging was not focusing on the right health threat: The messaging needed to focus on the impacts of smoke inhalation. Working with public health medical doctors, messages began to focus on the potential health impacts from inhaling wildfire smoke. For example, wildfire smoke contains a type of particulate matter called PM2.5, and if these particles get into a person's lungs, they can cause cardiovascular and respiratory issues.[20] Individuals with lung conditions or other underlying medical conditions can become very ill when exposed to wildfire smoke.[21]

Additionally, geographical location also posed a risk to the public's health. Two affected communities, Shady Cove and Glendale, are located in valley or bowl-like areas, so the smoke-contaminated air did not dissipate from these areas. Both communities were advised to evacuate. Some evacuees were able to head to the nearby Oregon coast. However, these communities included a large percentage of older people and people of lower socioeconomic status, and evacuation was less feasible or realistic for these individuals.

Through working with the local community health department, the federal Forest Service, the local forest service, and the local environmental health department, the

CERC toolkit began to adapt the messages to contain what was needed regarding the health threat of smoke inhalation. Coordinating public messaging became a joint effort among local and state agencies, including multiple disciplines and multiple jurisdictions. Additionally, the US Forest Service developed and monitored a blog that became the "go-to" source of public information about health impacts from wildfire smoke. The health agencies provided the US Forest Service with health information and proactive steps people could take to protect their health.

During an AAR, emergency risk communicators learned that the CERC toolkit for wildfires needed to be edited and revised to focus on the impacts of smoke inhalation. The updated CERC manual has been used in subsequent wildfire smoke responses and continues to be edited and adapted based on lessons learned through each wildfire smoke response.

Overview of Message Testing and Developing Consensus Recommendations

The CDC CERC model[22] and the National Center for Food Protection and Defense's Best Practices for Risk and Crisis Communication[23] both advocate that, during the precrisis phase, emergency risk communicators create and test messages that could be used during a health emergency. Additionally, communicators should work with other agencies and coordinate these messages to ensure coordinated and consistent public messaging is achieved.

Creating messages can be an easy task: Identify what information is available, work with subject matter experts to ensure the information is scientifically accurate, and format the information according to the communication channel that will be used to disseminate it. Message testing and coordinating with partner agencies take message development further and will require more time and additional coordination.[7,22]

Message Testing and Consensus Recommendations

Message testing emerged in the 1970s as a form of public relations evaluation and measurement. Message testing provides an opportunity to determine whether messages will persuade individuals to take an action, but often message testing does not occur because it can be expensive and time-consuming.[24] Developing consensus recommendations differs from message testing in that consensus recommendations for public health emergencies are agreed upon by subject matter experts regarding the health, medical, and other strategic recommendations to mitigate health threats.[25] Consensus recommendations bolster future emergency response efforts. These recommendations ensure that agencies will engage in similar response activities and achieve consistent public messaging regarding these activities. Gathering key leadership, subject matter experts, and communication officers from multiple disciplines and jurisdictions – especially those with shared media markets – to discuss consensus recommendations is a key preparedness activity; however, during the COVID-19 pandemic response – due to the novel virus and its global impact – consensus recommendations were developed during the emergency response.[24,25,26] When agencies come together to discuss similarities and differences in activities and messaging, they ultimately must agree upon consensus recommendations. After agencies are clear on response activities and recommendations, message testing can occur.

To engage in message testing, first assess whether there is a budget for message testing. If there is a large budget available, your health agency may consider hiring a public relations firm, communication consultants, or university researchers to conduct formal message testing. If there is a smaller budget or no budget available, there are two options to consider: (1) Assess whether there is any opportunity for pro bono work with public relations firms, communication consultants, or university researchers or (2) if there is no budget, identify partner agencies and stakeholder groups who might be willing to donate some of their time to assist with a scaled-down version of message testing.

Many health departments do not have budgets for formal message testing, so the following recommendations are for real-world applications of message testing with a small or no budget. Even without a budget, low- to no-cost message testing provides the opportunity to get outside of your organizational bubble, check your messaging assumptions, and learn more about the people you are trying to communicate with.[27]

Steps to Take When Planning for Message Testing

1 *Identify if there are evaluation experts within your own health department, neighboring health departments, or state health department.* If there aren't any evaluation experts in the public health system, consider working with evaluation partners from universities or other government agencies who would be willing to donate their time.
2 *Work with evaluation subject matter experts to develop a basic evaluation plan to test messages.* Identify what messages you want to test, the metrics to test them, and ways to analyze the data. When testing messages, consider the following factors: the values of the people you are trying to reach, whether they trust or like the official spokespeople, and aesthetics like images, colors, words, and phrasing.[27] Ensure the messages being tested are based upon the consensus recommendations regarding response activities.
3 *Identify the method you want to use.* Different methods of collecting data include focus groups, semistructured interviews, online surveys, or "ask a friend."[27] Consider the target audience of the messages and invite individuals who can do so to provide feedback to ensure the messages will resonate with the target audience. Again, if you have a small budget, offering incentives such as a gift card or another form of payment will be appreciated by the participants.

Two common ways with which to engage in message testing are to gather input and feedback on the messages, including text, wording and phrases, and images.[24] The goal of message testing is to ensure the message will resonate with the target audience and that this audience will be motivated to take an action. Ideally, surveys are then used as mini-field tests to gather feedback from a large population of people.[24] Since surveys gather information from a larger population of people, the quantitative data can be analyzed to provide additional information about the likelihood that individuals will take an action.

Many health departments will create plans to utilize focus groups and qualitative methods in order to gather and analyze information. While these findings will not be generalizable to a larger population, they often provide valuable information regarding language (including wording and phrasing), images, and color, and they even provide information on dates to avoid when disseminating messages. For

example, there may be events, holidays, or religious observances that are occurring, and information shared during these times will likely not be read or acted upon.
4 *Collect and analyze the data.* After outlining methods, start collecting data. After collecting data, analyze them using the appropriate methods and tests. If qualitative methods are used, consider following up with the focus groups or stakeholders to gather more information or to clarify the information they provided.
5 *Update the communication materials as needed.* Using the data that were gathered, begin a systematic process of updating existing materials based upon feedback. If qualitative methods were used, share the edited material with the focus groups and stakeholders to ensure the edits match their feedback.
6 *Finalize the materials and share them.* After editing and reviewing the materials through the agency's internal review and clearance procedures, begin to share the materials as outlined in the CERC plan.

Mini-Case Study: Middle Eastern Respiratory Syndrome

In the spring and summer of 2014, Saudi Arabia experienced a large outbreak of Middle Eastern respiratory syndrome coronavirus (MERS-CoV), which generated some concern of a larger outbreak occurring during Hajj in October.[28] In Oregon, the state health department engaged in public health preparedness activities to educate individuals who were traveling to the area about the risk of MERS-CoV. They created a fact sheet with known information about the virus, about risks of getting ill, and about what to do upon return from the area.[29,30]

To ensure that the fact sheet and key messages would resonate with the intended audience, the communication materials were shared with different nongovernmental organizations to obtain feedback. Through the feedback process, the health department learned that the two images originally included in the fact sheet would not resonate with the audience. For example, one image constituted a map that incorrectly identified the area impacted by the MERS outbreak. The other photo was of a person whose image did not resonate with the intended audience. By engaging with groups that work with the intended audience to check messaging assumptions, the health department received feedback that helped them to update the images and change some of the text. This provides a basic example of informal message testing conducted by a health agency in anticipation of an emerging health emergency.

Theory Callout: CERC Framework

The CERC framework provides emergency risk communicators with an integrated approach to using strategic communications approaches to communicate health and risk information during a health emergency. Leveraging the six principles of Be First, Be Right, Be Credible, Provide Empathy, Promote Action, and Show Respect coupled with the crisis communication lifecycle phases of precrisis, initial, maintenance, recovery, and evaluation, CERC is a robust framework that can guide novice and seasoned emergency risk communicators before, during, and after a health emergency.

As a theoretical framework, CERC offers six propositions[31]:

1 Risks and crises create uncertain conditions that produce unique information needs among the public, stakeholders, and partners.

2   Two-way communications are needed to reduce uncertainty and promote action to mitigate health threats.
3   As the health threat evolves, communication will undergo a particular life cycle based on the crisis phases. Leveraging different communication channels to communicate throughout the crisis is critical.
4   The way information is communicated can influence the development and mitigation of the health emergency.
5   Proactive messages, or messages of self-efficacy, help reduce health risk during health emergencies.
6   Crisis communication requires message senders to consider a diverse audience.

More research is needed to analyze and test these propositions before the CERC framework can become more established as a theory. See Chapter 10 for more details on the current academic literature evaluating the CERC framework.

Derailment of Norfolk Southern Train in East Palestine, Ohio: An Analysis of CERC
Laura Herrmann, MPH

Overview of the East Palestine Train Derailment
East Palestine, Ohio, is a small village located near the Ohio–Pennsylvania border, about 45 miles northwest of Pittsburgh, Pennsylvania. On February 3, 2023, a Norfolk Southern train derailed east of the town, less than 1 mile from the Pennsylvania border. A total of 38 cars derailed, 11 of which contained hazardous materials.[32] Norfolk Southern officials and local emergency response crews became concerned about rising temperatures in five of the derailed cars containing hazardous materials, including vinyl chloride. Major concerns emerged in the days following the derailment of the risk of an imminent and potentially catastrophic explosion.[33]

A joint decision was made by Ohio and Pennsylvania state officials, the private Norfolk Southern rail company responders, and the public first responder response crews to conduct a controlled release of the chemicals to limit the possibility of an explosion. On February 5, residents within 1 mile of the derailment site were evacuated, and 5,000 other residents were put under a shelter-in-place order. On February 6, a controlled release, also sometimes called a "controlled burn," was conducted.[34] This caused large black plumes of smoke to be released and raised immediate concerns about air quality. Shortly after the controlled release, residents were also noting effects on wildlife, such as observing dead fish. Officials noted on February 15 that three waterways that are tributaries of the Ohio River were contaminated.[35]

On February 8, the evacuation order was lifted. Residents began to return home. By February 10, residents began to report symptoms such as rashes and nausea.[36] There are ongoing concerns about the possible health effects on humans, wildlife, and the quality of the air, water, and soil. In the time since the controlled release, many local, state, and national leaders and agencies have been involved in the response to the crisis. National and international interest in the story and concern over the derailment have led to calls for national policy change to improve rail safety. As of September 2024, the US Environmental Protection Agency (EPA) continues with testing and clean-up efforts in the area.[37] Additionally, a class action lawsuit was filed in 2024 seeking a $600 million settlement in economic damages to individuals and business affected by the disaster.[38,39] Furthermore, the US Department of Justice and EPA are seeking a $310 million consent decree. If the degree is approved, "Norfolk Southern will be required to take measures to improve rail safety, pay for health monitoring and mental health services for the surrounding communities, fund long-term environmental monitoring, pay a $15 million civil penalty and take other actions to protect nearby waterways and drinking water resources."[37,40]

Timeline of Key Events
- February 3, 2023, 8:55 p.m. EST: 38 cars derailed, 11 of which were carrying hazardous materials including vinyl chloride, benzene residue, and butyl acrylate.
- February 4: The EPA arrived in East Palestine.
- February 5: Ohio Governor Mike DeWine activated the Ohio National Guard; 5,000 residents were put under a shelter-in-place order; residents within a 1-mile radius in both Ohio and Pennsylvania were given an evacuation order.
- February 6, 3:30 p.m. EST: A controlled release of five cars contained vinyl chloride was conducted to prevent explosion. Governor DeWine gave a press conference prior to the controlled release.
- February 8: The evacuation order was lifted, and residents began to return to their homes.
- February 10: Some residents who returned home reported developing a rash and nausea within half an hour of returning.
- February 14: Governor DeWine gave a press conference with updates about concerns regarding air quality, water quality, and impacts on wildlife.
- February 16: An EPA administrator arrived to assess Norfolk Southern's response; Governor DeWine asked CDC for assistance in assessing residents experiencing symptoms.
- February 21: Ohio State Health Department set up a clinic to assess symptoms in residents.
- February 22: Former president Donald Trump visited and hosted a press conference.
- February 23: Secretary of Transportation Pete Buttigieg visited and hosted a press conference.

Overview of CERC Principles and Phase-Based Messaging
CDC has outlined six key principles for CERC. These six overarching CERC principles, as well as the specific phase-based messaging guidance, will serve as the basis for the following analysis of the messaging during the Norfolk Southern train derailment in East Palestine, Ohio.

The six CERC principles are Be First, Be Right, Be Credible, Express Empathy, Promote Action, and Show Respect. Additionally, the CERC principles outline the goals for messaging during different phases of a crisis response. The initial phase of crisis and emergency response is typically characterized by uncertainty during the first 24–72 hours of an event, while the maintenance phase typically lasts much longer and constitutes the bulk of the risk communication effort. Resolution- or recovery-phase messaging comes much later, when the community has fully dealt with the impacts of the event and is starting to move toward a new normal.[6]

According to CERC guidelines, each phase has specific communication needs to be addressed. In the initial messaging phase, expressing empathy, establishing credibility, and explaining what is known about the risks are the focuses of these communications. Other important practices for initial-phase messaging include the CERC principles of Be First and Promote Action. In the maintenance phase of messaging, more emphasis is placed on deeper risk explanations, answering questions, and addressing misinformation. This is also a time for risk communication that those promotes actions that can move the community toward risk mitigation and resolution. In the resolution phase, risk communicators seek to express a need to establish a new normal and to help both the public and organizations involved in the response to learn from the crisis in order to be better prepared for similar crisis events in the future.

Introduction to the Analysis of CERC Principles in the East Palestine Train Derailment Response
To analyze the emergency and risk messaging that emerged after the train derailment in East Palestine, I focused on the Ohio state government communication responses through the lens of the office of the Governor, Mike DeWine. I was interested in leadership responses to the crisis. In particular, I was interested in how Governor DeWine performed as a spokesperson while coordinating with many local, state, and national agencies as well as the private rail company Norfolk Southern. The analysis is focused on two press conferences that occurred during different phases of the crisis that both featured Governor DeWine as the spokesperson. The first press conference analyzed was conducted during the initial phase of the crisis, less than 72 hours after the original event and before the controlled release was executed. The next press conference analyzed was conducted during the early maintenance phase of the crisis, about 9 days after the original event and approximately 1 week after the controlled release.

In addition to these press conferences, I analyzed some of the Ohio state government's written press releases and website updates that were hosted on the Governor's website as well as the Ohio Emergency Management Agency (EMA) website.

In May 2023, the crisis was still in the maintenance phase, and little clear recovery messaging has been put forward by the state of Ohio, the office of the Governor, or other national leaders. That being the case, I took the opportunity to also perform a comparison analysis of two other prominent national leaders who visited the area and conducted maintenance-phase press conferences: Donald Trump and Pete Buttigieg. It was interesting to see how different leadership responses did or did not follow CERC phase-based messaging principles and how this might yield insights into being an effective crisis event spokesperson and risk communicator.

Analysis of Initial-Phase Messaging
On February 6, 2023, Ohio Governor Mike DeWine appeared as the spokesperson at a press conference in East Palestine. This was at the end of the initial phase of the crisis, within the first 72 hours of the initial event and just before the controlled release of the five cars that were considered explosion risks. According to the CERC principles for initial-phase messages, Governor DeWine did several things well. Governor DeWine came across as a credible source of accurate information, fulfilling the CERC requirements of being right and being credible. He was straightforward, honest about what he did and did not know, and deferred to experts when they had answers that he did not. He gave facts, communicated risk, and described a life-or-death situation.

In addition to being right and being credible, Governor DeWine is also "first" in the sense that he gave a formal press conference within a reasonable amount of time after the crisis and before next major steps were taken. Some attendees questioned whether Governor DeWine could have responded sooner than 2.5 days after the event. When questioned directly about the timing of the press conference, the Governor cited that the level of threat was being continuously assessed. As soon as the threat of rising temperatures in five cars escalated, he went to East Palestine to address the situation, and once a decision was reached between the rail company and the Pennsylvania and Ohio governments, he shared that information.

Finally, Governor DeWine promoted action, which is an important CERC principle for the initial phase of messaging. Namely, he issued an evacuation order in stark terms.

He explained that this emergency evacuation was necessary due to the imminent controlled release and the threat this posed to residents in the immediate vicinity.

While Governor DeWine did an admirable job of meeting many of the CERC initial-phase messaging criteria, there were also areas that could have been improved. One area that could have been significantly improved was expressing empathy, a key principle of CERC messaging, especially in the initial phase of a crisis response. There was no real acknowledgment of the fear and confusion residents may have been feeling, nor any acknowledgment of the risks being taken by those individuals who were directly responding to the crisis. Another area where there was room for improvement was showing respect. Governor DeWine's tone was very matter-of-fact, perhaps reflecting his exhaustion. This tone verged on lacking showing of respect for residents and the media, though it was not outright disrespectful. Despite the lack of empathy and the potential for improvement in the tone of the delivery, this was a solid initial-phase message overall, with most of the content that would be expected according to CERC principles.

In addition to this initial-phase press conference, I also looked at press release statements issued by the Governor's office, which are currently housed on the Ohio EMA website. During the emergency response, the Governor's website had a banner at the top of the page linking to these Ohio EMA resources. To analyze press releases written during the initial phase, I look at two of the earliest from the days of February 5 and February 6.

Similar to the Governor's delivery as spokesperson at the press conference, these press releases met a number of key CERC principles for initial-phase messaging. They were "first" in the sense that they were written in the early days of the crisis response and contained explanations of the emerging threat of rising temperatures in several of the rail cars. They promoted immediate emergency action in the form of evacuation. They also established credibility by containing accurate information delivered in a matter-of-fact tone.

Just as these strengths were similar to those of the Governor's press conference, these press releases also shared the press conference's weaknesses. These statements lacked any expressions of empathy regarding the fear, confusion, and disruption to the lives of residents, nor any empathy or shows of respect for first responders who had been at this dangerous scene for several days. The inclusion of a statement of empathy would have made these press releases stronger initial messages.

Analysis of Maintenance-Phase Messaging
On February 14, Governor DeWine was again the spokesperson during a follow-up press conference addressing maintenance-phase concerns in East Palestine following the train derailment. Governor DeWine once again presented himself as a credible spokesperson who delivered accurate information, meeting the criteria of being right and being credible. In this press conference he did a much better job of showing respect to conference attendees and the media, other experts, and the general audience. Governor DeWine also delivered more in-depth risk explanations and coordinated with many field experts, who also gave in-depth risk explanations. He explained in greater detail what had gone into the decision to conduct the controlled release. He talked about what was within his power to prevent something like this from happening in the future and discussed policy changes for the transportation of hazardous materials. He also made a strong commitment to the community of stakeholders, stating: "We'll be here until everything in East Palestine is done."[35]

Governor DeWine and the panel of experts also spent about half of the press conference addressing questions and misinformation. Many of the questions they addressed had been topics of speculation and misinformation circulating on the internet. These topics included: the possibility of contaminated waterways and drinking water sources; the possibility of air contamination; and the impacts on human health and wildlife health. The team did a fairly good job of addressing these questions by presenting facts first. Especially regarding waterways and drinking water sources, in-depth explanations of what was being done and what was known were given.[41]

Despite meeting many of the CERC principles and guidelines for maintenance-phase messaging, there was room for improvement in this press conference in a few areas. Once again, there was a complete omission of any kind of statement of empathy for East Palestine residents or for the people working in response to the crisis. In addition to not making a statement of empathy, Governor DeWine made no attempt to explain how the derailment happened mechanically or how to prevent a derailment like this from happening in the future outside of promoting policy change. It is possible that this was not addressed because the National Transportation Safety Board (NTSB) had not yet concluded its investigation into what had caused the derailment. Finally, while many concerns and areas of misinformation were addressed, there were also some confusing and contradictory messages. For example, confidence in the message that the drinking water supply was likely to be safe was tempered by, and possibly undermined by, recommendations to drink bottled water and seek private well water testing. Despite these opportunities for improvement, this was a solid maintenance-phase response, and Governor DeWine performed admirably as a spokesperson.

Looking at press releases and website updates from the same time period of February 15 and February 16, the analysis of maintenance-phase print messaging once again reflects the press conference analysis. The press releases and website updates adequately provided detailed risk explanations about multiple subjects, many of which also helped to mitigate the impacts of rumors and misinformation. There were also links and phone numbers provided to many different resources, including well water testing, air quality testing, a care line for mental health resources, and descriptions of future plans for health clinics. However, once again, these press releases and website updates lacked messages of empathy for residents and first responders.[42]

Comparison with Maintenance-Phase Messages from Other National Leadership Figures
I decided to look at two more press conferences with national leaders to assess their responses according to the CERC principles for maintenance-phase messages. The first is a press conference delivered by former president Donald Trump, and the second is a press conference that was delivered by Secretary of Transportation Pete Buttigieg. Comparing these responses to each other as well as to press conferences lead by Governor DeWine yielded valuable insights into the strengths and weaknesses of leadership responses to crisis events.

On February 22, 2023, former president Donald Trump visited East Palestine and delivered a press conference. In contrast to Governor DeWine, Trump expressed empathy for residents and first responders. Empathy was probably the strongest part of his emergency and risk communication. He also made a commitment statement, but it was not firm and made use of if/then statements, such as: "We're gonna find time to come back, if necessary. If they don't give you the treatment that you need, we will be back."[43] Finally, Trump explained that he had brought bottled water with him on his plane, and that his team had helped coordinate other water deliveries for the East Palestine community.

While Trump's message delivered empathy, made an attempt at commitment, and mentioned one action step that residents could potentially take (to acquire bottled water), it lacked many other components of CERC maintenance-phase messaging criteria. For example, it did not give any risk explanations pertinent to the situation, as would be expected in a maintenance-phase message. Outside of the mention of bringing bottled water, Trump did not offer an explanation of what else was being done to help the community or where to seek resources (including this bottled water). This means that there were no actionable steps residents could take based solely on this message. Furthermore, he did not show respect to political rivals who had responded to the crisis, such as the Governor of Ohio and the federal agencies who responded to the event. Finally, he spent a good deal of time speaking about topics that were unrelated to the crisis event entirely, such as the COVID-19 response under his presidential administration, Big Ten football, and the war in Ukraine. These omissions and detractions made this message a poor maintenance-phase message overall according to CERC principles.

On February 23, the Secretary of Transportation Pete Buttigieg visited East Palestine and delivered a press conference. This was the same day that NTSB released its initial report.[44] Buttigieg expressed empathy for the people of East Palestine as well as first responders, particularly calling attention to a recent loss that a specific first responder group was experiencing that day. Buttigieg also showed respect to local officials and to those attendees who asked questions. He appeared to be a credible source of information, giving coherent answers to questions within his sphere of influence. He gave a firm commitment to safety assessment and described what he was doing regarding policy that could improve safety standards for the transportation of hazardous material. He was the only leader to specifically name and thank public health officials and to address the mental health of residents. He also gave an in-depth explanation of the current hazardous train risk designations, which helped to explain both how this crisis could have happened and why the proposed policy changes would help to prevent something like this from happening in the future.

While Buttigieg got a lot of things right in this maintenance-phase message, one thing he missed as a risk communicator was being first. While this is more important as a part of initial-phase messaging, many questions that he fielded during the press conference were about why this response, 3 weeks after the incident, was the first response. Essentially, the questions were: Why did you fail to deliver an initial message? And why are we only just now hearing from you with a maintenance-phase message? While the maintenance-phase message itself was good, it seems that the impact of this message was blunted by Buttigieg's lack of an initial-phase message.

Buttigieg acknowledged he could have said something sooner and explained that he intended to defer to the NTSB report, which had been released that same day. My critique of this situation is that Buttigieg should have immediately offered an initial message of empathy that showed respect for residents and first responders, as well as citing that more information would be available after NTSB had had time to complete its investigation. Had he delivered an initial message to that effect, the impact of his maintenance-phase message would have been stronger.

Recovery-Phase Messaging
Recovery-phase messaging is characterized by helping the public to move on from the crisis and to learn from past mistakes to better prepare for future similar emergencies. Although much of this case study analysis is focused on initial and maintenance messaging, as of November 2024 the following information provides insights regarding recovery messaging.

Recovery Messaging
Ohio Governor Mike DeWine's website signals a shift to the recovery phase of crisis messaging with the last press release regarding East Palestine dated February 1, 2024.[45] The EPA website also suggests a shift from the maintenance phase to the recovery phase,

shifting from weekly updates on the East Palestine remediation and testing efforts to "as-needed" messaging as of June 28, 2024.[46] The final phase of CERC phase-based messaging also appears to be on the horizon. As of February 2024, the National Institute of Environmental Health Sciences awarded six grants to conduct research and community engagement in East Palestine.[47] The findings of these research endeavors may help contribute to future evaluation of messaging regarding the Norfolk Southern derailment.

Water and Soil Testing Updates
The Ohio Environmental Protection Agency currently reports no risk to the municipal water supply and continues to conduct monthly testing of surface water impacted by the derailment. This testing does not include private wells, but residents who are concerned about their private wells are encouraged to request free testing.[48] The last surface water sampling test report is dated September 3, 2024, showing alternately nondetectable, decreasing, and/or low levels of chemicals (vinyl chloride, benzene, acrylates, and glycols) from the derailment-affected waterways in and around East Palestine. The report also notes that levels may increase after rainfall.[49] The Pennsylvania Department of Environmental Protection has stated its intent to continue testing residents' private drinking well water within 1 mile of the derailment site for up to 10 years. Its August 27, 2024, update also confirmed that the EPA has finished its soil remediation efforts.[50]

Public Health Impacts Research
Independent researchers have found both more chemicals and more widespread contamination than officials originally stated. Researcher Andrew Whelton states that "We found contamination more than two miles downstream of the derailment site. At the time, officials were telling people that had all been contained at the derailment site. But we found, when we initially arrived, contamination openly flowing in the creeks farther downstream than officials were claiming it was."[51] The research team also found that the evacuation order may have been lifted too soon from a public health standpoint. While the interiors of buildings in East Palestine were tested, the devices approved for this testing were incapable of detecting contamination.[51,52] Independent research and testing are ongoing, including at the nearby University of Pittsburgh Department of Public Health, where two groups of researchers are looking into impacts on residents, crops, and livestock and are conducting soil sampling and water testing.[47,53]

Discussion of Implications
The first major implication of these findings is that selection of a spokesperson who can deliver a detailed explanation of the crisis as well as express empathy is crucial to executing messaging according to CERC principles. While Governor DeWine successfully included many of the key CERC principles of both initial- and maintenance-phase messaging, his omission of empathy in both phases left something to be desired in his role as spokesperson. By contrast, Trump's message had little substantive content that would be expected of effective CERC maintenance-phase messaging but did effectively express empathy. This empathy alone would probably be compelling to some people who were directly affected by this disaster. This brings me to the conclusion that an otherwise effective message can be strengthened quite a lot by including even a simple expression of empathy, and an otherwise ineffective message, lacking grounding in CERC principles, might be well received solely because of its inclusion of empathy. Empathy is an important component of crisis messaging that should not be overlooked. If the office of the Governor asked for just one piece of feedback that could improve overall messaging, I believe implementing empathy would have allowed the Governor's messaging to have had a greater impact.

The next implication of the analysis of this messaging is that timing matters. Being first – or at minimum being present early on or as soon as possible – is important. Of all the press conferences analyzed, Buttigieg's met the greatest number of CERC principles for maintenance-phase messages, but the impact of this otherwise strong example of a leadership response was blunted by his failure to be first. Had he delivered an initial-phase message, his maintenance-phase message would have been stronger. Governor DeWine encountered similar questions in his initial-phase message on why he had not spoken to the public sooner. While his answer seemed coherent and logical, he could nevertheless have made a public statement sooner expressing empathy and stating what was known and what officials were doing to learn more. The overarching implication is that it is never too early to express empathy and state that you are looking into the situation as it emerges, at a minimum. In this example of a train derailment, I would have suggested that the Governor issue a response of some kind within the first 24 hours rather than waiting almost 3 days to respond.

Another finding of this analysis is that consistency across platforms increases credibility. The Governor and his team did well in this area, presenting consistent messaging across the press conferences, written press releases, and website updates regarding the train derailment. One critique I would offer regarding this area is that the consistent omission of any empathetic messaging reduced organizational credibility and might have led the public to have a negative perception of the Governor.

Even issuing just one message of empathy in the initial phase or including one or two solid lines of empathetic messaging throughout the message campaign would have gone a long way.

Another important observation that arose from this analysis is that accuracy requires coordination with many experts, organizations, departments, and levels of government. To be right and to be credible, leaders and spokespeople must coordinate with many experts while remaining within the scope of their own professional expertise. This also highlights the necessity of showing respect to other experts and leaders, since so much coordination is required for an effective response. I thought the Governor did an exemplary job in this regard and would only recommend that he continue to do this well.

A final observation that emerged from this analysis is that strong emergency and risk communication in all phases requires the practice of deep listening. Taking ample time to adequately address all questions, or as many as possible, leads to more successful messaging and more effective spokespeople. The press conferences that more successfully followed the CERC principles for phase-based messages but also gave ample time for questions demonstrated respect to those asking the questions and provided the time for thorough responses to those questions. This format also gave opportunities to address misinformation, to give more detailed risk explanations, and to explain next steps and calls to action with greater specificity. While Governor DeWine did a reasonably good job at this, he could have used these questions to show respect and perhaps express empathy rather than merely answering them in a matter-of-fact tone.

End-of-Chapter Reflection Questions

1 Reflect on your health department's readiness to communicate during an emergency. Can you identify who develops messages during emergencies? Do you know your agency's policies regarding social media and the role of spokespeople?

2 Review your agency's crisis communication plans. Do you have plans in place to respond to a variety of public health threats? Do these plans include sample

messages based on consensus recommendations from partners and stakeholders? Do you have vendors identified who are approved by the business office to receive contracts quickly to support marketing campaigns?

3. If you could change one thing about how your agency communicates during an emergency, what would it be?

4. How does your agency communicate internally with its employees during an emergency? How do you keep your employees updated on public health emergencies that the agency is responding to?

5. Do you know how your agency communicates with community-based organizations and partner organizations? Name three ways your agency communicates with external partners during an emergency.

References

1. Seeger M, Reynolds B, Day AM. Crisis and Emergency Risk Communication: Past, Present, and Future. In: Finn F, Winni J, editors. *Crisis Communication.* Berlin, De Gruyter Mouton, 2020; 401–18.

2. Public Health Emergency Preparedness and Response Capabilities: National Standards for State, Local, Tribal, and Territorial Public Health. *Centers for Disease Control and Prevention.* 2021. www.cdc.gov/orr/readiness/capabilities/index.htm (Accessed January 11, 2024).

3. Public Health Emergency Preparedness and Response Capabilities: National Standards for State, Local, Tribal and Territorial Public Health. In: CDC, editor. *Prevention.* Washington, DC, US Department of Health and Human Services, 2018. www.cdc.gov/readiness/media/pdfs/CDC_PreparednesResponse Capabilities_October2018_Final_508.pdf (Accessed April 1, 2024).

4. *Study Guide for the Examination for Accreditation in Public Relations.* New York, Universal Accreditation Board/Public Relations Society of America, 2021.

5. Houser RS. The Role of Public Health Emergency Management in Biodefense: A COVID-19 Case Study. *Disaster Med Public Health Prep* 2023;17:e185.

6. CDC. *Crisis and Emergency Risk Communication October 2017.* Atlanta, GA, CDC, 2018.

7. CDC. *Crisis and Emergency Risk Communication October 2014.* Atlanta, GA, CDC, 2014.

8. Nelson C, Lurie N, Wasserman J, Zakowski S. Conceptualizing and Defining Public Health Emergency Preparedness. *Am J Pub Health* 2007;97: s9–s11.

9. *National Incident Management System Basic Guidance for Public Information Officers.* Washington, DC, US Federal Emergency Management Agency, 2020.

10. Appendix G1: Fact Sheet Joint Information Center. In: CDC, editor. *Prevention.* Washington, DC, US Department of Health and Human Services, 2005. https://archive.cdc.gov/www_cdc_gov/sars/guidance/g-education/app1.html (Accessed April 1, 2024).

11. Conley C. The JIC Never Sleeps. *Centers for Disease Control and Prevention.* 2011. https://blogs.cdc.gov/publichealthmatters/2011/03/the-jic-never-sleeps (Accessed April 1, 2024).

12. Partners and Collaborators for Emergency Preparedness and Response. *Rural Health Information Hub.* 2024. www.ruralhealthinfo.org/toolkits/emergency-preparedness/1/partners-collaborators#:~:text=Working%20with%20community%20partners%20and,other%20response%20and%20recovery%20activities (Accessed April 1, 2024).

13. Zafari K, Biggemann S, Garry T. Mindful Management of Relationships during Periods of Crises: A Model of Trust, Doubt, and Relational Adjustments. *Indus Mark Manage* 2020;**88**:278–86.

14. National Response Framework: Emergency Support Functions. *Federal Emergency Management Agency*. 2021. www.fema.gov/emergency-managers/national-preparedness/frameworks/response#esf (Accessed April 1, 2024).

15. *Emergency Support Function 8: Public Health and Medical*. Washington, DC, Federal Emergency Management Association, 2021.

16. Section 508 of the Rehabilitation Act of 1973. *General Services Administration*. n.d. www.section508.gov/manage/laws-and-policies (Accessed March 27, 2024).

17. Douglas Fire Conflagration Update. *Stayton Fire District*. n.d. www.staytonfire.org/News.asp?NewsID=251 (Accessed April 1, 2024).

18. Templeton A. Wildfire Smoke in Southern Oregon Leads to Emergency Room Visits. *OPB*. 2013. www.opb.org/news/article/smoke-from-southern-oregon-fires-affect-health-of-/ (Accessed April 2, 2024).

19. Metcalfe J. Clouds of wildfire smoke are choking Southern Oregon. *Mother Jones*. 2013. www.motherjones.com/politics/2013/08/air-quality-wildfire-southern-oregon (Accessed April 2, 2024).

20. Wildfire Smoke and Your Patients' Health. *United States Environmental Protection Agency*. 2023. www.epa.gov/wildfire-smoke-course/why-wildfire-smoke-health-concern#:~:text=Fine%2C%20inhalable%20particulate%20matter%20(PM2,may%20even%20enter%20the%20bloodstream (Accessed April 2, 2024).

21. Gan RW, Liu J, Ford B, O'Dell K, Vaidyanathan A, Wilson A, et al. The Association between Wildfire Smoke Exposure and Asthma-Specific Medical Care Utilization in Oregon during the 2013 Wildfire Season. *J Expos Science Envir Epidemiol* 2020;**30**(4):618–28.

22. Reynolds B, Seeger M. Crisis and Emergency Risk Communication as an Integrative Model. *J Health Comm* 2005;**10**(1):43–55.

23. Seeger M. Best Practices in Crisis Communication: An Expert Panel Process. *J Appl Commun Res* 2006;**34**(3):232–44.

24. Kim M, Cappella JN. An Efficient Message Evaluation Protocol: Two Empirical Analyses on Positional Effects and Optimal Sample Size. *J Health Commun* 2019;**24**(10):761–69.

25. Lazarus JV, Romero D, Kopka CJ, Karim SA, Abu-Raddad LJ, Alemida G, et al. A Multinational Delphi Consensus to End the COVID-19 Public Health Threat. *Nature* 2022;**611**:332–45.

26. Marie G, Thomas K, Cassandra R, David T, Loth VdA, Eva P. The European Union and Public Health Emergencies: Expert Opinions on the Management of the First Wave of the COVID-19 Pandemic and Suggestions for Future Emergencies. *Front Public Health* 2021;**9**:698995.

27. Sanderson B. *How to Test Your Communications*. Machynlleth, Public Interest Research Centre (PIRC) and ILFA-Europe, n.d.

28. Lessler J, Rodriguez-Barraquer I, Cummings DAT, Garske T, Van Kerkhove M, Mills H, et al. Estimating Potential Incidence of MERS-CoV Associated with Hajj Pilgrims to Saudi Arabia, 2014. *PLoS: Current Outbreaks*. 2014. https://currents.plos.org/outbreaks/article/estimating-potential-incidence-of-mers-cov-associated-with-hajj-pilgrims-to-saudi-arabia-2014/index.html (Accessed April 1, 2024).

29. *CD Summary: Middle East Respiratory Syndrome*, 11th edition. Portland, OR, Oregon Health Authority, 2014.

30. *Coronavirus Infections: MERS-CoV (Middle Eastern Respiratory Syndrome Coronavirus)*. Portland, OR, Oregon Health Authority, Public Health Division, 2014.

31. Veil F, Reynolds B, Sellnow T, Seeger M. CERC as a Theoretical Framework for

Research and Practice. *Health Promot Pract* 2008;9(4):26S–34S.

32. Ebrahimji A, Yan H. It's been more than a month since a freight train carrying hazardous chemicals derailed in Ohio. Here's what's happened since. *CNN*. 2023. www.cnn.com/2023/02/23/us/east-palestine-ohio-train-derailment-timeline/index.html (Accessed March 13, 2023).

33. Watch | Ohio governor Mike DeWine discusses Ohio train derailment in Columbiana County. *YouTube*. 2023. www.youtube.com/watch?v=aaG5vpsgc1I (Accessed March 13, 2023).

34. Orsagos P. Crews release toxic chemicals from derailed tankers in Ohio. *AP News*. 2023, www.news-herald.com/2023/02/06/crews-release-toxic-chemicals-from-derailed-tankers-in-ohio-2 (Accessed March 13, 2023).

35. Watch: Ohio Gov. Mike DeWine gives update on East Palestine train derailment. *YouTube*. 2023. www.youtube.com/watch?v=iux2SeIjdNo (Accessed May 19, 2024).

36. Salahieh N, Yan H, Sutton J. Evacuation order lifted for residents near where train carrying hazardous chemicals derailed. *CNN*. 2023. www.cnn.com/2023/02/08/us/east-palestine-ohio-train-derailment-fire-wednesday/index.html (Accessed May 19, 2024).

37. Newsletter: East Palestine Train Derailment Response. *United States Enviromental Protection Agency*. 2024. www.epa.gov/east-palestine-oh-train-derailment/newsletter-east-palestine-train-derailment-response-10-31-2024 (Accessed November 11, 2024).

38. Bronstad A. Norfolk Southern's $600M Class Settlement Gets Final Approval. 2024. www.law.com/2024/09/26/norfolk-southerns-600m-class-settlement-gets-final-approval/?slreturn=20241111133742 (Accesssed November 11, 2024).

39. Funk J. Judge approves $600 million settlement for residents near fiery Ohio derailment. 2024. https://apnews.com/article/east-palestine-derailment-norfolk-southern-settlement-d08463bd83c5dc19f89719d04747d98c (Accessed November 11, 2024).

40. United States Reaches Over $310 Million Settlement with Norfolk Southern to Address Harms Caused by East Palestine Train Derailment. *United States Deparment of Justice*. 2024. www.justice.gov/opa/pr/united-states-reaches-over-310-million-settlement-norfolk-southern-address-harms-caused-east (Accessed November 11, 2024).

41. Fortin J. Ohio train derailment: Separating fact from fiction. *New York Times*. 2023. www.nytimes.com/2023/02/28/us/ohio-train-derailment-east-palestine.html (Accessed May 19, 2024).

42. Information & Resources. *Ohio Emergency Management Agency*. n.d. https://ema.ohio.gov/media-publications/east-palestine-derailment-info/information-resources (Accessed March 13, 2023).

43. Former president Trump visits East Palestine, Ohio following toxic train derailment. *C-SPAN*. 2023, www.c-span.org/video/?526220-101/president-trump-visit-east-palestine-ohio (Accessed May 19, 2024).

44. Transportation secretary Pete Buttigieg visits East Palestine, Ohio. *YouTube*. 2023. www.youtube.com/watch?v=zF9KPEZuN38 (Accessed May 19, 2024)

45. East Palestine Train Derailment: News. *Mike DeWine, Governor of Ohio*. 2024. https://governor.ohio.gov/priorities/east-palestine-train-derailment/news/ (Accessed November 5, 2024).

46. US Environmental Protection Agency. East Palestine, Ohio Train Derailment. Operational Updates. 2024. www.epa.gov/east-palestine-oh-train-derailment/operational-updates (Accessed November 5, 2024).

47. National Institute of Environmental Health Sciences. Research. East Palestine (Ohio) Train Derailment Research

48   Response. 2024. www.niehs.nih.gov/research/programs/east_palestine (Accessed November 5, 2024).

48   Ohio Environmental Protection Agency. Pollution Issues: East Palestine Train Derailment Information. 2024. https://epa.ohio.gov/monitor-pollution/pollution-issues/east-palestine#:~:text=Ohio%20EPA%20independently%20tests%20the,call%20330%2D849%2D3919 (Accessed November 5, 2024).

49   Ohio Environmental Protection Agency. Reports & Data: East Palestine Surface Water Results. 2024. https://epa.ohio.gov/divisions-and-offices/surface-water/reports-data/ep-surface-water-results (Accessed November 5, 2024).

50   Pennsylvania Pressoom. Shapiro Administration Continues to Advocate for Western Pennsylvania Residents, Announces Plans to Test Drinking Water Near East Palestine Train Derailment Site for Ten Years. 2024. www.media.pa.gov/pages/dep_details.aspx?newsid=1929 (Accessed November 5, 2024).

51   Grant J. New studies shed light on the contamination and response to East Palestine derailment. *The Allegheny Front*. 2024. www.alleghenyfront.org/new-studies-contamination-communication-east-palestine-derailment/ (Accessed November 5, 2024).

52   Whelton AJ. Environment: Toxic chemicals from train derailment lingered in buildings for months – findings in East Palestine, Ohio. 2024. https://phys.org/news/2024-10-toxic-chemicals-derailment-lingered-months.html (Accessed November 5, 2024).

53   East Palestine Train Derailment Health Studies at the University of Pittsburgh. *University of Pittsburgh School of Public Health*. 2024. www.publichealth.pitt.edu/east-palestine-train-derailment-health-studies-university-pittsburgh (Accessed November 5, 2024).

Part I Precrisis Planning

Chapter 3

Identifying Who Needs to Know What and When
It's Not a Surprise What Your Audiences Need to Know

Chapter Objectives
- Describe the differences between partners and stakeholders.
- Identify audience segments during a health emergency.
- Compare and contrast stakeholder types of advocates, ambivalents, and adversaries.
- List different information needs for audience segments.
- Recall how public health law impacts emergency risk communication.
- List at least three laws or statues that impact emergency risk communication.
- Describe public health legal powers.

Emergency Risk Communication Messaging Starts with Precrisis Planning

During precrisis planning, emergency risk communicators have the opportunity to consider the unique information needs of the general public audience, stakeholders, and partners, and what each of these groups will want to know during a health emergency. With strategic planning, emergency risk communicators can identify and prepare content during the precrisis phase that can be adapted and tailored for audiences, stakeholders, and partners during a health emergency. Discerning between audiences, stakeholders, and partners is necessary for emergency risk communicators to ensure the right message gets to the right audience at the right time.[1]

Identifying audiences starts with understanding who needs to receive information from the health agency about the health emergency. Any person or group receiving information during a health emergency makes up an audience. Audiences can also be identified as internal or external. *Internal audiences* include those people and groups who are considered within the health agency. For example, employees of a health department make up an internal audience. Sometimes, state health departments will consider county health departments to be an internal audience as they are found within the public health system for the entire state. *External audiences* are those people and groups who are outside the health agency or the public health system. For example, elected officials, community-based organizations, private companies, or educational systems can be external audiences as they are outside the health agency.

To further differentiate audiences, it is important to understand the audiences' relationships or network affiliations to the health agency. An audience's relationship or network affiliation can give it a unique label of a stakeholder or a partner. *Stakeholders* are individuals or groups that have a special connection to the health agency or are involved in the health emergency and are very interested in how the incident will impact them.[1] Stakeholders can include cases or ill individuals, family members of cases or ill individuals, elected officials, or businesses. In contrast, *partners* have a working relationship with the health agency. Partners collaborate in an official capacity during the health emergency response. They play an official role within the incident management team or incident command structure; often partners have a legal responsibility to be involved in the health emergency response. Partners include other government agencies such as emergency management, environmental health, or transportation. Depending on how state and local government manages emergencies, some nonprofit organizations, like the local Red Cross chapter or the nonprofit 2-1-1, may be official partners and have a designated role in the health emergency response.

As outlined in Chapter 2, multiple public health emergency preparedness (PHEP) capabilities specifically identify stakeholders and partners who are essential to supporting a health emergency response. Although there are 15 PHEP capabilities, emergency risk communicators need to take particular note of the following capabilities that impact emergency risk communication messaging and activities:

- Capability 1: Community Preparedness
- Capability 3: Emergency Operations Coordination
- Capability 4: Emergency Public Information and Warning
- Capability 6: Information Sharing
- Capability 11: Nonpharmaceutical Interventions

Table 3.1 is based upon the Centers for Disease Control and Prevention (CDC) Office of Readiness and Response's PHEP capabilities and identifies partners and stakeholders by PHEP capability.[2]

Including the identification of stakeholders and partners in the PHEP capabilities demonstrates the importance of understanding audiences and discerning whether the audience is a stakeholder or partner. Audiences, stakeholders, and partners will have unique information needs, and emergency risk communicators need to be prepared to respond to inquiries and provide these groups with the right message at the right time.

Identifying Audience Segments and How They Are Different from Each Other

Internal Audiences

Internal audiences include those people and groups who are considered within the health agency or public health system. Internal audiences for health emergencies include employees of the health agency responding to the incident. Depending on the organization of the public health system within the state and location, county health agencies could also be considered an internal audience. For smaller health departments, many employees will be involved with the emergency response, so internal communication will be easier since most of the health department staff will be involved in the response. But for larger health departments that provide many health programs and services, public health services will continue even during a health emergency. When this occurs, it is important that staff who are not working on the emergency response are aware of what is happening. This is crucial because even though they are not working on the response or

Table 3.1 Identification of partners and stakeholders that would support activities related to Public Health Emergency Preparedness capabilities

Capability	Partners	Stakeholders
Capability 1: Community Preparedness	Emergency management, emergency medical services (EMS), environmental health agencies	Media organizations, volunteer organizations, childcare organizations, health care systems and providers*
Capability 3: Emergency Operations Coordination	Emergency management, public health agencies, public health laboratories, tribes and native-serving organizations	Volunteer organizations, advisory councils
Capability 4: Emergency Public Information and Warning	Emergency management, EMS, 911 authority, poison control centers*	Media organizations, community and faith-based organizations
Capability 6: Information Sharing	Emergency management, EMS, environmental health agencies, tribes and native-serving organizations, hazardous material regulators and responders	Pharmacies, private-sector organizations, health care coalitions*
Capability 11: Nonpharmaceutical Interventions	Environmental health agency, law enforcement, legal authorities, mental/behavioral health agencies	Businesses, community and faith-based organizations, school districts, travel and transportation agencies, groups representing and serving populations with access and functional needs

* Depends on how state and local governments manage health emergencies through the incident command structure.

serving as spokespeople, they are likely to be asked questions by friends, neighbors, their family, and other people in their personal networks.

External Audiences

External audiences are people and groups who are outside the health agency or the public health system. External audiences will be made up of stakeholders and partners who will have information needs. Audience segmentation can help emergency risk communicators differentiate among segments of external audiences, identify their information needs, and create messaging that resonates with each audience segment.

Audience Segmentation

The general public constitutes several different types and groups of people with their own ways of relating, communicating, and sharing information. To ensure messages reach and resonate with an audience, it is important to identify different audience segments and create messages designed for that audience. During an emergency, early

Table 3.2 Variables that need to be considered for audience segmentation

Variable	Consideration
Risk level	Determine who is most at risk based on current health threat
Location or proximity	Determine who is closest to the risk or health threat
Health condition	Determine who has current health conditions that may put them at a heightened risk (e.g., age, underlying medical conditions, pregnancy)
Mobility	Depending on socioeconomic status, age, and/or health status, some people may not be able to leave an impacted area as easily as others
Visual/auditory/English proficiency	Determine who may need to receive the information in multiple media formats or languages
Employment	Determine whether there are particular industries that are affected by the health crisis
Education level and health literacy	When dealing with health emergencies it is important to use plain language for nonmedical audiences
Values	Determine what the audience segment values, believes in, and supports
Organizational affiliations	Determine what organizations individuals in this segment belong to or associate with
Media and technology access	Determine in what ways this group communicates and how can they be reached

messages will often focus on those most at risk based on health risk, the location of the health emergency, and underlying or chronic medical conditions. The development of emergency messages is discussed in detail in Chapters 6–9.

Audience segmentation has its roots in social sciences and social philosophy, with modern influences from psychology and marketing.[3] Public relations scholar James E. Grunig offers a basic definition of audience segmentation: "divide a population, market, or audience into groups whose members are more like each other than members of other segments."[4] The rationale for is that audience segments are more definable, accessible, reachable, and large enough to communicate with in an efficient way.[4]

To apply this thinking to emergency risk communication, "segments should be homogeneous with respect to patterns of variables (and values on those variables) determining the attitude and behaviors targeted by a communication effort."[3] The idea is that if audience segments can be identified, messages can be tailored for those groups.

Basic audience segmentation can begin with variables such as demographics, including age, race, gender, education, socioeconomic status, and geographic location.[5] Additionally, you should identify channels and ways to reach these individuals as well as determine how likely or able they are to take an action.[3,5] When identifying and grouping segments, it is key to ensure that the segments are distinct from each other, are related to the communication strategy, and are large enough to justify the time and effort required to target them.[5]

Understanding who is receiving your information is a critical factor in emergency risk communication planning and in strategic communications planning in general. Identifying audience segments during a health emergency draws upon basic audience segmentation variables as well as other variables unique to a health emergency (see Table 3.2).

Mini-Case Study: Audience Segmentation for Outbreaks

Applying audience segmentation is necessary in order for emergency risk communicators to get the right message to the right people at the right time. The following examples are of actual public health outbreak investigations, and they provide an opportunity to consider audience segmentation in small and large emergencies. These examples are real public health investigations that have been shared through the International Outbreak Museum (www.outbreakmuseum.com).

Case Study 1 (Reprinted through the International Outbreak Museum licensed under a Creative Commons Attribution-Noncommercial 4.0 International License)

On May 16, 2012, a local auto dealership called the Washington County (Oregon) Health Department to report a potential foodborne illness outbreak among employees who had attended a staff meeting on May 13. The meeting was held in an open space off the showroom floor. Submarine sandwiches, chips, and condiments from a nearby fast-food restaurant had been provided to attendees.

Environmental health staff conducted an onsite environmental inspection of the restaurant and its operations. Food handlers and restaurant managers reported no recent gastrointestinal illness (within the previous 2 weeks). No other patrons had complained of illness. The restaurant was cited for two violations defined by environmental health staff as critical: presence of potentially hazardous food not maintained at proper hot or cold holding temperatures; and presence of open beverages on the food preparation table. During interviews with dealership employees, one recalled that a customer with a sick child had used the diaper-changing station in the women's restroom before the lunch. When the woman and toddler left, the restroom was a mess. The employee cleaned it up as best she could with dry paper towels. She didn't wear gloves or use bleach but did wash her hands. She left the restroom, opened the dealership's front door for another employee carrying the food, and was the first to take a sandwich from the platter.

Applying Audience Segmentation
To identify audience segments in this outbreak, let's narrow in on three variables: risk level, location, and organizational affiliation (see Table 3.3). Using these three variables, we want to look at who is at risk of getting ill, what is their physical location with regard to the health threat, and what organization affiliations are present. First, those at risk include anyone who ate at the auto dealership. Second, anyone who was located within the auto dealership is also a potential audience segment – so here, we would include the mother who used the restroom. Next, in addition to the auto dealership, the other organization involved is the Washington County Health Department. For this small outbreak we have three potential audience segments: those who made the food, those who were physically located at the auto dealership, and those in the health department handling the investigation. Although this is a small outbreak, each audience segment will have its own information needs for this outbreak investigation.

Table 3.3 Risk by audience segment in Case Study 1

Variable	Audience segment
Risk level	Anyone who ate at the auto dealership
Location or proximity	Anyone who was at the auto dealership (including woman and toddler)
Organizational affiliation	Restaurant who supplied food, auto dealership employees, and Washington County Health Department employees

Mini-Case Study 2 (Reprinted through the International Outbreak Museum is licensed under a Creative Commons Attribution-Noncommercial 4.0 International License)

On May 27, 2007, Lane County Health and Human Services (LCHHS) received a report of a possible measles case admitted to a local hospital. The index case was in his 20s, unimmunized, and had been in Japan during his putative incubation period. A second case was identified later. The cases lived in a midsized urban community (population: 200,000) and, as was determined later, had active social lives. On May 31, Lane County officials confirmed the diagnosis of measles in the index case by polymerase chain reaction testing. His prodrome began on May 20. He flew on May 21 from Tokyo to San Francisco, and thence on May 22 to Eugene. His rash was first noted on May 25. He spent time at a local hospital emergency department (ED) and visited a health food store, naturopath, and Japanese restaurant during his communicable period.

The patient was not given a mask while in the ED waiting for his initial evaluation; rather, he was placed in a regular-airflow room and then wheeled through the hospital without wearing a mask and ultimately put in a taxi for the ride home. A review of the hospital's airflow system revealed that air from the emergency room (where the case had been housed but not isolated) was shared with the coronary care unit and mother and baby unit. The circulated air had a mixture of about 20% outside air and 80% recycled indoor air with 90–95% effective filtration and no high-efficiency particulate air (HEPA) filter.

During the investigation, the index patient refused to identify household contacts and did not respond to LCHHS phone calls, making contact investigation difficult. An unannounced home visit helped to clarify the situation and obtain new information.

Information regarding four persons exposed on airline flights was not received until 2 weeks after the likely exposure. A week later, health officials were informed of two additional persons considered to have been exposed, having sat next to or in front of the case, but phone numbers were not provided, and they had common last names. It also transpired that the case provided an incorrect seat number, and the model of the airplane was different from that listed on the airline's website, further confusing attempts to identify exposed persons.

A second, unimmunized case, who had socialized with the index patient on the night he arrived home from Japan, developed a febrile prodrome on May 30 and a rash consistent with measles on June 1. Koplik spots were visible. He declined lab testing.

Although nurses advised Case 2 to stay home to avoid spreading the disease, he went to public places. On May 29, Case 2 went to a hip-hop show at a local concert hall and then to a downtown bar. On the next night, he went out for sushi.

Table 3.4 Risk by audience segment in Case Study 2

Variable	Audience segment
Risk level	Ill individuals and individuals exposed to index case
Location or proximity	Local hospital, natural foods store, naturopath office, Japanese restaurant, concert venue, and airport
Organizational affiliation	Local hospital, natural foods store, naturopath office, Japanese restaurant, concert producers/venue organizers, and airport and airlines

Three bands that played at the hip-hop concert were on a national tour. During these shows, attendees typically stand, dance, and mingle, the band is on a stage just above the floor, and the band members often venture into the audience. The band members were in Utah when they were notified about their possible exposure, and specimens to verify immunity were collected in Colorado. The testing was performed at CDC in Georgia, and after the tests proved negative, the band members were vaccinated while performing in Iowa.

Applying Audience Segmentation
To identify audience segments in this outbreak, let's narrow in on three variables: risk level, location, and organizational affiliation (see Table 3.4). Looking at risk level, the first audience segment would include those who were ill (i.e., cases) and those who were exposed. For location, the second audience segment would include people at the local hospital, health foods store, naturopath office, Japanese restaurant, concert, and airport. For organizational affiliation, the third audience segment would include employees at the hospital, health foods store, naturopath office, airport and airlines, and the concert producers. This outbreak, although small, is complex because of the multiple locations the person with measles went and traveled to. There are multiple audience segmentation variables present in this case, but for ease we chose three to focus on for this activity.

Audience Segmentation: Stakeholders, Partners, and the Media

External audience segmentation can be further refined through differentiating stakeholders and partners. When emergency risk communicators identify audience segments that are stakeholders and partners, more clarity is achieved regarding message needs. As described earlier in this chapter, *stakeholders* are individuals or groups that have a special connection to the health agency or are involved in the health emergency and are very interested in how the incident will impact them.[1] Stakeholders can include cases or ill individuals, family members of cases or ill individuals, elected officials, or businesses.

The origins of understanding stakeholders are found in the field of business, emphasizing the interconnectedness of relationships between a business and its customers, suppliers, employees, investors, and communities and arguing that a business should create value for all stakeholders, not just formal shareholders.[6] Stakeholder theory provides a framework for management to consider regarding how to work with groups that are interested in and impacted by an organization even if they are not formal members of an organization.[7,8]

There are three important reasons why engaging with and tailoring messaging to communication stakeholders are important during health emergencies. First, stakeholders have information that you don't know because they are outside your organization and can provide you with a point of view or information that you may not have access to. Second, stakeholders may have resources they could provide to aid the health agency's response. For example, a retailer might have access to bottled water and could provide this during an emergency response. Third, and finally, stakeholders can help communicate a health agency's message. They can help amplify the key emergency risk messages from the health agency through their own internal and external communication channels.

When engaging with stakeholders, it is important to identify the stakeholder type. The Crisis and Emergency Risk Communication (CERC) manual outlines three types of stakeholders:

- Advocates
- Ambivalents
- Adversaries

Advocates are stakeholders that are aligned with the health agency's mission, purpose, and overall messaging. Advocates will freely amplify the health agency's messages as they agree with and see mutual benefits to be gained from aligning with the health agency. Advocates are those who are already supporting your agency's mission and are on board with your agency's emergency response. When a health agency engages with advocate stakeholders, the key communication objectives are: (1) Maintain their trust; (2) follow through on any commitments the agency has made to the stakeholders; and (3) provide an opportunity to receive feedback from the stakeholders.

Ambivalent stakeholders are neutral stakeholders that do not fall on either side of an issue. Stakeholders in this realm generally neither agree nor disagree with the health agency; essentially, they are neutral. Ambivalent stakeholders observe, monitor, and watch the situation unfold. They will not be likely to take a public position on, amplify, or negate the health agency's messaging. When the health agency engages with ambivalent stakeholders, the key communication objectives are: (1) Maintain their neutral position and (2) engage with ambivalents when there is an opportunity to move them toward changing into the advocate stakeholder type. Ambivalents are often called the "moveable middle" by political strategists.

Adversary stakeholders do not agree with the health agency's mission, vision, or purpose and often actively work against the health agency's public messaging. When a health agency engages with adversary stakeholders, the key communication objective is to discourage any negative action they could take against the health agency. Table 3.5 provides a comparison of advocates, ambivalents, and adversaries.

Understanding stakeholder types and the relationships stakeholders have with a health agency is important for strategic communication planning and emergency risk communication. By understanding what stakeholders will help amplify the health agency's emergency risk communication, emergency risk communicators can work to ensure advocates receive the latest communication materials and products that can be shared with multiple audiences. In contrast, by identifying adversary stakeholders, emergency risk communicators can strategically prepare for when adversaries may troll public online social media posts and provide negative comments, or for what additional resources may be needed for an upcoming in-person public event that may be protested by adversary stakeholders. Finally, emergency risk communicators can also determine

Table 3.5 Comparison of stakeholder types

Type	Definition	Communication objectives
Advocate	Stakeholders that are aligned with the health agency's mission, purpose, and overall messaging	Maintain trust, follow through on commitments, and provide opportunities for feedback
Ambivalent	Stakeholders that do not fall on either side of an issue	Maintain their neutral position or engage when there is an opportunity to move them toward changing into the advocate stakeholder type (i.e., "movable middle")
Adversary	Stakeholders that do not agree with the health agency's mission	Discourage any negative action they could take against the health agency

what energy and resources to expend on ambivalent stakeholders and whether there truly is a moveable middle that could be persuaded to support the health emergency's operations. See also Chapter 8 on using health communication campaigns to promote action during long-term health emergencies.

As outlined earlier in this chapter, *partners* have a working relationship with a health agency. Partners collaborate in an official capacity during a health emergency response. They play an official role within the incident management team or incident command structure; often partners have a legal responsibility to be involved in a health emergency response. Partners include other government agencies such emergency management, environmental health, or transportation.

Partners have unique information needs during health emergencies because they play an official role in the emergency response. The information needs of partners often fall under PHEP Capability 3: Emergency Operations Coordination and Capability 6: Information Sharing. First, partners need to understand their response role based on the incident type and what they need to do to support the health emergency. This information is based on the emergency support functions located within the health agency's emergency operations plan. Examples of partners include but are not limited to emergency management, emergency medical services, environmental health agencies, tribes and native-serving organizations, and hazardous material regulators and responders. Second, partners need to be able to receive and send epidemiological data, resources and supplies, and other operational information about the health emergency response. Partners need to know meeting frequency, be given organization charts for response staff, approved talking points, schedules of media briefings, and reporting templates, and be told which internal systems and processes will be used to share data.

The media has a unique relationship with health emergencies as they constitute stakeholders with interests in the health emergency, but they can also be unofficial partners during the initial stages of a health emergency to help amplify emergency risk communication messaging, including on what people can do to protect their health. Over time, the media will shift from being unofficial partners to being more like vested stakeholders and watchdogs. For example, while initially the media will freely report what the public needs to do to stay safe from a health threat, over time the media will shift their focus to determining who is responsible, why the health emergency occurred, what are the long-term impacts to the community, what are the solutions, and who is ultimately going to cover the costs and expenses to ensure this type of health emergency does not occur again in the future.[9] The media will use particular frames, or editorial lenses, to present the story. Common media frames used to report on disasters and emergencies include attribution of responsibility, human interest, conflict, morality, and economics.[10] Media frames will change over time throughout the life cycle and phases of a health emergency (see Chapters 6, 7, and 9). For example, during the initial and maintenance phases of the health emergency, media stories using the human interest frame will focus on who is impacted by the health emergency, such as highlighting fatalities and survivors. Human interest frames will also include stories about heroes and those who are going above and beyond to help those affected by the emergency. Over time, as the health emergency moves from the initial phase into the maintenance and then recovery phases, media frames of attribution of responsibility and economic impact will emerge.

Information Needs during a Health Emergency

This chapter so far has used audience segmentation to define and identify internal and external audiences through a set of variables including but not limited to health risk, location, and organizational affiliation. To further differentiate external audience segments, we identified whether the audience segment is classified as a stakeholder or partner. The media was discussed as a unique stakeholder. The current section outlines the information needs of internal audiences and external stakeholders and partners with consideration of their relationship to the health emergency.

Common Information Needs for Internal Public Health Audiences

- General information about the health emergency, approved talking points, and hotline numbers.
- If they are asked questions by stakeholders, where should they direct them? What are the key points of contact for the emergency response?
- What is the likelihood they may be pulled in as surge staff?
- How often will information be updated? Where can they find this information?
- Are there any upcoming media briefings?
- Media and social media policies.
- Human resources and staffing policy changes for health emergency work.

Common Information Needs for Stakeholders

- Best sources of official information about the health emergency.
- Health risk information (what is it, what signs and symptoms to look for).
- What to do to protect health – specific action steps.
- Where to find more information and contact information (website URLs, social media, and hotline/call centers).
- Upcoming media briefings and schedules.
- Upcoming town hall or public input sessions.
- How to provide feedback.

Common Information Needs for Official Partners
- Organizational chart of emergency staff with key contact information.
- Incident command structure meeting frequency.
- Reporting templates.
- Situational awareness information.
- How to report data.
- Approved talking points.
- Joint Information Center contact information.

Common Information Needs for the Media
- Latest information on health emergency (what happened, who is affected, what is the health risk).
- Statistics (fatalities, cases, hospitalizations).
- Costs and expenses related to emergency response activities.
- Attribution of responsibility.
- What the health department is doing to find the source of the outbreak.
- Name and title of spokesperson.
- Upcoming media briefings.
- Opportunities for interviews.
- B-roll related to the health emergency.
- Stock images of the virus (if applicable).

Five Common Mistakes Made with Stakeholders and Partners
Through strategic planning and open engagement, health agencies can develop empowered and mutually beneficial relationships with stakeholders and partners. However, there are five common mistakes that health agencies make with stakeholders and partners during health emergencies. By identifying and understanding these common mistakes, emergency risk communicators can work to prevent these actions from occurring and to effectively communicate with stakeholders and partners.

The five common mistakes that are made with stakeholders and partners are[1]:

- Inadequate access
- Lack of plain language
- Lack of empathy
- Timeliness
- Lack of input

Inadequate access means that the health agency has not provided access to key stakeholders and partners about the health emergency or emergency operations. A key function of PHEP planning is to identify stakeholders and partners, understand how the organizations will work together during a health emergency, and assign specific roles and responsibilities based upon emergency support functions. However, during fast-moving emergency responses and with novice emergency response staff, providing access to stakeholders and partners early in the response is often overlooked. It is important for emergency risk communicators and incident command staff to ensure stakeholders and partners have access to health emergency information and emergency response operations and activities.

Lack of plain language means the health agency responding to the health emergency is using jargon and terminology that are unfamiliar and unknown to the audiences receiving the health messaging. The National Assessment of Adult Literacy revealed the following findings[11]:

- 53% of American adults have intermediate health literacy, meaning they can find the age range for a particular vaccine from a childhood vaccination chart.
- 22% of American adults have basic health literacy, meaning they can identify two reasons why a person should be tested for a disease based on an information pamphlet.
- 14% of American adults have below basic health literacy, meaning they can read instructions and take an action based on short instructions.

In short, 89% of the American adults are not proficient in health literacy. In this study, health literacy is determined by familiarity with everyday health-related words, having experience of the type of written material, and having knowledge of how the health care system works. This study revealed that only 11% of the American public is proficient in health literacy, meaning they are able to define a medical term.

For emergency risk communicators, it is important to remember health literacy when engaging with nonmedical audiences, including the general public, stakeholders, and even response partners. Using medical terms and government jargon with the majority of audiences during a health emergency will not effectively communicate important health and risk information. Instead, leverage plain-language techniques such as organizing information to serve the audience, choosing words carefully, and making information easy to find.[12] The US federal government has multiple resources to assist health communicators in using plain language.[12]

Lack of empathy means the health agency is unable to identify with, understand, or acknowledge the emotions experienced by stakeholders and partners. Often, working in organizations and businesses can feel impersonal and mechanical, as if the individual is a cog in a machine. This lack of personalization and connection to the human experience negatively impacts interactions and dialogue between health agencies and stakeholders and partners. The CERC principles outlined in Chapter 1 include the use of empathy during health emergency responses. Using empathy is not restricted to health leaders or spokespeople. Instead, any person working for a health agency or within the health emergency response can use empathy to humanize the experience, engage in active listening with stakeholders and partners, and acknowledge what the other person or group is experiencing. Empathy is a key ingredient to building and maintaining trust during health emergencies.

Timeliness is often tied to withholding information until more certainty is available. The CERC principles outlined in Chapter 1 include Being First with emergency risk communication. Being First means the health agency claims responsibility and authority for releasing official health emergency information as soon as possible. Often, agencies will want to wait to release information until they have complete certainty regarding its validity; unfortunately, this is often an unaffordable luxury during emergencies. Addressing uncertainty is a key component of emergency risk communication, and this is explicitly addressed in Chapter 6. Even if a health agency is not yet certain about a health emergency, by communicating early and addressing the uncertainty of a health emergency, a health agency can build credibility, authority, and trust with stakeholders and partners.

Lack of input means that the health agency is not engaging with stakeholders and partners and is primarily internally focused. This includes making decisions about the health emergency without input from key stakeholders or response partners. By not providing adequate access for stakeholders and partners regarding decision-making, the health agency will be perceived at best as inaccessible and at worst as arrogant and paternalistic. Inadequate access can impact trust and damage relationships between a health agency and its stakeholders and partners. While some decisions will need to be made specifically by the lead responding agency, allowing opportunities for stakeholders and partners to provide input and feedback will ultimately serve the health agency in the long run. Empower stakeholders and partners to engage in decision-making and support their agency to provide input and feedback. By working together, the whole is often greater than the sum of its parts.

Mini-Case Study: Odwalla Juice Outbreak

On October 30, 1996, Odwalla, Inc. – a fresh juice company – was notified by the Seattle King County Health Department, based in Washington state, of a link between its unpasteurized apple juice and an outbreak of *E. coli* O157:H7.[13] The company immediately issued a voluntary recall and included 12 other juices in its recall. Although the company's product distribution was limited to six states in the United States (California, Colorado, New Mexico, Texas, Oregon, and Washington) and one province in Canada (British Columbia), the rise of online media and newswire services heightened global media attention. Odwalla issued refunds to customers and offered to pay for medical expenses associated with the outbreak.[13] Unfortunately, the outbreak led to the death of a 16-month-old and sickened 60 other children. Odwalla ultimately included a flash pasteurization process in its production procedures. This process kills bacteria within the juice but retains the flavor and freshness of the product.

Applying Audience Segmentation

To identify audience segments in this outbreak, let's narrow in on three variables: risk level, location, and organizational affiliation. Using these three variables, we want to look at who is at risk of getting ill, what is their physical location or proximity to the health threat, and what organization affiliations are present.

First, those at risk include anyone who drank the implicated juice. Second, location or proximity includes anyone who produced or sold the juice, anyone who bought the juice, and the government authorities who regulated food products. Next, the other organizations involved include consumers, grocery stores, suppliers, juice manufacturers, and the Odwalla company.

Understanding Information Needs

To identify information needs, emergency risk communicators need to understand the health risks and the audience segments. Using these two variables, emergency risk communications can identify what information these groups will need and provide each audience segment with the appropriate emergency risk communication messages. Table 3.6 shows the risk variables by audience segment and information needs.

Table 3.6 Risk variable by audience segment and information needs

Variable	Audience segment	Information needs
Risk level	Anyone who drank the implicated juice	Product lot numbers, how to dispose of product, obtaining a refund, and signs and symptoms of illness
Location or proximity	Anyone who produced the juice, anyone who sold the juice, anyone who bought the juice, and food regulators	Product lot numbers, location where juice was produced, source of fruit, how to dispose of product, obtaining a refund, and signs and symptoms of illness
Organizational affiliation	Consumers, grocery stores, suppliers, juice manufacturers, Odwalla, and the media	Product lot numbers, how to dispose of product, obtaining a refund, source of fruit, location where juice was produced, ongoing investigation: new processes to ensure bacteria are killed, when product can be sold again, situation overview, who is responsible, what is being done to stop the health threat, and signs and symptoms of illness

Understanding How Public Health Law Impacts Emergency Risk Information

Public health law is a field that focuses on legal practice, scholarship, and advocacy on issues involving the government's legal authorities and duties to protect the health and safety of individuals while balancing individual rights of autonomy and privacy. Public health law issues range from narrow questions of legal interpretation to complex matters involving public health policy, social justice, and ethics.[14] Public health law impacts emergency risk communication in two key ways:

1. Ensuring transparent communication and information sharing about risks to the communication
2. Protecting the autonomy and privacy of individuals impacted by the health threat

There are six key areas where public health and emergency risk communication intersect. These areas include defamation, the Privacy Act of 1974, the public's right to know, the Freedom of Information Act, 508 compliance, and public health legal powers. The following paragraphs highlight each of these key areas and its relevance for emergency risk communicators.

Defamation is exposing an individual or an organization to hatred or contempt. Defamation can lower the esteem of an individual in the eyes of others, and it causes an individual to be shunned and injures an individual in their business. There are two different forms of defamation: slander and libel. The spoken form is referred to as "slander," and the written form is called "libel." The key takeaway for emergency risk communication is the interplay between defamation and the right to privacy.

For example, statements warning the public about a specific individual who is spreading an infectious disease or a business location that has been contaminated by a toxic substance can give rise to libel allegations. Warning statements about someone who is sick or statements about a business that might be contaminated by a toxic substance need to be discussed with the health agency's attorney before releasing any public information. Due to the Privacy Act of 1974, health agencies should never give out a patient's private information, including their name or personal address. Instead, aggregate the data and deidentify the person; simply provide information on the *case*, or ill individual. Reporters will always ask for information about the cases and will want the health agency to give as much information as possible.

The Privacy Act of 1974 prevents disclosure by government agencies of personal data about employees and others. These data include age, race, sex, and medical information. Additionally, the Health Insurance Portability and Accountability Act of 1996 (HIPAA) ensures personal medical records and individually identifiable health information cannot be released by a medical institution without the consent of the patient or the patient's legal guardian. For example, when a person visits the doctor, they will sign a HIPAA form to provide consent for a sample of their blood to be used in a research study, but the patient's personal identity will not be revealed in that study.

For emergency risk communicators providing information about an evolving outbreak, the media will ask about ill individuals affected by the health emergency. The health agency can provide general information such as their sex, age, and general location, but the health agency cannot release that their name, what their status is, or what hospital they are receiving treatment at unless the hospital has approved that information to be released publicly.

In contrast to private health information, there are some public health records that can be given to anyone. This means that everyone has a right to access such public records, including journalists. Examples of public records include birth and death certificates, accident reports, and complaints filed with the police. In Oregon, the state releases birth data on an aggregate basis. No individual birth data are provided that would allow someone to be identified as a particular individual, but rather the data are aggregated and deidentified.

Each state has enacted its own public records and public release laws. It is important for emergency risk communicators to be aware of public records laws in the state where they are working. These laws will dictate what types of information and data can and cannot be released during health emergencies.

The public's right to know is based on legislation related to hazards involving chemicals, transporting chemicals across state lines, and locations where chemicals are being stored. The legislation outlines that people have a right to know where these chemicals are being stored in their communities. For emergency risk communicators, it is important to keep this legislation in mind regarding potential environmental hazards and health emergencies. Additionally, while not specifically related to communicable or infectious diseases, emergency risk communicators can consider what the public wants to know about what the health agency is doing to respond to and mitigate health emergencies. Further, any documents produced after a health emergency to outline what the health agency learned ought to be released and posted to the health agency's website.

The Freedom of Information Act and state public records laws constitute federal and local legislation that gives the public the ability to request government files and government information.[15,16] Since the Freedom of Information Act is focused on the US federal government, each state in the United States will have its own public records laws.[16] The terminology at the state level includes but is not limited to Open Records

Laws, Public Records Laws, Public Record Disclosures, Freedom of Information, and the Public Information Act.

There are limitations on what can be accessed, but generally these acts and laws are established to ensure transparency in government decisions and use of resources. For government workers, this means that any emergency responses, emails, meeting minutes, and certain kinds of documents could be requested and released to the public.

508 compliance (Section 508 of the Rehabilitation Act of 1973) requires US federal agencies to provide accessible information to people with disabilities when using electronic and information technology.[17] Many state governments have passed local legislation requiring information and technology accessibility.[18] Government employees who create, review, or revise content need to ensure that such content is accessible to those with disabilities. Content includes documents, electronic signatures, PDFs, presentations, software and websites, spreadsheets, videos, audio files, and social media. For emergency risk communicators, accessibility not only includes those with disabilities but also those with limited English proficiency. Ensuring audiences can receive and understand emergency risk communications is critical to successfully sharing this information.

Public health legal powers relate to the authority that state and local health agencies have to manage health emergencies, communicable disease outbreaks, and other states that threaten public health. There are two ways in which public health authorities have power. First, power comes through the state health department via what are called *police powers*. Police powers are granted by the 10th Amendment to the Constitution. Under these police powers, states have the authority to enact and enforce public health law, and this is often delegated to the state health department. This means that the health department must undertake reasonable attempts to protect and promote the public's health, safety, and general welfare. This is the basic mission and legal authority of a state health department. In a health emergency, the authority of a public health agency can be more broad, such as through the enactment of the Model State Emergency Health Powers Act.[19] Within this Act, during a public health emergency, the state government and often specifically the Health Officer has the authority and power to enact certain activities to protect the public's health. For example, in Oregon, if a public health emergency is officially declared by the governor, the state health director becomes the lead person in responding to the emergency, has the lead authority in responding to the event, and gets to decide on how restrictive public health intervention measures can be with regard to isolation and quarantine.

The second way in which health authorities have power is through delegation of authority to local health departments. This occurs via how the state government manages the administrative functions of the public health code. For example, state creates legal codes and statues to establish a local government's authority, which is called *home rule*. Most states have given local health departments the right of local self-governance, which means that the local health departments have the right to make decisions concerning their own welfare.[20] This means that local health departments can make decisions without requiring approval from the state government.

It is important for emergency risk communicators to understand the scope of the authority and independence of state and local health departments when planning for and responding to public health emergencies. If local authorities are able to act without approval from other health authorities, then county Health Officers can make decisions in one county that may differ from a Health Officer's decisions in a neighboring county.

This can cause complications when counties share news media markets or counties include high numbers of commuters who live in one county and work in another. Risk communicators need to ensure coordinated and consistent emergency risk communication messages are produced. This often occurs during precrisis planning when health departments come together to discuss how they will manage a health emergency. Additionally, depending on the scope and scale of the health emergency, the state health department may be able to step in and manage a heath emergency that spans multiple jurisdictions (i.e., a multicounty outbreak) requiring the coordination of resources and communications in order to effectively respond.

A major challenge in the United States regarding public health authorities is the friction between the benefit to the community and individual liberties. As outlined earlier, during large-scale health emergencies, public health may be given to the health authority to restrict activities in order to protect the public's health. During COVID-19, health authorities implemented strict isolation and quarantine activities advising no travel and requiring telework and online education for children.[21,22] However, the longer the COVID-19 outbreak went on, the less willing some of the American public was to continue with such strict public health interventions, including the wearing of masks and receiving multiple vaccinations.[22] In response to the COVID-19 outbreak, some state legislatures are working to restrict the power of health authorities to protect the public's health.[22,23]

Theory Callout: Stakeholder Management Theory

Stakeholder management theory developed out of the business and management field by discerning the differences between shareholders and other individuals or businesses that might have nonmonetary interests in a company.[6] When this theory was developed, it was novel for a company to consider the interests of people or businesses that were not directly monetarily benefiting by the company.[7,8]

Using stakeholder management theory, emergency risk communicators can consider the level of influence each stakeholder has with the health agency. The amount of influence and the prominence of the stakeholder within the public health system (i.e., their networks and presence) can affect what and how the health agency manages the health emergency. As described earlier in this chapter, *stakeholders* are individuals or groups that have a special connection to the health agency or are involved in the health emergency and are very interested in how the incident will impact them.[1] Stakeholders can include cases or ill individuals, family members of cases or ill individuals, elected officials, or businesses. Emergency risk communicators need to consider the unique information needs of each stakeholder and to develop messaging that resonates with each stakeholder.

> **Case Study: The Water Crisis in Jackson, Mississippi**
> Jaime Jimenez, MPH
>
> Overview of the Water Crisis in Jackson, Mississippi
> Ensuring people have access to clean water for drinking, domestic use, food production, or recreational purposes is critical to maintaining public health.[24] When water is not properly treated or poor sanitation develops, preventable diseases can occur, such as cholera,

diarrhea, dysentery, hepatitis A, typhoid, and polio.[24] When there is inadequate management of urban, industrial, and agricultural wastewater, the drinking water of hundreds of millions of people potentially becomes dangerous.[24]

Jackson, Mississippi, experienced intense rain in late August 2022. This led to the compromising of the city's primary water treatment facility: the O.B. Curtis Water Plant.[25] The city declared a water crisis between August 30 and September 15, impacting 150,000 residents. In Jackson, one in four people live in poverty, making conditions even worse for the number of these individuals who rely on tap water.[25] Jackson's Mayor, Chokwe Antar Lumumba, was pivotal in communicating with residents. The mayor leveraged the City of Jackson's communication resources and social media account to reach the city.

Timeline of Key Events
- August 26: Residents are updated on the recent flooding; the City of Jackson advises those that were impacted by the 2020 flooding to make evacuation plans in the next 48 hours.
- August 29: Flooding affects the O.B. Curtis Water Plant; water is not being treated.
- August 29: Mayor Lumumba declares a water system emergency in Jackson.
- August 30: Boil water notice is still in effect; water distribution sites are opened in partnership with the Jackson Municipal Airport Authority.
- August 31: A water system update was provided and noted that the overall water pressure had decreased to 40 PSI.
- September 1: A water system update is provided, and the O.B. Curtis Water plant makes progress but still experiences problems.
- September 2: A water system update is provided, and the plant output increases to 80 pounds per square inch (PSI). The ideal pressure is 87 PSI to adequately supply the entire system.
- September 3: A water system update is provided, and the plant output increases to 86 PSI; challenges are still present.
- September 4: A water system update is provided, and the plant output increases to 90 PSI; challenges are still present. All of Jackson should have some pressure and most resident should have normal pressure. A tool was provided to report discolored water and pressure issues at https://arcg.is/0LDmjb.
- September 5: A water system update is provided, and all of the residents in Jackson should have some pressure and experience normal pressure. The plant output is meeting the goal of 87 PSI.
- September 6: A water system update is provided, and the plant remains at a steady pressure; water distribution sites are updated.
- September 7: A water system update is provided, and all storage tanks have stable water levels.
- September 8: A water system update is provided, and the plant remained at a steady pressure over the past 24 hours and overhead storage tanks were maintained overnight.
- September 9: A water system update is provided, the plant remains at steady pressure, and pressure should be stable throughout the city; water production continues to improve.
- September 10: A water system update is provided, and the plant is working at 88 PSI, pressure should be stable throughout the city, and the water production continues to improve.

- September 12: A water system update is provided, and the plant is working at 88 PSI, pressure should be stable throughout the city, and the water production continues to improve.
- September 13: A water system update is provided, and the plant is working at 89 PSI, pressure should be stable throughout the city, and water production continues to improve; discolored water and reduced pressure have been reported – these issues were related to routine water leaks or meter issues.
- September 14: A water system update is provided and the plant is working at 89 PSI.
- September 15: The boil water notice for all City of Jackson water customers is lifted; per the Mississippi State Department of Health, residents are advised to run their faucets to clear any old water.

Note: This timeline was compiled based on announcements made from the City of Jackson media news website using the keyword "water."[26]

Overview of CERC Framework
The CDC's CERC principles provide a framework for communicating on behalf of an organization responding to a public health emergency.[1,27,28]

Phase-Based Messaging
The CDC has broken messaging in public health crises into a series of five phases: the precrisis, initial, maintenance, resolution, and evaluation phases. During the precrisis phase, also called the "preparation phase," background information may be developed, draft messages are designed, partnerships can be established, plans can be documented, and approval processes can be developed.

The initial phase marks the beginning of an official situation of a public health emergency. This time is crucial for acknowledging the event with empathy and providing messages that explain the situation using common language. Providing messages with action items will help reduce feelings of anxiety and stress.

The maintenance phase increases the public's knowledge of the risks associated with the crisis, as well as that of the stakeholders involved, and involves adjusting messages to improve their utility.

The resolution phase involves reinforcing positive behaviors that the public can implement to prevent future events and encourages the public to support those who are most vulnerable.

The evaluation phase allows time to document the challenges and successes and the strategies for communicating more effectively using the CERC principles. Throughout all phases, CERC encourages communicators to engage with communities and empower them to make decisions that will improve or maintain positive health.

CERC Principles
The CERC principles form a guide for creating messaging in a time of disaster. Following each principle will allow you to create a message that will result in the public making the best decisions while acknowledging the ever-changing situation that a disaster creates. According to the CDC's CERC 2018 Introduction,[27] the six principles are:

- *Be First:* Time is an important variable in a public health emergency. Ensuring that information is communicated as fast as possible is critical. Once the information reaches a public audience, the first source becomes the preferred source.
- *Be Right:* Correct information builds credibility. Communicating what is known, what is unknown, and what actions are being done all contribute to an accurate communication message.

- *Be Credible:* During public health crises, the pillars of honesty and truthfulness should be prioritized. Ensuring messages contain these components is important.
- *Express Empathy:* Public health crises create mixed emotions. Messages that acknowledge the spectrum of emotions and the challenges that are being combatted build trust and rapport with the public.
- *Promote Action:* Messages that describe actions that people can take will calm anxiety, restore order, and promote a sense of control, which can be beneficial to members of the public.
- *Show Respect:* Crises can exacerbate feelings of vulnerability as well as highlight instances that create trauma. Respectful communication promotes cooperation and rapport.

CERC Analysis of the Messaging in the City of Jackson, Mississippi

To identify how the City of Jackson effectively or ineffectively used the CERC principles, example messages are critiqued on how well they aligned with the noted principle. Overall, the City of Jackson produced updates on the status of the O.B. Water Treatment Plant daily and ensured that residents were aware of where to find water distribution sites. These two types of information drove much of their messaging. The City of Jackson's website and Twitter (now X) profile were pivotal in communicating with the public on updates.

Be First

The pre-initial phase included a boil water advisory that was issued a month before this water crisis.[29] Boil water advisories and other media releases were key communication channels for notifying residents regarding water updates. During the last week of August, the city communicated the impacts that flooding could have on the area before the declaration, which highlighted that close monitoring and open channels of communication were being displayed.[30] The initial phase was instigated on August 29 with the official announcement of the water crisis via Twitter and the official webpage data.[31] The city was the first to declare the situation as an emergency, ahead of Governor Tate Reeves by 72 hours.[32] This provided the city with a strong point in its messaging. The rollout of this information was timely and followed the first CERC principle of being first.

Be Right

The City of Jackson communicated every day for 2 weeks. Any information that may have been of concern was brought up the next day. This was consistent through every phase of the disaster cycle. In the report that declared the official water system emergency, there was the following clarification:

> **Contrary to some reports, the City is NOT cutting off water to residents.** The City remains in contact with the state Department of Health and the EPA [Environmental Protection Agency] over continued issues with the system. Residents are advised to call the City's **311 line** for additional information. The City will resume water distribution and update the media on times and locations. A PDF copy of the emergency order can be found under the "Mayoral Executive Order" tab on the City website.[33]

This message did an excellent job of correcting misinformation early in the process. By addressing incorrect information on the same day when the incident was declared a disaster, the city showed a commitment to being right. There was a reference to the City's

311 number and coordination with the state Department of Health and the EPA. These two organizations were used throughout the process, ensuring information was fact-checked by two credible sources. A recommendation to improve this messaging would be to include information about the health impacts of consuming contaminated water.

Be Credible
The corrections that Mayor Lumumba was willing to make to the media regarding his provision of accurate information about the city's condition demonstrated credibility. He criticized television stations for continuously using clips of dark, muddy water coming from faucets. The mayor corrected these portrayals, stating that "the dark water was likely a localized problem and not representative of water being treated at Jackson's two primary water plants."[34] By confronting this misinformation and in being willing to bring in testimonials from the US Department of Justice and the EPA, he was able to create credible messages. The delivery of these messages when on camera facilitated to the mayor's – and thus the overall City of Jackson's – communication.

Express Empathy
The CERC principle of expressing empathy was not explicitly achieved in the messages produced. Many statements were curt and lacked emotive language. For example, the following is the whole message released on September 10:

> (Jackson, Miss.) – The O.B. Curtis Water Plant remained at a steady pressure over the past 24 hours and is currently working at 88 PSI. All tanks are currently maintaining good margins for overhead storage and made gains overnight. Pressure should still be stable throughout the city.
> Overall water production continues to improve. Yesterday, the membrane plant production remained steady and the conventional side increased significantly. The team continues to work to increase production capacity.
> The repaired raw water pump #4 has arrived at the plant. It has been placed back on the pump platform by crane this morning. Work is ongoing to place the raw water pump back in service.
> Investigative sampling will continue to monitor water quality. At this time the distribution system is not ready for full sampling to clear the boil water notice. We will continue to evaluate when full sampling can begin. This is contingent upon sustained pressure. We will need two rounds of clear samples to be able to remove the boil water notice.
> If you are experiencing discolored water or no pressure please report using this tool https://arcg.is/0LDmjb. This will allow us to track any remaining issues and address them. We are currently monitoring this information to respond as needed.[35]

The benefit of this style of message is that it is straight to the point. It addresses the water treatment plant. It addresses the precautions and the type of sampling being completed to ensure safety. The end of the message concludes with an action a person can take to report water issues. The last sentence details that this information is being monitored. However, there is a lack of emotional language or signs of sympathy for the public who are living in these conditions. If the message had included acknowledgments of living through a hard or stressful time, a more complete message would have been delivered. These types of messages were consistently deployed through the initial, maintenance, and resolution phases.

Promote Action

A clear example of messaging that promoted action was given on September 4, when concerns regarding discolored water and low pressure were noted. The City communicated via its website and Twitter account how to report those concerns. Those messages included a link to an online reporting tool that mapped out areas of concern.[36] This link was active through the entire crisis and now takes visitors to a webpage for all Jackson water concerns. An additional example is a community meeting invitation that was disseminated on the City's Twitter account.[37] This invitation was grounded in a discussion with the mayor and welcomed the participation of local, state, and federal officials. This event occurred between 6:00 and 7:30 p.m. at the College Hill Baptist Church. Holding the event after business hours allowed people to participate after work. Hosting the event at a faith-based institution in a city that is close to 55% religious was a strategic way to increase attendance.[38] This represented an important way of allowing residents to act on the experiences they were having and of allowing them to be heard.

Show Respect

The final phase of this crisis can be marked by the lifting of the boil water notice and the reassurance by the Mississippi Emergency Management Agency on September 15 that the situation was safe and residents no longer needed to be concerned.[39] This message could have been delivered with more empathy, but it was timely and brought a sense of relief to the public. The message was respectful because it provided relief to the public while not promising too much. As the goal was to fix the O.B. Water Treatment Plant and lift the boil water advisory, this message did not go beyond this promise, which is important.

Implications for Organizations

In using the City's website and Twitter account, there was a limit to the length and type of messages being sent out to the public. Both communication channels require internet access, which is limited to certain populations. The City also has an Instagram account and a YouTube account that were not active during this process. Those two resources would have provided methods for capturing and disseminating press briefings. This disaster impacted the daily lives of 150,000 people, yet the emphasis was on the water treatment plants. Instead of including photos of individuals who were directly affected by the water crisis, the city focused on images of buildings. This suggests the City prioritized getting the water treatment plants up and running without considering the personal nature of the water crisis and how people were directly affected by it. Another implication of the use of these media is the lack of personal interaction that they allow. Many tweets provoked questions and comments but lacked responses. Or in the case of the webpage that posted updates, there were few methods for interacting further with the actual information being stated. There was a phone number and a link for addressing water needs but not for addressing the needs of day-to-day survival. This research found many published news articles bringing up concepts of disinvestment and environmental racism. The City's webpage and Twitter account never addressed those sentiments. The consequences of this communication style might be seen in the future if another such water crisis occurs. There are long-term solutions that were not discussed during this period, which has left many questions unanswered in the evaluation and recovery stages of this event. Going forward, Jackson has a lot of work to do to follow CERC principles more effectively.

Recommendations

At the city level, partnerships between the Mississippi Emergency Management Agency and the Mississippi Department of Health need to be strengthened. If more messages had contained quotes from high-level officials, the credibility of messages sent out by the City of Jackson would have been increased. Messages across organizations at the state and city level lacked empathy. In the future, during times of crises, this CERC principle needs to be followed to a greater extent. The approach taken might also have been considered disrespectful because the incident and the individuals were not fully acknowledged. Few to no messages expressed understanding of people's situations, vulnerable populations, or ensuring equity in more marginalized neighborhoods. This created a barrier between City officials and residents, who may have been experiencing a worse situation than the City realized.

Communication at the state and city level entailed different messages with various levels of empathy. In a conference 1 day after the official ending of the water crisis in Jackson, Governor Reeves commented, "I've got to tell you; it is a great day to be in Hattiesburg. It's also, as always, a great day to not be in Jackson."[40] This type of messaging highlights the reality that the failure of the O.B. Water Treatment Plant was due to decades of disinvestment in the water infrastructure in the city. The city of Jackson has repeatedly sought funding from the state to address water system issues, but the Governor continues to deny the city additional funds.

It was interesting that this crisis occurred when Jackson had been operating under a boil water advisory weeks before the official water crisis was declared. Boil water advisory notices provide residents with succinct messages that certain neighborhoods need to boil their water before consuming it, and they include lists of "dos" and "don'ts" to ensure people do not become sick from contaminated water. Due to the perfunctory nature of these notices, empathetic messages are not included. This might also have contributed to why some of this messaging lacked empathy, due to a reliance on maintaining the same structure to these messages.

Going forward, if Jackson includes more empathetic messages within its current approach, this could generate trust from those communities that are impacted. Encouraging partnerships and clearer lines of communication at the city level is crucial for empowering the community. Additionally, Mayor Lumumba was used as a spokesperson for this crisis, but incorporating a larger team at the city level would have allowed him to draw on greater information resources instead of deferring to communications from the state level.

End-of-Chapter Reflection Questions

1 What are your agency's policies regarding community-sensitive public health information during outbreaks? For example, does your agency have a policy about naming businesses during foodborne illness outbreaks?

2 Think back to a recent disease outbreak. Name some of the audience segments that needed information. Were you able to meet their communication needs?

3 Identify stakeholders and partners in a disease outbreak. What are their information needs? What would be the best way to share information with them?

4 Review your agency emergency response plans with a focus on how epidemiologists and public health preparedness staff work together. What are the strengths of the plan? What gaps need to be addressed?

5 Field trip: Relationships are vital before and during health emergencies. Set up an in-person meeting with a community-based organization you haven't met yet or haven't seen in a while to discuss the current status of emergency risk communication in your agency.

References

1. CDC. *Crisis and Emergency Risk Communication October 2014.* Atlanta, GA, CDC, 2014.
2. Public Health Emergency Preparedness and Response Capabilities: National Standards for State, Local, Tribal, and Territorial Public Health. *Centers for Disease Control and Prevention.* 2021. www.cdc.gov/orr/readiness/capabilities/index.htm (Accessed January 11, 2024).
3. Slater MD. Theory and Method in Health Audience Segmentation. *J Health Commun* 1996;1(3):267–83.
4. Grunig JE. Publics, Audiences and Market Segments: Segmentation Principles for Campaigns. In: Salmon CT, editor. *Information Campaigns: Balancing Social Values and Social Change.* Thousand Oaks, CA, Sage Publications, 1989; 199–228.
5. Smith RA. *Audience Segmentation Techniques.* Oxford, Oxford Research Encyclopedias, 2017.
6. Freeman RE. About Stakeholder Theory. 2018. http://stakeholdertheory.org/about (Accessed March 24, 2024).
7. Freeman RE, Harrison JS, Wicks AC, Parmar BL, De Colle S. *Stakeholder Theory: State of the Art.* Cambridge, Cambridge University Press, 2010.
8. Freeman RE, Harrison JS, Zyglidopoulos S. *Stakeholder Theory.* Cambridge, Cambridge University Press, 2018.
9. Covello VT. Risk Communication. In: Frumkin H, editor. *Environmental Health: From Local to Global.* New York, Jossey Bass/John Wiley and Sons, Inc., 2005; 988–1009.
10. An S-K, Gower KK. How Do the News Media Frame Crises? A Content Analysis of Crisis News Coverage. *Public Relat Rev* 2008;35:107–12.
11. Whitehurst R. *The National Assessment of Adult Literacy: Health Literacy Results.* Bethesda, MD, National Institutes of Health, Office of the US Surgeon General, 2006.
12. Plain Language Materials and Resources. *Centers for Disease Control and Prevention.* 2023. www.cdc.gov/healthliteracy/developmaterials/plainlanguage.html (Accessed March 4, 2024).
13. Martinelli KA, Briggs W. Integrating Public Relations and Legal Responses During a Crisis: The Case of Odwalla, Inc. *Public Relat Rev* 1998;24(4):443–60.
14. Hoke K. *What Is Public Health Law?* Washington, DC, American Public Health Association: Network for Public Health Law, n.d.
15. Freedom of Information Act (FOIA) webpage. *Office of Information Policy.* n.d. www.foia.gov/about.html#:~:text=Since%201967%2C%20the%20Freedom%20of,the%20know%20about%20their%20government (Accessed March 4, 2024).
16. Public Records Laws and State Legislatures. *National Conference of State Legislatures.* 2023. www.ncsl.org/cls/public-records-law-and-state-legislatures (Accessed March 4, 2024).
17. Section 508 of the Rehabilitation Act of 1973. *General Services Administration.* n.d. www.section508.gov/manage/laws-and-policies (Accessed March 4, 2024).
18. State-level accessibility law and policy. *General Services Administration.* n.d. www.section508>.gov/manage/laws-and-policies/state/#:~:text=Government%20Code%20Section%207405%20directs,of%20electronic%20and%20information%20technology (Accessed March 4, 2024).
19. Gostin L. *The Model State Emergency Health Powers Act.* Washington, DC, Center for Law and Public's Health at Georgetown and Johns Hopkins Universities, 2001.
20. McCarty KL, Nelson GD, Hodge Jr. JG, Gebbie KM. Major Components and Themes of Local Public Health Laws in Select U.S. Jurisdictions. *Public Health Rep* 2009;124(3):458–62.
21. Impact of opening and closing decisions by state. *Johns Hopkins University.* 2022. https://coronavirus.jhu.edu/data/state-timeline (Accessed March 4, 2024).
22. Nair S, Davis M. Isolation, Quarantine, and Public Health Authority Beyond the

Pandemic. *ASTHO*. 2022. www.astho.org/communications/blog/isolation-quarantine-and-public-health-authority-beyond-the-pandemic (Accessed March 4, 2024).

23. Zhang X, Warner ME, Meredith G. Factors Limiting US Public Health Emergency Authority COVID-19. *Int J Health Plan Manage* 2023;**38**(5):1569–82.

24. Drinking water. *World Health Organization*. 2022. www.who.int/news-room/fact-sheets/detail/drinking-water#:~:text=Safe%20and%20sufficient%20water%20facilitates,and%20numerous%20neglected%20tropical%20diseases (Accessed March 4, 2024).

25. Berlow J. The water crisis in Jackson follows year of failure to fix an aging water system. *NPR*. 2022. www.npr.org/2022/08/31/1120166328/jackson-mississippi-water-crisis (Accessed August 31, 2022).

26. News. *The City of Jackson, Mississippi*. n.d. www.jacksonms.gov/news?filter_keyword=water (Accessed August 31, 2022).

27. CDC. *Crisis and Emergency Risk Communication October 2018*. Atlanta, GA, CDC, 2018.

28. Veil F, Reynolds B, Sellnow T, Seeger M. CERC as a Theoretical Framework for Research and Practice. *Health Promot Pract* 2008;**9**(4):26S–34S.

29. Boil water notice remains in effect. *The City of Jackson, Mississippi*. 2022. www.jacksonms.gov/boil-water-notice-remains-in-effect (Accessed August 31, 2022).

30. Flood Update: Friday August 26. *The City of Jackson, Mississippi*. 2022. www.jacksonms.gov/flood-update-friday-august-27 (Accessed August 31, 2022).

31. @CityOfJxnMS. The City of Jackson is NOT cutting off water to residents due to complications from the Pearl River flooding. X/Twitter. 2022, August 29.

32. Jackson, Mississippi Water Crisis. *Center for Disaster Philanthropy*. 2022. https://disasterphilanthropy.org/disasters/jackson-mississippi-water-crisis/ (Accessed November 11, 2024).

33. Mayor Lumumba declares system emergency. *The City of Jackson, Mississippi*. 2022. www.jacksonms.gov/mayor-lumumba-declares-water-system-emergency (Accessed August 31, 2022).

34. Inman E. Lumumba tells residents at town hall meeting not to trust the state on water system issues. *Clarion Ledger*. 2022, September 28.

35. Water system update: Saturday, September 10. *The City of Jackson, Mississippi*. 2022. www.jacksonms.gov/water-system-update-saturday-september-10 (Accessed September 10, 2022).

36. @CityOfJxnMS. If you are experiencing discolored water or no pressure, please alert us using this online reporting tool. X/Twitter. 2022, September 4.

37. @CityOfJxnMS. Mayor Chokwe Antar Lumumba will hold a community meeting Tuesday night to provide updates on the status of the water. X/Twitter. 2022, September 19.

38. Popular religions in Jackson, MS. *Facts by City*. 2018. www.factsbycity.com/popular-religions/Jackson-MS/statistics.html (Accessed August 31, 2022).

39. @CityOfJxnMS. The boil water notice for ALL City of Jackson water customers HAS BEEN LIFTED, per the Mississippi State Department. X/Twitter. 2022, September 15.

40. Williams A. "A great day to not be in Jackson," governor says during Hattiesburg event. *WAPT*. 2022. www.wapt.com/article/a-great-day-to-not-be-in-jackson-mississippi-governor-says-during-hattiesburg-event/41252344 (Accessed September 16, 2024).

Part I Precrisis Planning

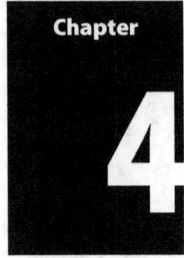

Addressing the Information Needs of the Public and Medical Community during a Public Health Emergency

Chapter Objectives
- Describe two types of information that epidemiologists and emergency risk communications cocreate.
- Identify three unique information needs of the medical community.
- Explain how the information needs of the medical community are different from those of the general public.
- List two ways hospital and other medical facilities can leverage the Crisis and Emergency Risk Communication (CERC) framework to communicate with staff and patients.
- Explain the Elaboration Likelihood Model.

Cocreating Emergency Risk Communication Messages with Epidemiologists

Collaboration among emergency risk communicators, epidemiologists, clinical experts, and other subject matter experts is critical to the development of scientifically accurate and credible emergency risk communication messages. Being able to create emergency risk communications that demonstrate the Crisis and Emergency Risk Communication (CERC) principles of Be Right, Be Credible, and Promote Action requires the scientific data being gathered and analyzed by epidemiologists and other subject matter experts within the health agency.

"Epidemiology is the branch of medical science that investigates all the factors that determine the presence or absence of diseases and disorders."[1] Epidemiologists collect and analyze data from people affected by a health emergency to identify the threat and develop a plan to respond to and manage it. Using quantitative and qualitative methods, epidemiologists gather data to understand the context in which a disease exists and progresses, rates of new illness (i.e., incidence rates), and the number of existing cases (i.e., prevalence). Understanding exposure to the infection is key to developing a public health intervention that will protect people's health. Additionally, epidemiologists seek to understand people's responses to the illness, including mild or typical symptoms, current immunity, classical clinical features of the illness, and even death.[2]

Chapter 2 outlined the key roles to include in a crisis communication team for a health agency and advocated for ensuring subject matter experts serve on the crisis communication team. Subject matter experts such as epidemiologists can be included in the communication team to ensure the development of accurate emergency risk communication messages based on the available science and epidemiological data. While emergency risk communicators understand how to write health messages for a health emergency, the scientific content of the messages will come from the epidemiologists who are collecting the data about the evolving health emergency and its impacts on the community. The following sections outline how epidemiologists and emergency risk communicators cocreate emergency messages that are actionable, understandable, and data-driven.

Message Content: Health Risks and Interventions

Epidemiologists can provide two important types of message content: health risks and interventions. As emergency risk communicators develop messages for the initial, maintenance, and recovery phases of an emergency, the health risk will change as new data become available. Working with epidemiologists ensures emergency risk communicators will have the most accurate and up-to-date information about the health threat, including signs and symptoms, level of risk based upon exposure, level of risk based upon age or underlying health conditions, and what interventions are available to mitigate or prevent the health threat.

Using the 2015–2016 Zika outbreak, let's review how message content is cocreated between epidemiologists and emergency risk communications. The information gathered by epidemiologists creates a profile of the illness and identifies who is most at risk. Through descriptive and analytic epidemiology, the following information describes the health risks associated with the Zika virus.

Health Risk

In 2016, the World Health Organization (WHO) declared Zika a public health emergency of international concern due to clusters of microcephaly cases and other neurological disorders reported in Brazil and in French Polynesia.[3] Epidemiological information helped health officials understand what the illness is, who is affected, how they are affected, and the location of the outbreak, and in turn develop health interventions to deal with the outbreak. Prior to the recent outbreak, Zika virus was primarily carried by monkeys with little "spillover infections in humans."[4] However, since 1952, public health officials have had evidence that Zika can infect humans. Early cases were found in Uganda and Nigeria and later in other African countries and Indonesia. By 2007, an epidemic occurred in Yap Island; another then occurred in French Polynesia in 2013, followed by others in Cook Island and New Caledonia in 2014.[4] By 2016, 60 countries were experiencing Zika cases, and by 2017 cities along the US–Mexico border also reported Zika cases. The Zika virus is transmitted to humans by the bite of a female mosquito. Humans spread it to other humans through sexual transmission. Additionally, there is perinatal transmission, meaning the Zika virus can be transmitted *in utero* to a developing fetus, causing microcephaly – a brain abnormality.[4] Zika can also cause Guillain–Barré syndrome. Symptoms of Zika in adult humans include mild fever, joint pain, headaches, rash, and pink eye.[4] Symptoms can last for up to 7 days and the incubation period is 3–12 days.

All of this information can be used to develop initial, maintenance, and recovery messages for audiences identified through the emergency risk communication plan. Chapters 6, 7, and 9 provide specific steps for writing and creating emergency risk communications during a health emergency. The following is a sample initial emergency risk communication message about Zika. More information about writing and creating initial messages is presented in Chapter 7.

Initial Messages: What They Are and How to Write Them

Communicating early during a health emergency manages the expectations of the public and stakeholders, establishes organizational credibility, establishes trust with those affected by the emergency, and provides actionable health information that people can act upon to protect their health. These first crisis messages are called "initial messages" and they are usually sent within the first 24–48 hours of a health emergency.

Initial message components include:

- Addressing uncertainty
- Making a commitment
- Providing messages of self-efficacy
- Expressing empathy

Incorporating these message components into emergency risk communication messages allows spokespeople and health agencies to follow the CERC principles.

Addressing Uncertainty and Making a Commitment

Addressing uncertainty focuses on what is known about the health threat, what is not known, and what public health officials are doing to learn more about the emerging threat. The following example of addressing uncertainty comes from Representative Eliot L. Engel, Ranking Member of the House Committee on Foreign Affairs, on January 28, 2016. Parentheticals are included to emphasize how the message addresses uncertainty (i.e., what is known, what is not known, and what health officials are doing to learn more) and what constitutes a commitment to the community.

> We shouldn't allow the ongoing uncertainty surrounding the Zika virus to spark a panic. *(what is unknown)* Domestic and international health experts are taking this issue seriously, and I'm committed to working in Congress to ensure that this outbreak is dealt with quickly and competently. *(what is known)*
>
> President Obama's recent meeting with top U.S. health officials and today's announcement by the World Health Organization (WHO) of an emergency meeting on Zika are good steps. *(what health officials are doing to learn more)* I encourage continued efforts to address the issue head-on. *(making a commitment)* This challenge will require enhanced research, substantial resources, interagency cooperation, and coordinated efforts to ensure that clear information reaches the public as quickly as possible. I have long called for increased engagement with our partners in the Americas, and at this difficult time, the United States must assist our neighbors as they continue to fight the Zika virus. *(making a commitment)*[5]

Providing Messages of Self-Efficacy

Providing messages of self-efficacy or promoting action, a CERC principle, means giving people a meaningful action they can take to protect their health and prevent illness. The following example comes from WHO regarding reducing sexual transmission of Zika:

> For regions with active transmission of Zika virus, all people with Zika virus infection and their sexual partners (particularly pregnant women) should receive information about the risks of sexual transmission of Zika virus.

WHO recommends that sexually active men and women be counselled and offered a full range of contraceptive methods to be able to make an informed choice about whether and when to become pregnant in order to prevent possible adverse pregnancy and fetal outcomes.

Women who have had unprotected sex and do not wish to become pregnant due to concerns about Zika virus infection should have ready access to emergency contraceptive services and counselling. Pregnant women should practice safer sex (including correct and consistent use of condoms) or abstain from sexual activity for at least the entire duration of pregnancy.

For regions with no active transmission of Zika virus, WHO recommends practicing safer sex or abstinence for a period of three months for men and two months for women who are returning from areas of active Zika virus transmission to prevent infection of their sex partners. Sexual partners of pregnant women living in or returning from areas where local transmission of Zika virus occurs should practice safer sex or abstain from sexual activity throughout pregnancy.[6]

Expressing Empathy

In July 2016, Ashley Young, a pregnant woman living in the United States, wrote then-President Barack Obama a letter about her Zika concerns and potential for getting sick and passing the illness to her child *in utero*.[7] President Obama replied to the letter, and his first paragraph is an example using empathy. He acknowledges her concerns and admits his own as a father. The rest of the letter outlines self-efficacy steps Ashley can take and the United States' commitment to addressing the Zika health threat through research on new vaccines and increased epidemiological surveillance to detect the disease. Parentheticals are included to emphasize how the message addresses empathy and uncertainty (i.e., what is known, what is not known, and what health officials are doing to learn more) and provides a message of self-efficacy.

Dear Ashley:

Thank you for writing me. Your email reached my desk, and as President and as a father, I want you to know I take your concerns very seriously. My foremost priority is the health and safety of Americans and my Administration is working around the clock to protect you and families across our country. *(express empathy)*

Most people who become infected with Zika will not even know it because the symptoms are usually nonexistent or mild. However, as you noted, scientists have established a link between Zika infections during pregnancy and poor birth outcomes. Our primary goal is to minimize these outcomes, and early in the year I instructed my staff to do all we can to respond to the Zika threat. *(address uncertainty – what is known)*

While we are still learning about Zika, we do know there are ways to minimize your risk if it does appear in your community, including protecting yourself from mosquito bites by wearing long sleeves and pants, staying in places with air conditioning and window and door screens, and wearing EPA-registered insect repellants. You can find more information and steps you can take to protect yourself and your family from Zika at www.CDC.gov/Zika. CDC regularly updates this information as we learn more, so I encourage you to check back often. *(address uncertainty – what is known; provide messages of self-efficacy)*

In the meantime, I have directed my team to accelerate research on new vaccines and methods of detecting the disease. Additionally, I've formed a coalition of experts and Federal, State, and local leaders to combat the spread of Zika so that we can identify any outbreaks in the continental United States early and contain them. To make sure our public health officials have the resources needed to prepare and respond to Zika, I've asked Congress to approve $1.9 billion in emergency funding to support and advance these efforts as quickly as possible. *(make a commitment)* Again, thank you for writing. Your message will remain on my mind. *(express empathy)*

Sincerely,

Barack Obama[7]

Interventions

The second message content area where emergency risk communicators and epidemiologists cocreate emergency risk communications is communicating health interventions, or the actions people can take to protect their health during a health emergency. Chapters 7 and 8 provide in-depth information about promoting health interventions during short- and long-term health emergencies. Let us continue reviewing the 2015–2016 Zika health emergency to understand how epidemiologists and emergency risk communications cocreate emergency risk communication messages about health interventions.

Since the Zika virus is transmitted by mosquitoes, looking at the physical environment would be a key intervention in stopping mosquito breeding. This intervention of addressing the environment is critical in reducing the spread of Zika because there is no vaccine available to prevent Zika. Strategies to address mosquito breeding include:

- Elimination of standing water containers
- Use of larvicides (biological or chemical) to disrupt mosquito development
- Chemical control: spraying or toxic baits of adult mosquitoes
- Physical control: trapping female mosquitoes to prevent egg-laying or capturing eggs

There are no specific treatments for Zika; nonpharmaceutical intervention, such as providing supportive care in the form of resting, increasing fluids, and taking medication to reduce fever and pain, are key action steps that can be taken. Additionally, to reduce sexual transmission, wearing condoms is recommended.

All of this information can be used to develop initial, maintenance, and recovery messages for audiences identified through the emergency risk communication plan. Chapters 6, 7, and 9 provide specific steps for writing and creating emergency risk communications during a health emergency. The following is a sample maintenance emergency risk communication message about Zika. More information about writing and creating maintenance messages is provided in Chapter 7.

Maintenance Messages: What They Are and How to Write Them

Maintenance messages are usually sent about 7 days into a health emergency, and this phase can last for weeks, months, or even years. There are four key message components of a maintenance message that will support the CERC principles of Be Right, Be Credible, Promote Action, and Show Respect. Incorporating these message components into emergency risk communication messages allows spokespeople and health agencies to follow the CERC principles.

Maintenance message components include:

- Deeper risk explanations
- Interventions

- Making a commitment to the community
- Addressing rumors and misinformation

Continuing with the Zika virus outbreak, the following sections provide examples of the maintenance message components listed above. In April 2016, CDC released a statement scientifically confirming the link between the Zika virus and microcephaly.[8] This confirming affirmed many of the health interventions the CDC was promoting for pregnant women. The following paragraphs outline maintenance messages used by the CDC to deepen the knowledge regarding the risks to pregnant women by the Zika virus.

Deeper Risk Explanations

The following text is taken from the CDC website "Zika during Pregnancy."[9] The intended audience is pregnant women in the United States.

> Zika During Pregnancy
>
> CDC recommends you take special precautions if you are pregnant to protect yourself from Zika virus infection.
>
> Because Zika during pregnancy can cause severe birth defects, if you are pregnant, you should not travel to areas with Zika outbreaks (as indicated by red areas on the Zika map). Before traveling to other areas with risk of Zika (as indicated by purple areas on the Zika map), you should talk to a healthcare provider and carefully consider the potential risks of Zika and other infectious diseases.
>
> The only way to completely prevent Zika infection during pregnancy is to not travel to areas with risk of Zika and to use precautions or avoid sex with someone who has recently traveled to a risk area.
>
> We do not have accurate information on the current level of risk in specific areas. The large outbreak in the Americas is over, but Zika is and will continue to be a potential risk in many countries in the Americas and around the world. No local spread of Zika virus has been reported in the continental United States since 2017.
>
> There is no vaccine to prevent or medicine to treat Zika. If you are considering travel to an area with risk of Zika, talk to your health care provider first. It is important to understand the risks of Zika infection during pregnancy, ways to protect yourself, signs of Zika, and the limitations of Zika testing upon your return.[9]

The CDC website content continued to deepen the risk explanation by including information about travel to and from an area with a Zika outbreak, risk of Zika to future pregnancies, and Zika test results. This information was given in English and Spanish.

Interventions

As discussed earlier, there are no vaccines or treatments for Zika. Instead, prevention activities are key. CDC outlines the following key nonpharmaceutical interventions in an infographic (see Figure 4.1):

1. Increasing awareness about sexual transmission.
2. Steps to take to prevent transmission: wearing insect repellant; wearing long sleeves and pants; staying indoors with air conditioning or using window screens; removing standing water around the home.
3. Increasing awareness about Zika and birth defects and encouraging condom use.

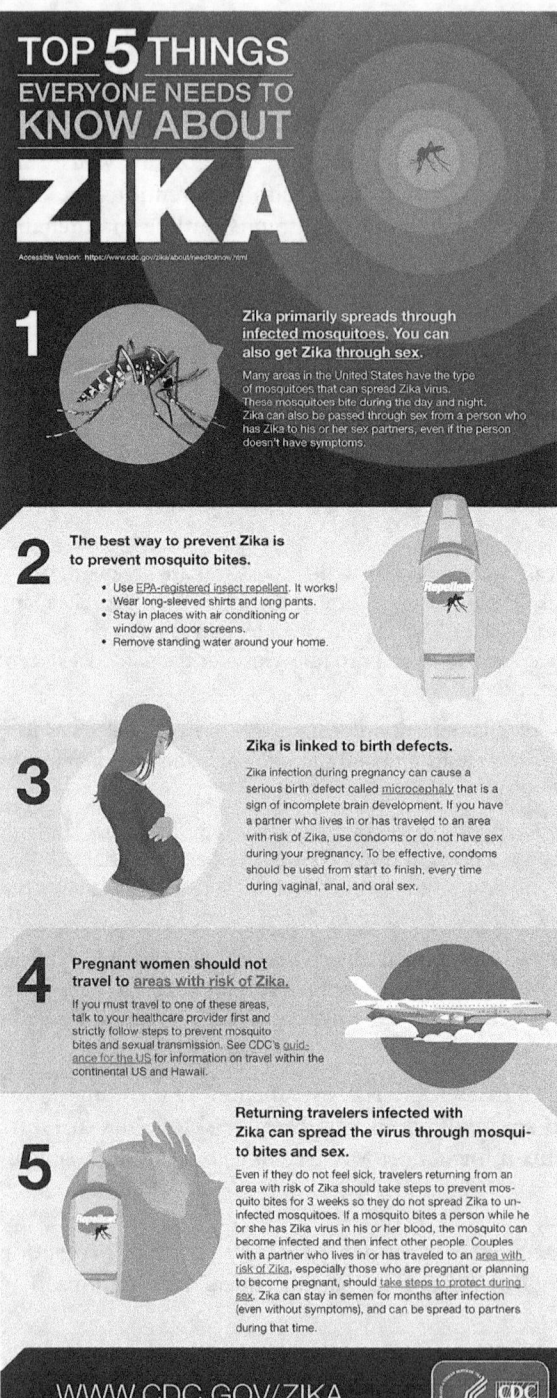

Figure 4.1 CDC infographic: Top 5 things everyone needs to know about Zika
CDC created this infographic to explain nonpharmaceutical interventions that the public can take to protect themselves from Zika. Providing information on interventions is a key message component of a CERC maintenance message.
Source: United States Centers for Disease Control and Prevention (CDC). The use of this material does not imply endorsement by CDC, Agency for Toxic Substances and Disease Registry (ATSDR), US Department of Health and Human Services (HHS), or the United States Government of the author. This material is available on the CDC website free of charge: www.cdc.gov/zika/about/needtoknow.html

4   Encouraging pregnant women to not travel to areas with Zika.
5   Monitoring return travelers and using safe-sex practices.

Making a Commitment to the Community

The following example message was sent out after the outbreak of Zika and shows how the Obama administration communicated a commitment to the community during the health emergency. This example demonstrates how the President make a commitment to the community to monitor the situation and mitigate the health threat to the public.

> The Zika virus is a disease spread primarily through the bite of an infected mosquito – the same type of mosquito that spreads other viruses like dengue and chikungunya.
>
> While most people have no symptoms at all, Zika causes mild illness in some. However, the Centers for Disease Control and Prevention (CDC) has established a link between Zika infection during pregnancy and serious birth defects and other poor pregnancy outcomes. We also know that there can be other serious neurological impacts in some people who are infected with Zika.
>
> We are closely tracking and responding to outbreaks of this virus across the Americas. We have seen transmission in Puerto Rico, the U.S. Virgin Islands, and American Samoa, in addition to cases reported in Mexico, Central and South America, the Caribbean, and the Pacific Islands. The Florida Department of Health is tracking cases of non-travel related Zika in one small area in South Florida and is closely coordinating with the CDC as they further investigate this ongoing situation.
>
> And we know that this particular mosquito lives in certain parts of the southern United States, and we now know that Zika can also spread in another type of mosquito that is present throughout much of the United States. So now is the time to prepare as the seasons change and weather gets warmer.
>
> As President Obama said, we all have to remain vigilant when it comes to combating the spread of diseases like Zika. That's why the President has called on Congress to provide emergency funding to combat this disease, including to
>
>   a. speed the development of a vaccine;
>
>   b. allow people – especially pregnant women – to more easily get tested and get a prompt result; and
>
>   c. ensure that states and communities – particularly those in the South that have experienced local outbreaks of dengue and chikungunya in the past – have the resources they need to fight the mosquito that carries this virus.
>
> Congress needs to act now to ensure that we have the resources we need to take every step necessary to protect the American people from the Zika virus.[10]

Addressing Rumors and Misinformation

In February 2016, *The New York Times* wrote an article outlining rumors associated with Zika and providing accurate information.[11] One of the rumors and information correcting this misinformation are provided in the following as an example of how to address rumors that emerge during a health emergency.

> **Are genetically modified mosquitoes the real cause of the birth defects?**
> That buzzing sound you hear is a "no."
> A British company, Oxitec, released genetically engineered mosquitoes in Brazil in an attempt to control dengue fever. But the later microcephaly outbreaks were far away. For

example, the largest mosquito release was in Piracicaba, which is 1,700 miles from Recife, where microcephaly was most common. The mosquitoes have also been released in the Cayman Islands, Malaysia and Panama without causing problems.

Mosquitoes fly less than a mile in their lifetimes. Also, only male mosquitoes were released. They do not bite humans or spread disease and were genetically programmed to die quickly.[11]

Data Graphics

Another important way for epidemiologists and emergency risk communicators to cocreate emergency risk communication messaging is through data graphics that are used on websites, social media channels, handouts, slide decks, or media briefings. As outlined in Chapter 5, multiple communication channels can be used to disseminate key emergency public health messaging. Each communication channel will have a corresponding communication product that can be created and tailored for that particular channel. For example, when engaging in a media briefing, incorporating data graphs and charts may help enhance messaging and further explain the health risk to the public.

Engaging the crisis communication team, including graphic designer, social media manager, and website administrator, will help ensure the usability of the graphics for multiple communication channels. For example, CDC created a data graphic that visually depicts the percentage of babies that are born to people infected with the Zika virus while pregnant (see Figure 4.2). The graphic shows that 5% of babies are Zika-associated birth defects if the mother was infected with Zika while pregnant. Using

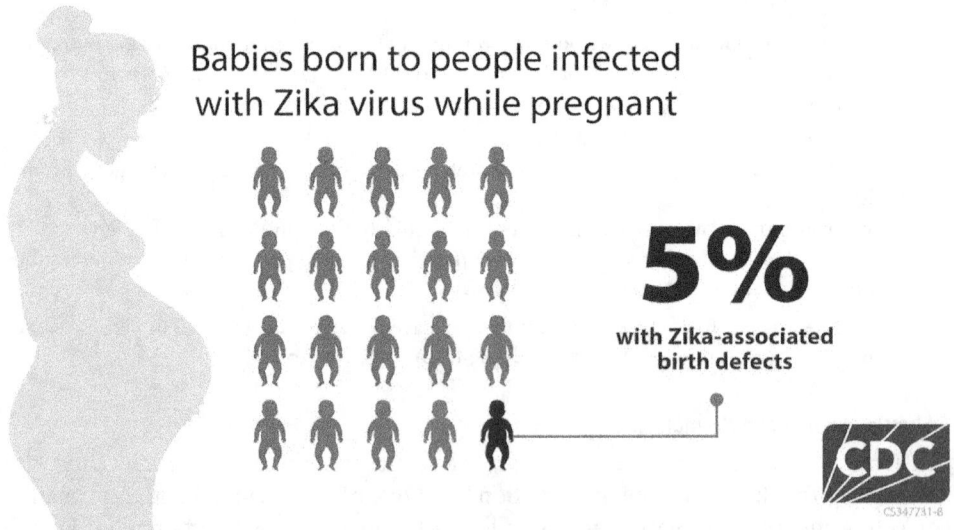

Figure 4.2 CDC graphic: Babies born to people infected with Zika virus while pregnant
CDC created this figure – a data graphic – that visually depicts the percentage of babies that are born to people infected with the Zika virus while pregnant. Data graphics are often cocreated by risk communicators and epidemiologists and are a visual way to explain the risk associated with a health threat.
Source: United States Centers for Disease Control and Prevention (CDC). The use of this material does not imply endorsement by CDC, ATSDR, HHS, or the United States Government of the author. This material is available on the CDC website free of charge: www.cdc.gov/zika/czs/index.html

contrasting colors and icons of infants, the visual depicts the low percentage of babies born with Zika-associated birth defects.

During the COVID-19 pandemic, CDC created a community-level map that would track data by county and provide a way for people to interpret the risk of getting COVID-19 in their own community (see Figure 4.3). Available epidemiological data

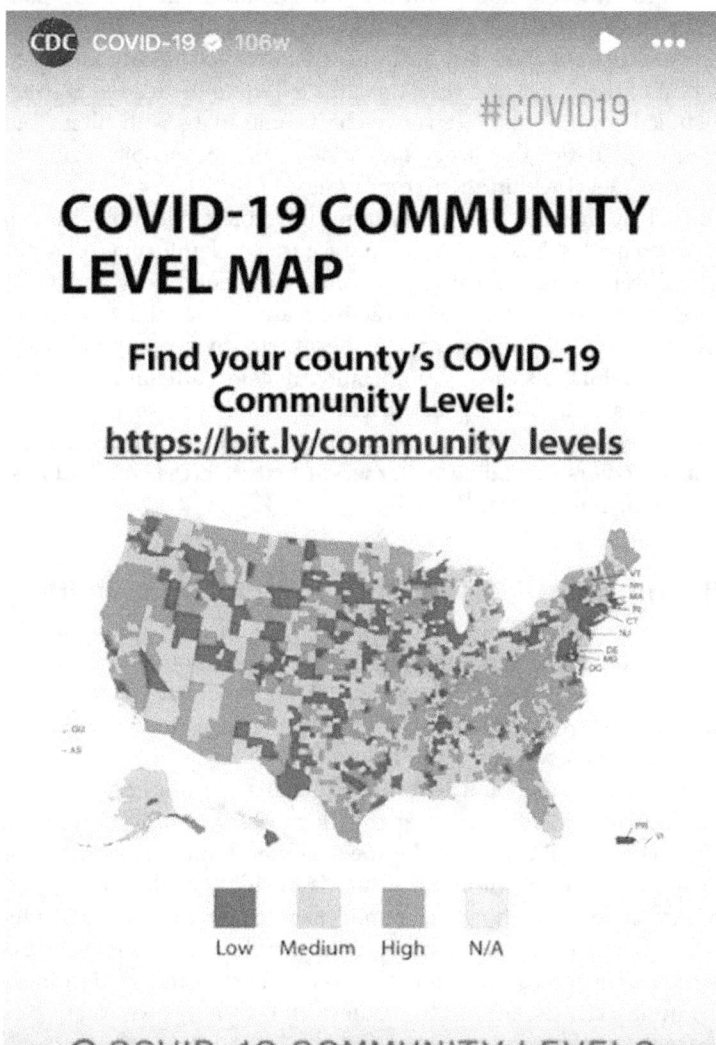

Figure 4.3 CDC Instagram post of United States COVID-19 community-level map
CDC created this figure – a data graphic – that visually depicts the risk of contracting COVID-19 in different communities across the United States. Data graphics are often cocreated by risk communicators and epidemiologists and are a visual way to explain the risk associated with a health threat.
Source: United States Centers for Disease Control and Prevention (CDC). The use of this material does not imply endorsement by CDC, ATSDR, HHS, or the United States Government of the author. This material is available on the CDC website and Instagram account free of charge: https://covid.cdc.gov/covid-data-tracker/#datatracker-home and www.instagram.com/CDCgov/?hl=en

about the number of cases and hospitalizations in the area were used to create the data graphic. The map included an image of the United States and incorporated assorted colors that corresponded to particular levels of risk: black was low level, light gray was medium level, and dark gray was high level.

The key for emergency risk communicators is to ensure that the health risk message can be succinctly explained and does not leave interpretation of the graphic up to the end user. A recent study revealed two common problems with public health graphics and data dashboards related to COVID-19.[12] First, in charts or graphs that focused on conveying risk, the color graduations were not prominent enough to indicate increased levels of risk. Interpretation of these data and risks was thus left up to the reader. Second, the data dashboards included case counts, interactive charts, and maps with filters, but there were limited to no explanations of what the data meant for people trying to understand their personal risk level within their community.[12]

Again, by working together, emergency risk communicators and epidemiologists can design website graphics and data dashboards that convey accurate risk information to the public through the use of trend lines, warning signs, and different colors and icons signaling increased or decreased threat. Create interactive features that allow people to select location information in order to understand the health risk by geographical area. Use "conventional urgency colors instead of non-standard color schemes (i.e., red, yellow, green, for high, moderate, and no urgency levels, respectively) so that the colors directly correspond to user mental models representing danger, moderate danger, and no danger. In addition to using colors, including patterned or texture areas could address accessibility concerns for color-blind users."[12]

Identifying Unique Information Needs of the Medical Community

So far, this chapter has examined how to communicate with the general public by cocreating emergency risk communication messages with epidemiologists. Another equally important set of people need to receive communications during an outbreak, and this group has different informational needs, requiring messages to be tailored to this unique audience. This unique audience is the medical community.

As outlined in Chapter 3, audiences and audience segmentation are important for emergency risk communicators to identify in order to tailor messages that will resonate with each audience. This section will highlight the medical community as a particular audience segment with a unique set of information needs during a health emergency. The first part of this section looks at how the public health community can better understand the needs of the medical community when developing emergency risk communication messages and materials for them. The second part of this section looks at how the medical community can use the CERC framework within its own health care system to communicate with its audiences.

Early coordination between public health, hospitals, urgent care clinics, skilled nursing facilities, and other organizations that provide health care is critical: "Improving response during this window requires acquiring the capability to execute three fundamental elements of early epidemic response: finding cases and identifying where infections are spreading, stopping or slowing community transmission, and supporting those infected or at risk for infection so that hospitals are not overwhelmed and mortality is reduced."[13]

Medical Community as Audience Segment

To understand how the medical community is integrated into public health emergency preparedness, it is helpful to look at the Administration for Strategic Preparedness and Readiness's (ASPR) Hospital Preparedness Program (HPP). The HPP is designed to support health care delivery system preparedness in the event of a large-scale health emergency and build collaborations between health care delivery and public health agencies.[14] Within the HPP, Health Care Coalitions (HCCs) are designed to bring together individual health care and response organizations such as acute care hospitals, emergency medical service (EMS) providers, emergency management agencies, and local and state public health agencies to prepare health care delivery systems to respond to health emergencies.

Similar to the Public Health Emergency Preparedness (PHEP) cooperative grants discussed in Chapter 2, HPP cooperative agreements require a particular set of reporting requirements to prepare the health care system for public health emergencies. These requirements include the following:

- Multiyear training and exercise plans
- Infectious disease preparedness surge annexes
- Infectious disease preparedness surge tabletop discussions/exercises
- Financial reporting, including budgets and spend plans
- Annual HCC work plans
- Annual HCC training plans
- Templates
- Annual joint HPP–PHEP vulnerable populations exercises
- Pandemic influenza planning requirements
- Joint exercises between HPP–PHEP partners
- After-action reports and improvement plans
- Crisis standards of care documents
- Hazard vulnerability assessments
- Attending particular public health preparedness conferences[15]

Since the HPP and HCC represent critical investments into a system's approach to preparing public and private health care organizations for health emergencies, it is equally critical for emergency risk communicators to consider the information needs of the medical community during a health emergency. As HPP requirements focus extensively on planning, exercising, and coordination between hospital preparedness and public health preparedness, emergency risk communicators also need to understand *what* to communicate with this particular audience. Additionally, it is important for emergency risk communicators to consider the information needs of the entire medical community. For example, there are health care providers who provide services outside of hospitals. While hospitals are an important partner in public health emergencies, primary and urgent care clinics often get overwhelmed with questions from their patients, and so they need the most up-to-date information. Including all medical providers on Health Alert Network (HAN) messages ensures the entire medical community will receive important emergency risk communication about a health emergency.

In contrast to the general public, the medical community has particular knowledge, skills, and job responsibilities that are technical, advanced, and treatment-focused. While public health is focused on preventing community health harms and carrying out government legislation to support the health of the community, the medical community is generally focused on treating and curing disease at the individual level.

Common Information Needs of the Medical Community during a Health Emergency

The following six information needs of the medical community are based upon systematic literature reviews of scientific research and personal interviews with members of the medical community.

Scientific Guidance

The medical community needs scientific, evidence-based guidance regarding the identification, collection, and reporting of disease data and data on the treatment of patients. Scientific guidance includes the following key information:

- Testing and testing priorities for suspected cases
- Handling, collecting, testing, and submitting requirements of clinical specimens
- Risk factors and symptoms of the illness
- How to prepare for receiving patients with the illness or disease[16]

Kattaryna Stiles, Oregon Health Authority Healthcare Preparedness Program liaison, explained that often scientific guidance documents can be written more abstractly to allow multiple types of health care organizations (urban health care systems, rural health care systems, small health care providers, etc.) to apply the guidance according to the size, scope, and resources available within the organization.[17] Further, Stiles suggested two challenges of providing scientific guidance during health emergencies: changing guidance and conflicting guidance between CDC and Oregon Health Authority.

First, during a health emergency, the evolving situation creates challenges when new information becomes available, especially when that new information directly impacts the scientific guidance that is currently available. By using dates, different colored fonts, and subheadings, health agencies can alert the medical community to new additions to the scientific guidance documents. Second, timing the release of scientific guidance can be challenging when state health departments are unaware of when CDC will release new scientific guidance. For example, a state health department may adapt CDC's scientific guidance to be more explicit regarding state and local statues. After releasing the adapted guidance, CDC may release a new document with new information. This can create challenges for the medical community as to which guidance ought to be followed.[17] Although issuing multiple editions of scientific guidance may feel redundant, medical providers agree that releasing scientific information early and often during a health emergency is important to enabling hospitals to manage response operations within their organizations.[18,19]

Data Reporting

The reporting of disease data is an important function hospitals and health care systems carry out because the more disease data public health epidemiologists have, the better they can identify the disease, its health effects, and who is at risk and so develop health interventions to mitigate impacts on the health care system responsible for treating the disease. Typically, the state government designates what diseases must be reported to the state health departments. A notifiable disease is a disease that "requires health providers (usually by law) to report to state or local public health officials. Notifiable diseases are of public interest by reason of their contagiousness, severity, or frequency."[20]

During COVID-19, hospitals had to report more than just cases of COVID-19; they also provided data on numbers of cases, deaths, new hospital admissions, numbers of hospitalized patients, and hospitalized patients in intensive care units. Some state and local health departments also tracked the number of available beds and ventilators within the health care system. Kattaryna Stiles suggested that during COVID-19 systems were used to track the data trends of hospitals regarding bed capacity. If beds were available, public health organizations could help coordinate information-sharing between hospitals, and patients were diverted to different hospitals as needed. These types of information-sharing and coordination were possible because hospitals reported key data regarding resource availability.[17] Juan Duchesne, Tulane School of Medicine Division Chief of Acute Care Surgery and Medical Director of the Trauma Center at University Medical Center New Orleans, agreed that data regarding resources (i.e., hospital beds, available ventilators, personal protective equipment [PPE]) were helpful, and he suggested that sharing data and models regarding viral replication rates and spread and hospital bed saturation would also help hospitals better manage their health care systems during a health emergency.[19]

Health Risk

Like the public, health care providers want to understand the health risk from a disease, including its signs, symptoms, incubation period, and treatment options. Providing more specific epidemiological information to determine risk and protective health actions is extremely helpful for medical providers. Genevieve Buser of Pediatric Infectious Disease for a large medical facility in Portland, Oregon, offered this insight: Alerting hospitals that "one case of measles was reported in Oregon" is unhelpful for understanding health risk or for taking action. In contrast, a better emergency risk message would say:

> One case of measles was identified in Portland Metro area (or county if can provide by law) in an unvaccinated adult with recent international travel. We suspect the infection was acquired internationally. Ongoing investigations are underway to determine exposures during the contagious period. General public risk is at baseline, and no action is needed at this time. Measles infection is spread through infectious droplets and aerosols. Two vaccinations or birth before 1957 are considered to give life-long protection against measles infection. More information to follow.[21]

Providing more information about the case, a descriptive epidemiology, and prevention and treatment information helps clinicians to determine whether their community is at risk or not.[21]

For medical providers, understanding the health risk, exposure risk, and symptomology is critical to determining the diagnosis, testing, and treatment of patients. In contrast, communicating health risks to the public gives them an opportunity to engage in behavior to prevent the threat from harming their health. If a person arrives at a hospital with illness or disease, it is often too late to prevent health harm, and the hospital or treatment facility must now contend with treating infectious exposures.

In addition to conveying information on risks to the general public, health care providers also need to understand how to treat and determine possible exposures to other patients and clinical staff. It is critical that health care providers know how the disease spreads so that health care facilities can take proactive measures to protect patients and staff from getting ill.

Information Relevant by Hospital Department or Medical Facility

In the United States, the private health care industry provides treatment in a variety of ways, including trauma care, hospital care including obstetrics and gynecology (OBGYN), cancer treatment and intensive care units, inpatient and outpatient surgeries, physical rehabilitation, assisted care living, nursing homes, and hospices. Each of these departments within a hospital or standalone health care facility requires specific information based upon its role and function in providing care. For health departments developing emergency risk communication, it is critical to understand the broad messages each health care facility needs (i.e., general prevention messages regarding nonpharmaceutical interventions) and more unique and tailored information regarding processes, procedures, and treatment.[17,18,19,21]

Personal Protective Equipment

The clinical community needs information about PPE and how to keep staff safe when handling specimens and when treating patients.[18,19] PPE keeps people safe from radiological and biological hazards.[22] Infection control practices like hand hygiene and PPE use are critical steps that support the prevention of illness spread.[22] PPE characteristics include design features, material performance, and use desirability. Design features include protection of mucous membranes, provision of a wide range of vision, and ability to communicate, and they are designed for the size of the person. Material performance includes durability over long shifts, ability to withstand repeated disinfection processes, and, in some cases, the ability to withstand tropical climate exposure. Desirability of use includes simple steps and procedures to don and doff the PPE and the ability to dispose of the PPE in an environmentally friendly manner.[22]

Interventions and Treatments

During a health emergency, interventions play a vital role in mitigating and preventing new cases of the illness through nonpharmaceutical and pharmaceutical activities and behaviors. Communicating health intervention information to the medical community is important so that health care providers can answer questions when asked by patients and work colleagues. Health care providers are often the first sources patients go to when seeking information about health risks. Additionally, when individuals become ill, they will seek out medical care, and the medical community needs to be prepared with clinical guidelines for treatment. During the COVID-19 health emergency, the US National Institutes of Health (NIH) developed COVID-19 treatment guidelines to provide clinicians with guidance for caring for patients with COVID-19.[23] To create the treatment guidelines, NIH convened a panel of medical experts to identify relevant information and published scientific literature related to COVID-19 and to create a systematic and comprehensive review of the literature. After synthesizing the information and discussing it, the panel recommended treatment guidelines based upon scientific evidence and expert opinion.[23] The guidelines created by NIH were also shared with the medical community on CDC's website, which provided specific information for health care workers.[24]

Understanding How Medical Community Audience Segments Are Different than the General Public

Chapter 3 of this book took an in-depth look at audiences and audience segmentation. It is important for emergency risk communicators to understand the information needs of the medical community and how they differ from the needs of the general public. This section outlines audience segments, key messages, channels, and communication products for the medical community.

Audience Segments

The medical community is made up of many distinct types of medical professional. These include primary care clinicians (i.e., medical doctors, nurse practitioners, physician assistants), pediatricians, osteopathy doctors, naturopaths, dentists, ophthalmologists, nurses, laboratorians, medical imaging technicians, anesthesiologists. There are also many different types of medical facility, including trauma care and hospital care, including pediatricians, neonatal, OBGYN, cancer treatment and intensive care units, inpatient and outpatient surgeries, physical rehabilitation, primary care, pediatrics, assisted care living, nursing homes, and hospices. It is important to outline the information needed by the various health care facilities.

Key Messages

As outlined earlier, there are six key information needs of the health care community. Ensure key messages to this audience include scientific guidance, data-reporting requirements to public health, epidemiological data, health risks, PPE, and health care interventions and treatments. In comparison, messages for the general public provide general overviews of the health emergency, including health risks and simple actions the public can do to protect their health.

Channels

Key channels to reach the medical community include Epi-X and the HAN. Specific webinars or conference calls can be hosted to share key medical information with the medical community. Additionally, leverage HCCs to share and amplify messaging for the medical community. For example, CDC hosts the Clinician Outreach and Communication Activity (COCA) call during health emergencies to share key information with the medical community.[25] In comparison with the general public, health departments are likely to use many channels, including news media and social media, to communicate with a broad audience. Specific channels for the medical community or secure channels like HAN and Epi-X may be used to communicate clinical information.

Communication Products

Based upon the key messages and channel identification, the following communication products will be needed to communicate with the medical community: (1) scientific guidance documents; (2) slide decks for webinars; and (3) handouts or videos as supplemental information for training or educational purposes. In comparison to the general public, communication products for the medical community need to include tailored and specific information. Often, emergency risk communicators develop educational materials like posters and infographics for the public and share those with the medical community. It is important for emergency risk communicators to realize that the medical community is looking for specific information from the health department about the health emergency. Often, HCCs will create public education materials that are of no use to the medical community. Instead, leverage preexisting materials from federal or state government agencies for public education and create and tailor communication materials that include key information that the medical community needs on:

- Scientific guidance
- Data reporting
- Health risks
- PPE
- Health care interventions and treatments

Mini Case Study: CDC COCA Call, COVID-19 Vaccines, December 30, 2020

This mini case study looks at information provided to the clinical and medical community from the CDC's COCA team. Read the following excerpt from the December 30, 2020, COCA call and answer the questions provided to further understand the importance of segmenting the clinical community as a specific audience with specific information needs.

> Good afternoon. I'm Commander Ibad Khan and I'm representing the COCA with the Emergency Risk Communication Branch at the Centers for Disease Control and Prevention. I'd like to welcome you to today's COCA call. COVID-19 vaccines: Update on allergic reactions, contraindications, and Precautions. Continuing education is not offered for this COCA call. All participants joining us today are in listen-only mode. After the presentations, there will be a Q&A session. Using the webinar system, you may submit a question at any time by clicking the Q&A button at the bottom of your screen, typing your question in the Q&A box, and submitting your question. The video recording of this COCA will be posted on COCA's webpage and available to view on demand a few hours after the call ends. If you are a patient, please refer your questions to your health care provider. For those who may have media questions, please contact CDC Media Relations at 4046393286 or send an email to media at CDC.gov. I would now like to introduce our presenters for today's COCA call.
>
> Our first presenter is Captain Tom Shimabukuro. Captain Shimabukuro is a medical officer and currently serves as the Veteran's Vaccine Safety Team lead for CDC COVID-19 response. Our second presenter is Commander Sara Mbaeyi. Commander Mbaeyi is a medical officer in the clinical guidelines team for CDC COVID-19 response. Captain Shimabukuro, please proceed.
>
> Thank you. I just want to make sure you can hear me before I start. (Yes, Captain.) Great. Good afternoon. And thanks for having me today. It's a pleasure to present to the group. I'm going to be talking about anaphylaxis following messenger RNA COVID-19 vaccination. I just want to note that some of the slides we'll be presenting today are adapted from a presentation at ACIP [Advisory Committee on Immunization Practices] on December 19th by Dr. Tom Clark. Next slide. So the first concern for anaphylaxis

Addressing the Information Needs of Public and Medical Community

following COVID-19 vaccination occurred in the United Kingdom, which initiated their vaccination program just prior to the US initiating its vaccination program. And on December 8 the UK started vaccinating with the Pfizer–BioNTech COVID-19 vaccine. On December 9, the UK authorities confirmed two cases of anaphylaxis after vaccination and promptly issued this press release from the MHRA [Medicines and Healthcare products Regulatory Agency]-based confirmation of guidance to vaccination centers on managing allergic reactions following COVID-19 vaccination with the Pfizer–BioNTech vaccine. Next slide. So as far as the US program, ACIP considered anaphylaxis risk during deliberations on the Pfizer–BioNTech COVID-19 vaccine during its December 11th and 12th meeting, it issued interim recommendations for the use of the Pfizer–BioNTech COVID-19 vaccine, and shortly thereafter, CDC issued interim considerations preparing for the potential management of anaphylaxis at COVID-19 vaccination sites. Next slide. So at an ACIP meeting on December 19th and 20th, CDC gave an update on anaphylaxis in the US following COVID-19 vaccination. And in this presentation, CDC had identified six case reports of anaphylaxis following the Pfizer–BioNTech vaccine that met the Britain collaboration criteria for anaphylaxis. All the cases occurred within the recommended observation window and were promptly treated, and all these suspected cases were notified through a CDC notification processes. And at that time, December 19, 272,000 doses of the Pfizer–BioNTech COVID-19 vaccine had been administered. Currently, there's over 2 million doses of the Pfizer vaccine that have been administered. Next slide. So seek actions to address. These reports of anaphylaxis include courses, close coordination with FDA on safety monitoring, and continued enhanced monitoring for anaphylaxis cases through the Vaccine Adverse Event Reporting System. This involves rapid identification and follow-up on suspected anaphylaxis cases and also case reviews and consultation with allergy immunology experts to provide guidance on evaluation of persons following anaphylaxis to COVID-19 vaccine. And I will say since the December 19th presentation, CDC and FDA through monitoring and various have continued to identify additional cases of anaphylaxis occurring following the Pfizer–BioNTech vaccination. Next slide. So I want to emphasize the role of health care providers in safety monitoring, specifically for monitoring for anaphylaxis.

And that primarily involves recognizing, responding, and reporting anaphylaxis cases following COVID-19 vaccination to VAERS [Vaccine Adverse Event Reporting System] and reporting adverse events to VAERS in accordance with the FDA Emergency Use Authorization reporting requirements and CDC guidance. I'll also mention participation in CDC's V-safe program, both for yourself when you get vaccinated and encouraging patients to participate in V-safe and finally communicating with patients on vaccine safety. Next slide. So VAERS is the nation's early-warning system for vaccine safety provides the quickest information on adverse events and the quickest information to allow us to characterize the safety profile of newly authorized vaccines when recommended in the population. It's comanaged by CDC and FDA. It's a spontaneous reporting or passive surveillance system, and it depends on individuals to send reports to viewers. So anyone can send a report to theirs. But health care provider reports are particularly valuable because we believe that the level of detail in the clinical information provided from health care providers in these reports is particularly useful for CDC and FDA. Next slide. The process for reporting adverse events to viewers is an online process. You go to the various websites at Verizon.gov and on the landing page you see here there is a link in the left-hand corner. You click on that link and it takes you to the electronic or the online reporting form and you can fill out a report.

Click "Submit" and then you get a notification that you have successfully completed a report for help. There's a 1-800 number and there's also an information email. And if you want to watch video instructions on submitting various reports, you can go to that YouTube link and view a video that's been created by CDC and FDA. Next slide. And I had mentioned previously – I just want to mention it again – V-safe is an active monitoring system that was stood up by CDC just for COVID-19 vaccination. And these are some resources on the program. Next slide. Right now, V-safe involves a manual registration process. Patients have to self-register. What I've shown you here on the on the right-hand side is a screenshot of the of the V-safe information sheet. The full sheet has a URL code and – I'm sorry – a URL and a QR code that you can scan to take you to the registration site. Patients have to enter a few data elements and register, and once you're in the system, then CDC begins sending text messages that involve health check-ins. And these messages have links to web surveys where individuals can report on their postvaccination experience.

And we are asking that health care providers help us get as many people to use V-safe as possible. And that primarily involves giving a one-page information sheet to patients at the time of vaccination or posting information in the clinic area or the area where individuals are getting vaccination posting so that individuals have access to the URL and the scannable QR code and also counseling patients on the importance of enrolling in V-safe. This just can be very quick and saying this is what the program is and we encourage you to participate. So we've created this electronic version of the V-safe information sheet as well, some promotional materials for distribution to public health and health care partners. Next slide. And I just want to wrap up with a reference slide here on information on how to report to viewers. The most important thing that health care providers can do, both to help us monitor for anaphylaxis and allergic reactions and to help us monitor vaccine safety in general, is to report adverse events to viewers and report them as quickly after they happen as possible and to be as complete on the report as possible. And then it has some safe resources and some general CDC vaccine safety information. Next slide. Thank you.[26]

Reflection Questions

Answer the questions provided to gain further understanding of the importance of segmenting the clinical community as a specific audience with specific information needs.
- Provide three examples of how these messages are designed for a clinical or medical audience based upon the common information needs of the medical community during a health emergency.
- How does the communication channel (e.g., webinar) support the intention of this being designed for a clinical or medical audience?
- How does the COCA call host and spokesperson support the intention of this being designed for a clinical or medical audience?
- Describe the role data play in this webinar and why this information about data is important for the clinical and medical audience to hear?
- How is this webinar different than a webinar planned for a general public audience?

Medical Community Using the CERC Framework for Its Audiences

In addition to the medical community being a message receiver of CERC messages, the medical community can also follow the CERC framework in communicating with its staff and patients. Specifically, the principles of Be First, Be Right, Be Credible, Provide Empathy, Show Respect, and Promote Action can help guide emergency risk communications with hospital and health care settings. A recent study developed a 13-question survey based on the CERC framework to analyze how hospital leaders in Singapore communicated emergency risk information to their staff members during the February 2020 COVID-19 response.[27] The research identified one key area where hospital leadership excelled in emergency risk communication and highlighted areas where improvements are needed.

The one area of strength of hospital emergency risk communication messaging was demonstrated by senior leadership. Senior leadership provided daily instructions that hospital staff felt were instructive and timely. Hospital staff also felt they were given enough information to stay safe. The following sections discuss the five areas for improvement discovered in the hospital study and how using CERC principles could have enhanced hospital emergency risk communication.

Middle Management

Although senior leadership demonstrated the CERC principles, hospital staff reported that middle management seemed to lack understanding of how to implement guidance from senior leadership within their teams. The inability to implement the guidance from senior leadership within teams left hospital staff feeling frustrated and unseen by their managers, and many hospital staff reported a lack of empathy from their immediate supervisor. By using the CERC principles of providing empathy and showing respect, middle managers could have better connected with their staff regarding the uncertainty of the emerging COVID-19 outbreak.

Resource Allocation and Logistics

Hospital staff reported a lack of clarity regarding new and emergent procedures regarding patient screening. The patient screening procedures and locations of patient screening would often change without staff being notified or receiving explanations as to why these changes had occurred. By engaging in the CERC principles of being right and credible and showing respect, hospital staff could have engaged in clear communication and information-sharing and established a communication protocol regarding the patient screening process. By establishing a communication protocol, the staff in charge of patient screening would be able to know how, when, and who to notify when changes were made to the screening process. This type of communication demonstrates the CERC principles by ensuring all staff have the most accurate information about patient screening, and it shows respect by ensuring that no one is left out of the communication loop, ensuring everyone is able to fully engage in their work and understand what is expected of them when carrying out their job responsibilities.

Human Resources and Staff Welfare

One of the biggest challenges staff within public health and the medical community faced regarding COVID-19 was the ability to personally process the evolving situation while simultaneously engaging in their professional work. Further, due to the workload increases, staff had to switch roles or take on other people's work throughout the outbreak. In the Singapore hospital study, staff reported a lack of empathy regarding their welfare during the outbreak. Further, staff felt that some of the human resources policies were communicated in an authoritarian and rule-based manner rather than with empathy and concern given the evolving health emergency. Engaging in empathy and showing respect to all staff are key CERC principles that can enhance internal human resource policy communications during health emergencies.

Information Overload

During health emergencies, in which uncertainty, stress, and anxiety are high, receiving information is helpful, but there also needs to be a balance in how and when information is shared. Sharing information too often or frequently changing processes or procedures can be hard for people to cognitively process. A balance must be struck regarding higher-priority and lower-priority communications. For example, hospital staff suggested that secure text messaging be used to communicate higher-priority alerts, while emails could be used to share lower-priority alerts. By sending secure text messages for higher-priority alerts, hospital staff could come to understand that a text message meant immediate action was required, while an email indicated action could be instigated later in time.

Audience Segmentation

The Singapore hospital study revealed that emergency communication within hospitals also requires audience segmentation. Specifically in this study, health care professionals who had worked more than 5 years at the hospital responded well to the senior leadership messages, while those who has worked less than 1 year at the hospital were often unsure of what actions to take during the health emergency. Other demographics, including age and job position, also affected how individuals processed information from senior leadership regarding the health emergency. Conducting audience segmentation and tailoring information within a hospital will ensure key health emergency messages are received and acted upon by all staff regardless of demographic differences.

Katrina Hurley, MD, chief of an urban emergency department in Canada, remembers wanting to receive transparent, frequent, and highly specific information about the emerging COVID-19 health threat.[28] For example, when guidance was being issued about PPE for hospital staff, she recalls wanting to receive specific evidence-based information that the recommended PPE would protect her and her staff from getting ill. She felt that evidence-based information would have enhanced her trust in these messages. Dr. Hurley also remembers receiving many questions from patients regarding information they had seen on social media or news media. While she didn't always know the social media post or news story to which the patient was referring, Dr. Hurley did her best to address patients' fears and combat misinformation. She even engaged in her own information-seeking, and she would share what she learned with colleagues and staff. A key takeaway here for hospital emergency risk communicators is to engage in news and social media monitoring to identify potential questions that patients might have based on trending news and social media posts. By reviewing these daily media reports, doctors can become more prepared to handle patient questions that arise from news and social media. See Chapter 10 for more information on news and social media monitoring.

Theory Callout: The Elaboration Likelihood Model

The Elaboration Likelihood Model (ELM) offers insights for emergency risk communicators on how to tailor messages for a specific audience and why tailoring messages can result in people taking a specific action.[29] The ELM, developed by researchers Richard Petty and John Cacioppo, explains how attitude change can persist over time or be relatively short-lived based on how messages are received and processed.[30] Using the lens of cognitive processing, Petty and Cacioppo suggested how people can be persuaded to change their mind or act through a continuum of thought processing. At one end of the continuum is low thought processing, and at the other is high thought processing. For those engaged in high thought processing about a message, such as considering the message sender, message content, and previous knowledge about the topic, it is possible that the individual may change their mind or be persuaded to look at the content differently.[31] Additionally, one's motivation and ability to process the information also play roles in how the information is received and processed. When motivation and ability are high, people engage a central route of processing and are likely to have their mind changed. In contrast, low thought processing may result in a short-term but not a permanent change of mind. For example, if motivation and ability are low or there is a lot of noise in the environment, the processing goes through a peripheral route and is not likely to result in a permanent change of mind. A temporary change of mind might occur, but not a permanent one.

Within the context of the Singapore hospital study and by applying the CERC framework within the hospital, the ELM can provide emergency risk communicators with additional understanding as to why it is important to tailor messages to the audiences. First, as discussed in Chapter 3, audience segmentation is important for understanding who the audience is and what characteristics and values are represented in each audience segment. Next, by considering the message sender, message content, channel, amount of noise or distraction in the media environment, and the audience's previous knowledge about the content, these messages can be tailored to resonate with each audience segment. Finally, infusing the tailored content with the CERC principles of being right, credible, empathetic, and respectful, the health emergency information is more likely to be received, processed, and acted upon by the audience segment receiving the tailored messaging.

Disaster Communications in Dallas, Texas: Using CERC Principles to Analyze CDC Communications When the Ebola Epidemic Came to the United States

Maxwell M. Leonhardt, MD, MPH

Introduction

On September 30, 2014, CDC Director Dr. Tom Frieden officially announced that the first case of Ebola virus disease (Ebola) to be diagnosed in the United States was being treated at Texas Health Presbyterian Hospital in Dallas, Texas.[32] Standing alongside Dr. Frieden was the Commissioner of the Texas Department of State Health Services, a hospital epidemiologist with the Texas Health Presbyterian Hospital in Dallas, and the Dallas County Health and Human Services Director.[32] This was the initial message of CDC's stateside response to the Ebola epidemic of 2014–2016. Ebola is an infectious disease, originating in Central Africa, which typically causes a severe – and often fatal – hemorrhagic fever, in which symptoms include malaise, vomiting, diarrhea, and internal as well as external bleeding.[33] Ebola virus is primarily spread via person-to-person transmission through direct contact with blood or bodily fluids of a symptomatic individual, such that a person is only able to spread the disease if they are also displaying symptoms.[33] Prior to

2014, there had been at least 20 outbreaks of Ebola, primarily occurring in West Africa, though none were as large as what was encountered in 2014.[33] During the 2014–2016 epidemic, Ebola was introduced to the United States for first time when a patient, who was likely exposed to Ebola in Liberia, traveled to Dallas, where he eventually developed symptoms and was diagnosed with Ebola.[34] A total of four cases of Ebola were eventually reported in the United States, three of which occurred in Dallas, and of those three, the second and third were nurses who had cared for the first case. The following analysis will outline the general timing of these cases and the three phases of disaster communications, and it will provide examples of how CDC positively or negatively highlighted the principles outlined in their own CERC manual.

Timeline of Key Events
In early 2014, Ebola was spreading rapidly around Liberia, Guinea, and Sierra Leone, and it was officially classified as a Public Health Emergency of International Concern on August 8.[34] On September 19 a man left Liberia, arrived in Dallas on September 20, and presented to the emergency room on September 26 with 2 days of symptoms, though was not admitted until September 28 when he returned to the emergency room a second time.[32] Two days later, on September 30, an initial message from CDC was given to the people of Dallas – and the United States as a whole – that the patient had been officially diagnosed with Ebola.[32] After over a week of caring for this patient, multiple press conferences, countless tweets, and quite a bit of discussion by local and national media and politicians, it was on October 8 that the first patient diagnosed in the United States with Ebola died.[35] On October 10, one of the nurses who had cared for that first patient was diagnosed with Ebola.[36] On October 14, a second nurse was diagnosed with Ebola, and it was reported that she had traveled on a commercial flight the night before.[37] The CDC Director told the public that she should not have traveled; however, it came out that she was unaware of this restriction, and she had at no point had a fever (temperature over 100.4°F). Even though she was under surveillance for symptoms, she had never been advised not to travel.[38]

These two cases led CDC to increase the personnel and equipment support it was sending to Dallas.[37] After these two cases in Dallas, which this analysis focuses on, there were no further diagnosed cases of Ebola in that region; however, there was another patient who was diagnosed in New York City after returning from serving as a volunteer health care worker in West Africa.[33] There were eventually seven other patients treated for Ebola in the United States; however, these patients were all diagnosed and underwent initial work-up outside of the country.[33] In mid-November, a press release from CDC stated that all patients and their contacts who were being monitored for possible exposures in Dallas and Ohio, where the third case had traveled, had all cleared the incubation period and these communities had no more active – or at the time potential – Ebola virus disease, and so the threat had been mitigated.

Initial Message
On September 30, the CDC Director, standing alongside representatives of local agencies, put out an initial message addressing the first patient to test positive for Ebola virus in the United States. This message came out soon after the results of the official CDC-sanctioned Ebola test.[32] The message was delivered in an even tone by the CDC Director. Everyone on stage was given an opportunity to share their experience in patient care or implementation of public health measures to mitigate the spread of Ebola, as well as to respond to specific media questions at the end. The press briefing began with an overview of the severity, route of transmission, incubation period, and symptoms of Ebola. Along with

confirming that there was a patient with Ebola in Dallas, the patient's journey through the symptoms of Ebola was explained. It was also detailed how he had been to the emergency room, been given antibiotics, and been discharged, returning to the hospital a few days later, before now testing positive.

The CDC Director was sure to remind everyone that patient care was the primary focus, and that CDC was supporting the hospital with this. He stressed that contact tracing was the second large focus, which CDC was supporting the city leadership with. There was reference to the Ebola treatment and contact tracing being done in West Africa and how the skills developed from that response could improve the care and strategies in the United States; however, it was stressed that the current case represented a very different situation and so required a different form of response. A message was directed at health care workers locally and nationwide to question patients as to whether they had been to endemic areas or had been exposed to anyone who may have themselves been exposed to Ebola. He stressed the necessity of adhering to proper PPE and hygiene practices and pointed out that nearly every hospital in the country had the capacity to properly treat and isolate Ebola patients. Following the CDC Director's message, the local epidemiologist clarified again how Ebola is spread and specifically acknowledged and addressed frequently misinterpreted science in this area. Before closing the press conference, the CDC Director reminded people that contact tracing and quarantine represented "core public health work" that CDC does well. He mentioned where and how to get more info, and he stated, "We will stop this in its tracks."[32]

Maintenance Message
Maintenance messaging by CDC was implemented over multiple platforms, including traditional as well as social media and, importantly, frequent in-person press conferences. Press conferences included updates on how the individual case (or cases) were progressing.[39] Another important element that was stressed in these press conferences was the frequently repeated concept that Ebola can only be spread by infected individuals who are symptomatic. There was also an online presence, with Twitter (now X) being utilized to share small pieces of information and with accessible educational materials being made available on the CDC website.[40] These online resources included information on the specifics of Ebola virus, reminders on handwashing, health care provider-specific instructions, frequently asked questions, and much more.[40]

When two of nurses, both of whom had treated the first case of Ebola, were eventually found to have the virus, CDC addressed their status and how they may have gotten Ebola. The messaging around the exposure focused on how poor adherence to proper donning and doffing of PPE by the poorly trained staff likely led to their exposure and eventual transmission.[37] They later rephrased this, as CDC received criticisms that this message put too much blame on the patients dealing with Ebola instead of CDC being accountable for not properly supporting these nurses dealing with the treatment of Ebola for the first time. More specifically regarding the third case, CDC reported that the nurse was diagnosed immediately after traveling from Dallas to Cleveland. Though the CDC Director stated the nurse should not have traveled, as she was considered an exposed contact, CDC later clarified that she had not been restricted from travel.[38]

Resolution Message
Though there was a fourth case of Ebola to be diagnosed in the United States during this crisis, the scope of this case study is on the situation in Dallas. The first resolution message from CDC came on November 14 after all the cases and contact tracing were resolved in Dallas. A press release was sent out in which CDC provided a quick synopsis of the four

cases, highlighted the work done by all health care and public health professionals, and confirmed that no individuals under 21-day quarantine had developed Ebola, which indicated that at that time Ebola had been contained.[41] A more robust official resolution message came in the form of a supplement, of over 100 pages, added to CDC's Morbidity and Mortality Weekly Report (MMWR) summarizing the outbreak.[33]

At this time, a digital and in-person exhibit on Ebola was established for a year, and it is still available online.[42] Both the MMWR supplement and the exhibit provided opportunities for CDC to provide the public with more information, to share lessons learned from the response, to acknowledge the lives lost, and to recognize the efforts put in by hundreds of people to combat the 2014–2016 Ebola epidemic.

CERC Principles
CDC created the CERC manual as a guide that they recommend using to direct communications in times of crisis.[43] The basis of the manual is six guiding principles that illustrate how to craft and deliver messages in emergencies. These are to be applied to messaging at every stage of a disaster response. In analyzing the messages delivered by CDC surrounding the cases of Ebola diagnosed in Dallas, six examples are identified and applied to each of the CERC principles. Each of these highlights how well or poorly the principles were followed at various stages of the messaging.

Be First
Being first sets the tone for the response messaging. It demonstrates that an agency is capable of putting together a message promptly, which in the eyes of the public may indicate that they can respond quickly as well. In this case, CDC, alongside local officials in Dallas, was able to host a press conference where it was stated: "We received in our laboratory today specimens from the individual, tested them and they tested positive for Ebola."[32] CDC was able to address the big-picture questions surrounding what Ebola is, how it arrived in Dallas, and what CDC and the city will be doing about it. CDC also addressed as many details as it legally could regarding the individual who was battling the virus. There was space for questions, which were all answered in the moment. Setting up a press conference rapidly, being sure to include local officials, and sharing all possible information up front are strong examples of how to be first in crisis communications. This approach showed the city and country that a response was underway, and it indicated how CDC would be conduct messaging regarding future positive cases in a prompt manner.

Be Right
Being first with initial and maintenance messages set the tone for how CDC was going to present information during this response, yet being sure that such information was right was important for continued community trust in the organization. Accurate information, especially in the case of an emerging virus that people are unfamiliar with, is important to eliminate confusion and keep people returning to CDC for guidance and assurance. CDC did a good job of sharing all it knew from the beginning, and to the fullest extent possible as each case was identified and treated within the legal and ethical bounds allowed with regards to patient privacy. The following quote from Dr. Frieden during his initial conference demonstrates how CDC is knowledgeable and a leader in the field by referring to the work that had already been done in West Africa, as well as the many organizations who work alongside CDC:

> While we do not currently know how this individual became infected, they undoubtedly had close contact with someone who was sick with Ebola or who had died

from it. In West Africa, we are surging the response not only of CDC where we have more than 130 people in the field, but also throughout the U.S. government. The president has leaned forward to make sure we are acting proactively there and the defense department is on the ground, already strengthening the response. We are working with USAID and other parts of the government as well as with a broad global coalition to confront the epidemic there. Ultimately, we are all connected by the air we breathe. And we are invested in ensuring that the disease is controlled in Africa, but also in ensuring that where there are patients in this country who become ill, they are isolated. We do the tried-and-true core public health interventions that stop the spread of Ebola.[32]

Be Credible
Being correct and accurate with information can help establish the credibility of an organization. However, that credibility, which takes so much effort to build, can begin to crack with only a few poor comments. When declaring the third case of Ebola to be confirmed in Dallas, CDC detailed where that individual had recently traveled in order to educate the public on who may or may not need to be concerned regarding possible exposure. This individual was one of the many nurses who had cared for the initial case of Ebola in Dallas. All of those who cared for the patient were considered possible exposures and told to monitor themselves for symptoms.[44] After caring for the first case, this nurse went to a family wedding in Ohio via plane, and though she was not symptomatic at the time of travel, all passengers on the plane were publicly asked to contact CDC and monitor themselves for symptoms.[44] In the initial messaging of the third case, the CDC Director saying that the nurse should not have traveled made it seem as if she had gone against the advice and authority of CDC.[38] When challenged further, it was revealed that the nurse had not been informed that her colleague had tested positive for Ebola, nor did she report a fever; therefore, she had been cleared to fly.[38]

This moment in the maintenance phase of messaging illustrated a lack of credibility. CDC thus lost some of the trust it had built up on multiple fronts. The initial fear that someone with Ebola had traveled when CDC was claiming to be tracking possible exposures and containing the spread demonstrated that it did not have as strong a grasp on the situation as it was letting on. This may have reduced CDC's credibility in the public eye; however, the primary loss of credibility occurred with the revelation that CDC had not been honest in what they had initially communicated to both the patient and the public. The message from CDC can be perceived as placing blame on the patient for traveling against advice, which will be addressed in the later subsection on the CERC principle Show Respect. By appearing to lie and place blame on the victim when CDC's efforts were being questioned and also appearing to have failed to contain the virus, this message from the CDC represents a poor example of being credible.

Express Empathy
When sharing the initial message, one of the first things said by the CDC Director was a great example of expressing empathy. After briefly explaining the background information on Ebola virus, Dr. Frieden revealed that there was a person who had tested positive in Dallas. Immediately after this he said, "First, to care for the patient. We'll be hearing from the hospital shortly, to provide the most effective care possible as safely as possible to keep to an absolute minimum the likelihood of the possibility that anyone would become infected."[32] This message shows a commitment to patient care and to protecting individuals in the community. Demonstrating this primary goal CDC's initial message expresses

empathy through its dedication to those individuals affected by Ebola instead of just focusing on population-level operations.

Promote Action
Throughout its messaging, CDC sought to promote action within the health care sector. This was done in maintenance messaging via its online platform as well as in press conferences. In one of the early press conferences, a week after the initial message, CDC directed a message at health care workers to "be on high alert and to identify individuals who have a travel history to the areas that are affected and that come in with any symptoms that could be associated with Ebola ..."[39] This is an example of the phrasing directed specifically at hospitals and health care workers that was used in many of CDC's messages. There were many of these targeted directions to health care workers advising them to question symptomatic patients as to whether they had been in a region where there was Ebola or had had contact with someone who may have been exposed. This messaging provided actions to those who were at the highest risk of being exposed to Ebola. It provided some sense of focus to the medical community and demonstrated this CERC principle well. The only criticism to be levelled in this area of health care-directed messaging is that there was not a lot messaging directed to the public on actions they could take.

Show Respect
As mentioned earlier, there were moments when the messaging took on a tone of blaming those who were exposed to and diagnosed with Ebola. The earlier example demonstrated how the message in question led to a loss of credibility. This message also failed to follow the sixth CERC principle of Show Respect. This message placed the burden of responsibility for exposure on the shoulders of nurses. These were nurses who had never cared for Ebola patients before and were not properly trained to do so. The following is the first thing the CDC Director said when announcing the first nurse to be diagnosed with Ebola:

> Good morning, everyone. And thank you for joining us. We're deeply concerned by the news that a health care worker in Texas has tested preliminarily positive for infection with Ebola virus. Confirmatory testing is underway at CDC and will be completed later today. We don't know what occurred in the care of the index patient, the original patient in Dallas, but at some point there was a breach in protocol and that breach in protocol resulted in this infection.[36]

This message begins not by acknowledging the challenges that this nurse has faced, but rather that there was a breach of protocol. Later, the CDC Director does demonstrate respect for what the nurse had gone through; however, beginning the message in this way came off as if the exposure had been the fault of those providing care. Respecting the communities at risk is important for maintaining their full participation and trust, and failing to do so at the beginning of the message may have caused people to dismiss the remainder of the message. This specific message demonstrates how CDC can inadvertently deliver messages that frighten the public by not embodying the principle of respect.

Lessons Learned
Based on this analysis, there are a few important lessons to be learned regarding disaster messaging. One of the clearest lessons from this case relates to the ways in which

accountability and blame can be perceived. When sharing its messages about the two nurses who had been infected with Ebola, the CDC messaging could have been perceived as being paternalistic to the point of blaming the victims. As mentioned earlier, this both damages the credibility of the messenger and fails to show respect to the local response. When describing the way in which the two nurses were exposed, CDC should have acknowledged that adapting to a new threat can be challenging and provided a supportive message. Addressing poor training represents an opportunity to be respectful and to state what could be improved.

The way CDC handled the situation of the nurse traveling was an extension of this paternalistic tone and could have been improved with more honesty up front. From the beginning, CDC should have acknowledged how it is challenging to adhere to quarantine policies. It is important also not to place blame before fully understanding what was told to whom.

Another lesson to be learned is that, when promoting action, it is important to address specific communities; however, specific actions need to be provided for the general public as well. CDC demonstrated good promotion of action in their online and in-person maintenance messaging to health care professionals. Much of the maintenance messaging was focused on how Ebola is only transmissible when an individual is infectious. Though this was meant to reassure the public, it did not provide any actions that people could implement to take some ownership in the campaign to prevent Ebola transmission. This was an opportunity to enlist the support of the public and decrease the amount of fear the public might feel and the unnecessary use of hospital resources by the public in anxious times.

Conclusion
Many lessons learned from the Ebola epidemic are still applicable. All organizations must continue to remember to provide less paternalistic messaging, to stress the importance of action in all communities, and to do everything possible to be honest and show respect to everyone. In the response to Ebola in Dallas in late 2014, CDC demonstrated three phases of disaster communication, and though positive and negative examples of each of the six CERC principles could be found in the messaging during each phase, this messaging was conducted at the high level that is expected of the federal agency responsible for infectious disease control in the United States.

End-of-Chapter Reflection Questions

1 Review your agency emergency response plans with a focus on how epidemiologists and public health preparedness staff work together. What are the strengths of the plans? What gaps need to be addressed?

2 Identify your health and medical partners for an infectious disease outbreak.

3 How do you communicate with these partners? What are the challenges with communicating with health and medical partners? Are you able to notify them of information prior to releasing information to the media?

4 Field trip: Relationships are vital before and during health emergencies. Set up an in-person meeting with a community-based organization or a medical professional you haven't met yet or haven't seen in a while to discuss the current status of emergency risk communication in your agencies.

References

1. What Is Epidemiology. *National Institutes of Health.* 2011. www.nidcd.nih.gov/health/statistics/what-epidemiology#:~:text=Epidemiology%20is%20the%20branch%20of,absence%20of%20diseases%20and%20disorders (Accessed March 4, 2024).

2. Brachman PS, Abrutyn E. Epidemiological Concepts. In: Brachman PS, Abrutyn E, editors. *Bacterial Infections in Humans.* Berlin, Springer, 2009; 1–50.

3. WHO statement on the first meeting of the International Health Regulations (2005) (IHR 2005) Emergency Committee on Zika virus and observed increase in neurological disorders and neonatal malformations. *World Health Organization.* 2016. www.who.int/news/item/01-02-2016-who-statement-on-the-first-meeting-of-the-international-health-regulations-(2005)-(ihr-2005)-emergency-committee-on-zika-virus-and-observed-increase-in-neurological-disorders-and-neonatal-malformations (Accessed March 2, 2024).

4. Ibrahim NK. Zika Virus: Epidemiology, Current Phobia and Preparedness for Upcoming Mass Gatherings, with Examples from World Olympics and Pilgrimage. *Pak J Med Sci* 2016;**32**(4):1038–43.

5. Engel Statement on Zika Virus [press release]. *House Foreign Affairs Committee.* 2016. https://democrats-foreignaffairs.house.gov/2016/1/engel-statement-zika-virus (Accessed March 4, 2024).

6. Zika virus: Key facts. *World Health Organization.* 2022. www.who.int/news-room/fact-sheets/detail/zika-virus (Accessed March 4, 2024).

7. Somanader T. Asked and Answered: President Obama's Letter to a Mother Concerned About the Zika Virus. 2016. https://obamawhitehouse.archives.gov/blog/2016/08/26/asked-and-answered-president-obamas-letter-mother-concerned-about-zika-virus#:~:text=I%20feel%20that%20something%20must,the%20rest%20of%20their%20lives (Accessed March 2, 2024).

8. Akpan N. It's confirmed. Zika virus causes microcephaly and other birth defects, CDC says. *PBS.* 2016. www.pbs.org/newshour/health/its-confirmed-zika-virus-causes-microcephaly-and-other-birth-defects-cdc-says (Accessed March 2, 2024).

9. Zika During Pregnancy. *Centers for Disease Control and Prevention.* 2023. www.cdc.gov/pregnancy/zika/protect-yourself.html (Accessed March 2, 2024).

10. Our response to the Zika virus. *Obama White House.* n.d. https://obamawhitehouse.archives.gov/zika (Accessed March 2, 2024).

11. McNeil DG. Zika Virus Rumors and Theories That You Should Doubt. *The New York Times.* 2016. www.nytimes.com/interactive/2016/02/18/health/what-causes-zika-virus-theories-rumors.html (Accessed March 2, 2024).

12. Momenipour A, Rojas-Murillo S, Murphy B, Pennathur P, Pennathur A. Usability of state public health department websites for communication during a pandemic: A heuristic evaluation. *Int J Ind Ergon* 2021;**86**:103216.

13. Bourdeaux M, Sasdi A, Oza S, Kerry VB. Integrating the US Public Health and Medical Care Systems to Improve Health Crisis Response. *Health Aff* 2023;**42**(3):310–17.

14. Hospital Preparedness Program (HPP). *Administration for Strategic Preparedness and Response.* n.d. https://aspr.hhs.gov/HealthCareReadiness/HPP/Pages/default.aspx (Accessed March 4, 2024).

15. Hospital Preparedness Program Cooperative Agreement FY2020. *Assistant Secretary for Preparedness and Response.* 2020. https://aspr.hhs.gov/HealthCareReadiness/HPP/Documents/Hospital%20Preparedness%20Program%20BP2%20Requirements%20At-a-Glance.pdf (Accessed March 4, 2020).

16. Testing and testing priorities for suspected cases. *American Hospital Association.* 2020. www.aha.org/news/headline/2020-03-26-cdc-updates-covid-19-testing-and-preparedness-guidelines (Accessed March 4, 2024).

17. Stiles K. Personal interview by Melville KGV, editor. 2023.

18. Aslam R. Written questionnaire provided to Melville KGV, editor. 2023.

19. Duchesne J. Written questionnaire provided to Melville KGV, editor. 2023.

20. Notifiable disease. *Centers for Disease Control and Prevention.* 2023. www.cdc.gov/nchs/hus/sources-definitions/notifiable-disease.htm (Accessed March 4, 2024).

21. Buser G. Personal interview by Melville KGV, editor. 2023.

22. What Is PPE? *World Health Organization.* n.d. www.who.int/teams/health-product-policy-and-standards/assistive-and-medical-technology/medical-devices/ppe (Accessed March 4, 2024).

23. Guidelines Development. *National Health Institutes.* 2024. www.covid19treatmentguidelines.nih.gov/about-the-guidelines/guidelines-development (Accessed March 4, 2024).

24. Interim Clinical Considerations for COVID-19 Treatment in Outpatients. *Centers for Disease Control and Prevention.* 2024. www.cdc.gov/coronavirus/2019-ncov/hcp/clinical-care/outpatient-treatment-overview.html (Accessed March 4, 2024).

25. COCA Calls/Webinars. *Centers for Disease Control and Prevention.* n.d. https://emergency.cdc.gov/coca/calls/index.asp (Accessed March 4, 2024).

26. Covid 19 vaccines: Update on allergic reactions, contraindications and Precautions. *Centers for Disease Control and Prevention.* 2020. https://emergency.cdc.gov/coca/ppt/2020/12.30.20-COCA-Call-Transcript.pdf (Accessed March 4, 2020).

27. Ow Yong LM, Xin X, Wee JML, Poopalalingam R, Chiang Kwek KY, Thumboo J. Perception Survey of Crisis and Emergency Risk Communication in an Acute Hospital in the Management of COVID-19 Pandemic in Singapore. *BMC Public Health* 2020;**20**:1919.

28. Hurley K. Personal interview by Melville KGV, editor. 2023.

29. Schmid KL, Rivers SE, Latimer AE, Salovey P. Targeting or Tailoring? Maximizing Resources to Create Effective Health Communications. *Mark Health Serv* 2008;**28**(1):32–37.

30. Petty RE, Brino P. The Elaboration Likelihood Model. In: Kruglanski AW, Higgins ET, Van Lange PAM, editors. *Handbook of Theories of Social Psychology, Volumes 1 & 2.* Thousand Oaks, CA, Sage Publications, 2011; 224–45.

31. The Elaboration Likelihood Model of Persuasion. *Behavior Works Australia.* n.d. https://prevention.nd.gov/files/bingedrinking/ELM%20-%20Australia.pdf (Accessed March 4, 2024).

32. CDC Press Conference: CDC Confirms First Ebola Case Diagnosed in the United States [press release]. *Centers for Disease Control and Prevention.* 2014. www.cdc.gov/media/releases/2014/t0930-ebola-confirmed-case.html (Accessed August 1, 2023).

33. Bell BP, Damon IK, Jernigan DB, Kenyon TA, Nichol ST, O'Connor JP, et al. Overview, Control Strategies, and Lessons Learned in the CDC Response to the 2014–2016 Ebola Epidemic. *MMWR Suppl* 2016;**65**(3):4–11.

34. Bedrosian SR, Young CE, Smith LA, Cox JD, Manning C, Pechta L, et al. Lessons of Risk Communication and Health Promotion – West Africa and United States. *MMWR Suppl* 2016;**65**(3):68–74.

35. Fernandez M, Philipps D. Death of Thomas Eric Duncan in Dallas fuels alarm over Ebola. *The New York Times.* 2014. www.nytimes.com/2014/10/09/us/ebola-us-thomas-eric-duncan.html (Accessed August 1, 2023).

36. CDC update on Dallas Ebola Response [press release]. *Centers for Disease Control*

and *Prevention*. 2014. www.cdc.gov/ media/releases/2014/t1012-ebola-reponse-update.html (Accessed August 1, 2023).

37. Texas Reports Positive Test for Ebola in One Additional Healthcare Worker [press release]. *Centers for Disease Control and Prevention*. 2014. www.cdc.gov/media/releases/2014/s1015-texas-second-healthcare-worker.html (Accessed August 1, 2023).

38. Schnirring L. Second Ebola-infected Dallas nurse triggers air passenger tracing. Center for Infectious Disease Research and Policy. *Center for Infectious Disease Research and Policy*. 2014. www.cidrap.umn.edu/ebola/second-ebola-infected-dallas-nurse-triggers-air-passenger-tracing (Accessed August 1, 2023).

39. CDC Telebriefing: CDC update on first Ebola case diagnosed in the United States [press release]. *Centers for Disease Control and Prevention*. 2014. www.cdc.gov/media/releases/2014/t1012-ebola-reponse-update.html (Accessed August 1, 2023).

40. Ebola Virus Disease: Factsheets and Posters. *Centers for Disease Control and Prevention*. 2022. www.cdc.gov/ebola/hcp/communication-resources/index.html (Accessed August 1, 2023).

41. CDC Releases New Reports on Ebola Cases in Liberia and the United States [press release]. *Centers for Disease Control and Prevention*. 2014. www.cdc.gov/media/releases/2014/p1114-ebola-liberia.html (Accessed August 1, 2023).

42. Ebola: People + Public Health + Political Will David J. Sencer CDC Museum. *Centers for Disease Control and Prevention*. 2018. www.cdc.gov/museum/exhibits/ebola.htm (Accessed August 1, 2023).

43. CDC. *Crisis and Emergency Risk Communication October 2014*. Atlanta, GA, CDC, 2014.

44. CDC and Frontier Airlines Announce Passenger Notification Underway [press release]. *Centers for Disease Control and Prevention*. 2014. www.cdc.gov/media/releases/2014/s1015-airline-notification.html (Accessed August 1, 2023).

Part I Precrisis Planning

Chapter 5

How to Get the Message Out
Understanding All of Your Communication Channels and When to Use Them

Chapter Objectives
- Describe how Media Richness Theory can guide the selection of communication channels.
- List two secure messaging systems used by public health agencies.
- List at least three internal communication channels that support collaboration.
- List at least three external communication channels that support public information.
- Describe how to organize a media briefing and town hall.
- Compare and contrast media channels, public alerting systems, mass communication channels, and digital media.
- Describe three ways to improve websites for emergencies.
- Describe the benefits and challenges of using social media.

Chapters 3 and 4 discussed identifying audiences, stakeholders, and partners who will be impacted by or involved with a health emergency response. In this chapter, the focus is on how information will be transmitted or disseminated to these various audiences through communication channels. Just as each audience group has its own information needs, identifying the best method to get information to each group is a critical part of emergency risk communication. This chapter will identify communication channels for transmitting information and highlight their corresponding tactics or communication products. In this way we identify the channel that could be used and also the corresponding tactics or communication products that will be need to be implemented to make use of that channel. For example, a media briefing or media interview is a communication channel, and the corresponding tactics or communication products are talking points. Another example is a website or web page communication channel, and the corresponding communication tactics or communication products are web page text (e.g., key emergency risk messages), data dashboards, and other relevant images.

Just as emergency risk communicators categorize audiences by identifying specific variables or characteristics about them, a similar process is used for channel selection. This process is guided by Media Richness Theory, which provides a helpful way to understand communication channels and their strengths and weaknesses for transmitting information.[1] There are four components outlined to aid in channel selection: the flow of information back and forth between the message sender and receiver; the inclusion of text and multimedia, including video, images, charts, and graphs; language variety; and personal focus.[2]

Table 5.1 Using Media Richness Theory to guide channel selection

Consideration	Media Richness Theory component
Is the audience internal to the agency or external?	Flow of information, language variety
Is feedback needed?	Flow of information
How much interaction is needed with the audience?	Flow of information, personal focus
Does the information need simply to be transmitted or transmitted and stored?	Flow of information
Does the channel need to transmit only text or do images, videos, and web links need to be included?	Inclusion of text and multimedia
Does the channel need to be private or password protected due to the sensitivity of the information that is being shared?	Flow of information
Does the channel provide a sense of personal connectedness?	Personal focus

Using Media Richness Theory, the questions in Table 5.1 can be used to aid in channel selection for communicating health information.

Much like a communications audit conducted to identify communication materials and decide on whether new materials need to be created (see Chapter 2), channel selection provides an opportunity to match the appropriate channel to the audience. This supports the purpose of emergency risk communication of getting the right message to the right audience at the right time.[3,4] The following sections outline the variety of communication channels and their corresponding tactics used in health emergencies and other types of emergency responses.

Internal Communication Channels

For the purposes of this book, internal communications focus on two components:
1. Employees of the health agency responding to the health emergency
2. Other health and government agencies involved in the emergency response

This distinction is important because of the secure messaging systems that are used by government agencies solely for information-sharing purposes, as outlined in PHEP Capability 6: Information Sharing. This section will look broadly at internal communications by first discussing secure alerting systems that federal and local health agencies use to communicate health information to government agencies and health care partners. We will then discuss business collaboration tools that are used to communicate with employees.

Secure Alerting Systems

Within the public health system, there are two specific communication channels – or secure messaging systems – that are used to communicate outbreak information between federal, state, and local health agencies. These are the Health Alert Network (HAN) and the Epi-X (the Epidemic Information Exchange).

Health Alert Network

The HAN is a secure messaging system used by federal, state, and local health agencies. The US Centers for Disease Control and Prevention's (CDC) HAN is CDC's primary method of sharing cleared information about urgent public health incidents with public information officers (PIOs); federal, state, territorial, tribal, and local public health practitioners; clinicians; and public health laboratories.[5]

Information shared through CDC HAN includes protocols and information about emerging health situations. There are three types of HAN messages:

- *Health Alert:* Conveys information of the highest level of importance about a public health incident.
- *Health Advisory:* Provides important information about a public health incident.
- *Health Update:* Provides updated information about a public health incident.

Under the federal HAN umbrella, state and local officials can also disseminate their own alerts to state and local partners.[5] The HAN is important because it provides a secure channel by which health departments can alert and warn partner agencies and health care systems about an emerging situation, asking them to notify the health agency if they see any suspect cases that might be related to the emerging situation. It provides an opportunity for information coordination and consistency from the health agency to multiple agencies and health care systems about an emerging or ongoing situation. The HAN is a one-way communication tool and does not provide interaction between agencies.

The communication tactic or product association with HAN is an alert message. The following is text from a sample HAN message that could be sent via HAN to health care providers regarding an emerging smallpox threat.

> **Scenario 1 Sample alert message for healthcare providers in an area without any cases of smallpox**
>
> On [date], the US Department of Health and Human Services (HHS) confirmed that [#] individuals in [city] have been confirmed to have smallpox. At this time, there are no suspected, probable, or confirmed cases within [area name].
>
> We do not know the extent or the source of the smallpox outbreak. Local, state, and federal officials, including public health and law enforcement, are working together to find these answers. They will update you as they learn more.
>
> Smallpox is a serious, life-threatening disease. There are no medications to cure smallpox, though medical care may help manage some of the symptoms. There are vaccines for smallpox. When given before exposure to the smallpox virus, vaccination can prevent the disease. When given within several days of an exposure to the virus, vaccination may prevent a person from developing smallpox, or may lessen the severity of disease.
>
> The [public health department] recommends that all medical providers and first responders in [area name] review the information for diagnosing and treating smallpox found on the Centers for Disease Control and Prevention (CDC) website at www.cdc.gov/smallpox. This website also provides information about the smallpox vaccines, vaccine administration, and vaccine adverse events.
>
> If you suspect a patient has smallpox, contact [local public health department] at [phone number] immediately for consultation. Follow guidelines for standard, contact, and airborne precautions to protect healthcare workers and other patients. If smallpox is diagnosed in the area, CDC will make the vaccine available.

[Public health department] will update the public and medical communities as the situation changes or more information is known. Contact [public health department] at [phone number] or for more information.[5]

Epi-X

Created in 2000, Epi-X is a secure network maintained and managed by CDC. Epi-X is primarily designed for epidemiologists, poison control centers, federal agencies, and other public health professionals involved in identifying, investigating, and responding to public health threats. It facilitates rapid reporting, immediate notification, editorial support, and coordination between public health professionals during public health investigations.[6] For example, events reported and shared on Epi-X include the 2002 West Nile Virus outbreak, the 2006 *Fusarium* keratitis outbreak, the 2009 H1N1 influenza outbreak, the 2014 Ebola outbreak, and the 2016 Zika virus outbreak. In contrast to the one-way channel of the HAN, Epi-X is designed to be a secure channel that allows for information-sharing and collaboration regarding emerging outbreaks and health threats.[7]

Epi-X is relevant to emergency risk communication because it provides a channel for rapid information-sharing across multiple jurisdictions to support nationwide disease tracking, investigation, and response as soon as officials detect a disease outbreak. "Epi-X was created to provide public health officials with a single source of up-to-the-minute alerts, reports, discussions, and comments – contributed by their peers, and moderated by Epi-X staff at CDC. The network's primary goal is to inform health officials about important public health events, to help them respond to public health emergencies, and to encourage professional growth and exchange of information."[6]

Partners who can participate in Epi-X include federal agencies such as CDC, the Department of Defense, the Department of State, the Department of Homeland Security, the Environmental Protection Agency, the Food and Drug Administration, the Department of Health and Human Services, the Department of Agriculture, and the Federal Emergency Management Association; state and local health departments; partner organizations; the American Association of Poison Control Centers; the Association of Public Health Laboratories; the Association of State and Territorial Health Officials; the Council of State and Territorial Epidemiologists; the National Association of City and County Health Officials; the National Association of State Public Health Veterinarians; and the Mexican and Canadian governments.[7] Private health practitioners are not given access to Epi-X unless they hold a government position.[8]

Epi-X is an important tool for emergency risk communication as it allows epidemiologists to gather and share information about an emerging threat with other health officials. This type of information-sharing can help identify potential links between cases across state lines and even across international borders. Epi-X can enable more robust investigation into the source of the outbreak as health officials work together to better understand the symptom profile, potential source, and risk factors related to the health threat. It can also help health officials with critical decision-making related to emergency response operations. For example, once the information from Epi-X is confirmed, that information can be used to alert the public about the health threat through public communication channels such as news media, social media, GovDelivery, and partner agency newsletters.

The communication tactic or product for Epi-X is a report. Such reports are used to seek cases of an infectious disease by including key information on what is currently known and by asking other epidemiologists for information and feedback.[8]

Hospital and Healthcare Information-Sharing

In addition to sharing information from emerging outbreak investigations, public health departments and emergency management coordinate with hospitals to determine the availability of hospital resources through an electronic database system.[9,10]

In Oregon, public health departments and hospitals coordinated efforts to develop the Oregon Capacity System, which was previously called HosCap. The intention of the system is to track hospital resources such as numbers of beds and ventilators. The system does not collect any patient-identifiable data. The primary benefit of this system is that it provides almost real-time data instead of requiring manual data entry. In Oregon, collaboration was achieved with nearly all institutions in the state, representing 90% of Oregon's hospital beds on the standardized, automatically updated electronic tracking dashboard.[9]

Another private-sector resource system used by health agencies and emergency management is called EMResource.[10,11,12] EMResource also tracks hospital beds, hospital and emergency medical services resources, and other emergency response data. In the United States, various states have adopted and implemented EMResource. For example, in Texas, emergency management monitors real-time communication to enhance responses to daily medical emergencies.[10] EMResource is used by health care, public health, first responder, and other government agencies. This system is utilized to monitor and provide notification of changes in resource statuses such as diversions, emergency operations center activations, resource availability, and other information. In Indiana, the data inputted into this system provide the Indiana Department of Health and health care coalitions with up-to-date information on capacity and needs.[11] EMResource is a tool to optimize communication and expedite patient care among health care facilities, public health, emergency management, and first responders. In Wisconsin, seven health care emergency readiness coalitions (HERCs) use EMResource to support hospital and emergency response information-sharing.[12] The data requested in EMResource are used to provide real-time updates on health care capabilities on a local, regional, and state-wide level. Through EMResource, partners can:

- Send time-sensitive alerts
- Review hospital diversion statuses
- Determine bed availability
- Share available resources to assist hospitals in need

The communication tactics EMResource or other hospital resource management tools include dashboards and graphs. These dashboards and graphs can be shared during partner webinars and meetings to provide situational awareness and support resource management and to support decision-making regarding health emergency operations.

Business Collaboration Channels

As outlined in Chapter 2 as part of Crisis and Emergency Risk Communication (CERC) planning and public health emergency preparedness (PHEP) Capability 4: Public Information and Warning, the crisis communication team needs to identify and use a notification system to inform staff and crisis communication team members of an emerging health emergency that will need crisis communication support. The notification system can use different communication channels such as business email or business text notifications. The following subsections outline how these internal notification systems can have multiple functions to support internal communication for public health departments.

Project Management Tools

To coordinate information-sharing with and among health department staff, a variety of methods can be used. Twenty years ago, whiteboards were used in small rural county health departments' conference rooms to communicate key updates and messages to employees about a meningococcal outbreak. Now there is a plethora of project management tools that can be used to store and share information internally with employees. Project management tools can also help you to organize emergency response operations, store key documents, and communicate with response operations staff. Many government agencies use Microsoft Office Suite as a tool to manage emails and documents and to support business administration.

SharePoint can provide a space for all employees to receive updates, share key messages on what information they can share with public, and identify what is going on in real time. Leverage SharePoint to create a space for internal updates about an emergency with health department staff. Emergency response staff will use secure and restricted files as working documents associated with an ongoing emergency.

Communication tactics or products associated with internal communications include status updates on the emerging health threat, key messages for the public, and points of contact for emergency response activities.

Microsoft Teams

During COVID-19, many government agencies and private health care systems needed to learn how to continue operations but adhere to the recommended physical distancing measures to mitigate the spread of the coronavirus between coworkers. In London, the National Health Service adopted the use of Microsoft Teams to support internal and external communications.[13] The National Health Service used Microsoft Teams in the following ways[13]:

- To deliver medical education sessions virtually, avoiding the need to meet in person
- To host non-face-to-face multidisciplinary team (MDT) meetings (e.g., lung cancer MDT meetings)
- To host frequently updated documents (e.g., staff rosters)
- To facilitate large group discussion forums (e.g., COVID-19 Journal Club)
- To collaboratively edit shared documents (e.g., research papers)
- To share data quickly using instant messages (e.g., oxygen usage in different wards)
- To host virtual meetings (e.g., board meetings)
- To broadcast live video streams (e.g., chief executive briefings)

For emergency risk communicators, using Teams represents a way to provide internal communications to health department employees. Having an informed workforce helps support emergency communication by ensuring all employees are sharing the same information, thereby improving message consistency.

The communication tactics or products associated with Microsoft Teams include creating a dedicated channel for questions and updates about the emergency response, weekly 15-minute "stand-up" meetings for all staff to update them on the emergency, or brief status updates or videos from the public health director or incident commander about the emergency.

Webinars and Conference Calls

Additional internal communication channels that help support the flow of information internally to employees and others in the public health system are webinars and conference calls. When done effectively, these channels can enable the sharing of key information and facilitate interaction between the message sender and the message receivers. The key to webinars and conference calls is to balance the amount of information that is shared, identify what is new information since the last time you met, and allow for people to ask questions.

During COVID-19, a study was conducted to determine the effectiveness of webinars for sharing information with hospital staff.[14] The webinars were used to educate clinicians about changes to clinical practice during health emergencies. Survey participants expressed dissatisfaction stemming from multiple potential issues. These included overall poor webinar quality, the repetition of information in multiple webinars, and a lack of sufficient tailoring of information to each audience.[14]

The study offered three lessons to be learned on how to make webinars more effective. First, planning through cross-agency coordination is necessary for communicating webinar topics and schedules and so avoiding repetition and scheduling conflicts. Second, content needs to be tailored appropriately to each intended audience. Third, webinars need to be more interactive.[15] The study's authors suggested four ways to improve interaction: allowing for questions to be asked throughout the webinar and not just at the end; providing live conversation or chat with the presenters instead of just sharing prerecording webinars; leveraging social media platforms to extend the interaction beyond the webinars and to post key highlights; and using a poll at the end to rate the webinar and reviewing the knowledge gained by attendees, their interests, suggestions, and challenges faced, which may help organizers to improve webinars in the future.[15]

Webinars require more communication tactics or products than conference calls. For webinars, visuals will be included, such speaker notes, slide decks, graphics, and charts. Speakers will also need a set of talking points and interactive questions to ask the audience. Organizers should ensure that a webinar host is able to post a polling question at the end of the webinar for feedback. It is also helpful to share the slide deck after the webinar or post it in a shared document repository where everyone will have access to the information.

For conference calls with large groups of people, which tend to be audio-only, the onus is on the speaker to reinforce key information that was shared during the conference call. For conference calls with smaller groups of people, it is helpful to identify who is on the call, who is taking notes, and who is responsible for sharing these notes

Zoom Fatigue

During COVID-19, government agencies, businesses, educational institutions, and health care providers were forced to move services online due to physical distancing requirements.[16] As a result of moving services and daily organizational operations online, people began to develop and experience "Zoom fatigue."

Zoom fatigue is defined as "somatic and cognitive exhaustion that is caused by the intensive and/or inappropriate use of videoconferencing tools, frequently accompanied by related symptoms such as tiredness, worry, anxiety, burnout, discomfort, and stress, as well as other bodily symptoms including headaches."[17]

Assessing Zoom fatigue through media naturalness theory helps to us understand how cognitive exhaustion and somatic exhaustion emerge.[17] First, as humans we are essentially hardwired to communicate by seeing and hearing each other. Zoom provides an opportunity for this, but ultimately, we do not achieve true eye contact via Zoom. To appear as if you are looking at someone on Zoom, you have to actually look at the camera, not the person.[16] Second, communication often occurs in real time via a back-and-forth flow between people with the ability to convey and listen to speech. With videoconferencing services there can often be delays in transmission or poor network connections that produce asynchronicities. "If a delay is perceived during videoconferencing (even if this perception occurs subconsciously in the range of milliseconds), the human brain works harder and thereby attempts to overcome the issue of asynchronicity, which is accompanied by increased cognitive effort to restore synchrony. Moreover, this effect is likely accompanied by enhanced frustration and stress."[17]

Third, when communicating with another person we often look for cues through facial expressions and body language to check whether the other person is understanding us. For audio-only situations such as a phone or conference call, we listen for verbal cues or long pauses to check for message understanding. Zoom provides audio and video options, but, depending on the individual's camera quality, lighting, camera angle, gaze direction, and whether they are sitting or not, it is hard to actually gage facial expressions and body language.[16]

Additionally, Canadian philosopher Marshall McLuhan famously wrote "... the medium is the message. This is merely to say that the personal and social consequences of any medium – that is, of any extension of ourselves – result from the new scale that is introduced into our affairs by each extension of ourselves, or by any new technology."[18] In the context of Zoom fatigue, McLuhan's words point to the consequences of new technologies for human interaction. Research on Zoom fatigue has highlighted that our brains are just not able to simultaneously cope with high information loads and electronic interaction.[17]

Thus, the very architecture of the technology that connects us during a health emergency can actually cause more stress, anxiety, and cognitive fatigue. The mirror effect is another phenomenon that disrupts our natural communication flow with another person through Zoom, because with Zoom, in addition to face-to-face human communication with another individual, we are also in face-to-face communication with *ourselves*. Our brains have yet to catch up with these developments, meaning our brains are not yet sure how to process this change in face-to-face communication. Since we can now see ourselves while communicating, we are now conscious of our own verbal and nonverbal feedback, causing us to engage in more controlled mental processes. This additional mental control leads to increased used of attention and working memory, which ultimately leads to cognitive exhaustion and fatigue.[17]

The pressures to multitask to complete tasks and deliverables during a health emergency are paramount. The emergence of videoconferencing as a main communication tool, constant instant messages, multiple observers, and the mirrored self – essentially the feeling of being stared at by others and of staring at one's own self – add to the fatigue and stress felt by videoconference participants.[17]

Information on Zoom fatigue has been included here because it points to two key factors for emergency risk communicators. First, public health emergencies can lead to stress and put pressure on the internal systems of a health agency to make decisions quickly in a context of uncertainty and unknowns and then communicate that information to the public, the media, stakeholders, and partners. Second, in a system that is already stressed, adding in Zoom and/or other videoconferencing tools can add to the stress and anxiety of those responding to the health emergency and those affected by it. The key takeaway here is to be aware and cognizant of potential information overload and to use Zoom and/or other videoconferencing tools effectively through clear meeting objectives, shorter update meetings, designating which meetings need to have participants' cameras on, and humanizing the experience for all involved. As we learn how to incorporate more technology into our workspaces, awareness of staff reactions to and willingness to adopt and adapt to using a new communication channel is important.

External Communication Channels

External communication channels are designed to inform audiences external to the agency and external to the emergency operations incident command structure. This section will include media relations channels, emergency wireless alerts, mass communication channels and digital and social media, and call centers and hotlines.

Media Briefings

Media briefings are created and organized by government agencies, organizations, and businesses to share a major news announcement with many members of the news media at once. Pre-COVID-19, most media briefings were held in person, but with the rise of streaming technology, online media briefings are now more common.

When organizing a media briefing, there are eight key steps to follow.

1. *Identify a location to host the media briefing.* If you are meeting at your agency's building, consider the size of the room, the accessibility of the room, lighting, audio, electricity, and Wi-Fi availability. If you are meeting online, consider what platform (e.g., Zoom, WebEx, Teams) and what meeting style (e.g., webinar, live meeting) you want to use. Next, consider the location where the spokesperson will give the announcement and consider camera angle, lighting, and audio. Specifically, you want to ensure that your spokesperson can be seen on camera with a professional background in a well-lit space that is free of external audio distractions such as barking dogs, construction work, sirens, etc.
2. *Identify team to support the event, including people and tools to support accessibility.* Managing a media briefing often requires a team including the media relations officer, the health emergency PIO, the spokesperson or spokespeople, tech support, and sign language interpreters. If your event is being held online, consider what tools are available to support closed captioning and ensure those tools are enabled on your account. A recent study of COVID-19 media briefings revealed that only 65% of countries across the world used a sign language interpreter.[19] This figure was lower in low-income countries (41%) and Sub-Saharan African countries (54%).

Surprisingly, no international organizations, including the World Health Organization (WHO), had a sign language interpreter present during COVID-19 press briefings.[19]

3 *Identify spokesperson or spokespeople.* Media briefings can be organized by one health department, but they may coordinate with other agencies to host their spokespeople as well. Hosting a coordinated media briefing ensures that each agency involved in the health emergency can provide an update on the key actions their agency is taking to support response operations. Ensure each spokesperson knows when to show up, where to go, and/or how to log on to the media platform.

4 *Review talking points and create visuals.* It is crucially important to take time with the spokesperson to review the current talking points and identify the key messages that need to be shared during the media briefing. Additionally, identify any visuals that may help communicate complex data or reinforce risk explanations. A study from the UK on visuals during health media briefings found that government officials included visual representations of data and infographic-style messages.[20] Visuals can help convey information on policy decisions, highlight available resources, and explain health risks. The most commonly used visuals by UK government officials during COVID-19 included the number of UK cases, and the number of hospital admissions, deaths, critical care beds, and mechanical ventilators, and a colored alert system. There are three key lessons to be learned from the UK study that emergency risk communicators need to consider[20]:

1 Have a plan for visuals that will be on your website and that will be used during the press briefing.
2 Ensure visuals convey the correct information, are easy to understand, and are accurate.
3 Explain risk levels and health threats and do not leave any information up to interpretation.

5 *Prep the spokesperson.* Next, prep the spokesperson by engaging in a mock media briefing, and practice questions you know the media are likely to ask. Go through the approved talking points multiple times. Provide feedback on the spokesperson's speed and tone of voice, which can boost trust and credibility with the audience. Ensure nonverbal communication (i.e., attire, physical space around the spokesperson) is aligned with and represents the values of the health department.

6 *Notify the media.* Send a media release announcing the media briefing to news organizations. Ensure they know the time, date, and location of the briefing. If the media briefing will be held in a physical space, make sure there is ample parking or let news crews know where the nearest parking is available. If the media briefing will be online, provide the meeting's details, including those of the spokespersons who will be attending.

7 *Prepare backup plans and process for troubleshooting technology issues.* When hosting the media, it is good practice to ensure there is a backup plan and you are ready to troubleshoot technology issues. Identify a second location in the event that your room or building is unavailable. Add signs and place greeters at the doors to ensure reporters get to the right location. Regarding technology issues, meet with your tech team early and ensure you have tech support on the day of the event. Work with the spokesperson on a backup plan in the event that their power goes down or their Wi-Fi drops; a good backup plan is to have them call into the media briefing instead of being on camera.

8 *Host the media briefing and debrief afterwards.* After the media event is over – whether in-person or online – it's a good idea to meet with the spokesperson, subject matter experts, and communications team to debrief. Make sure to highlight what worked well

and identify challenges that need to be addressed before the next media briefing. Debriefs can also increase trust and accountability among the communications team, facilitate organizational learning, and build institutional knowledge.

The communication tactics associated with media briefings are talking points. Talking points are sets of clear, easily remembered phrases that outline a proposal, project, or idea.[21] For emergency risk communicators, talking points include the emergency risk communication messages that will be delivered by the spokesperson. Once a set of talking points are developed, they can be tailored to be used on different communications channels (e.g., websites, social media) and by health department staff answering public inquiries or hotline or call center staff to support the development of preparedness responses.

Talking points keep the spokesperson on message whether they're giving a presentation, talking to a reporter, or in a meeting or elevator discussion. The purpose of talking points is to ease the verbal presentation, as it needs to be short and only to contain the most relevant information. Using bullet points can help condense and organize information.[21] Ensure the key emergency risk communication messages are included in the talking points. Keep in mind audience and information needs, the phase of the health emergency,[22] health risks, and the action steps people can take to protect their health. Weave in the CERC principles as appropriate.

Some agencies may have a teleprompter that you can make use of, or for online media briefings spokespeople can read their talking points directly from their computer. In that case, narrative talking points instead of bullet points are needed.

Public Alerting System: Wireless Emergency Alert System

The Wireless Emergency Alert (WEA) system is a partnership between FEMA, the Federal Communications Commission (FCC), and the nation's wireless service providers. Launched in 2012, the WEA system is designed to enhance public safety by allowing authorized federal, state, and local officials to send 90-character (recently increased to 360-character) geotargeted, text-like messages to the public's mobile devices during an emergency.

The WEA system is an essential part of US emergency preparedness and has been used more than 56,000 times to warn the public about dangerous weather, missing children, and other critical situations. The WEA system is designed to enable officials to send "imminent threat" alerts, as well as AMBER (America's Missing: Broadcast Emergency Response) alerts for missing and abducted children. A third type of alert – "public safety messages" – became available for alert originators in July 2019 (related messages include recommendations for saving lives and property). A fourth type of alert – a "presidential alert" – allows the President of the United States to send a message to the entire nation in the event of a catastrophic disaster, such as a nuclear attack.[22] The benefit of the WEA system over SMS text messages is the WEA system broadcasts use a "push" technology that sends messages to all enabled devices in a designated area, while SMS uses a point-to-point system and requires officials' prior knowledge of specific phone numbers.[22]

During the COVID-19 pandemic, no nationwide mobile alert was issued in the United States, but some state and local governments issued WEAs about the COVID-19 health emergency.[23] Specifically, governors in Colorado, Maryland, Michigan, New

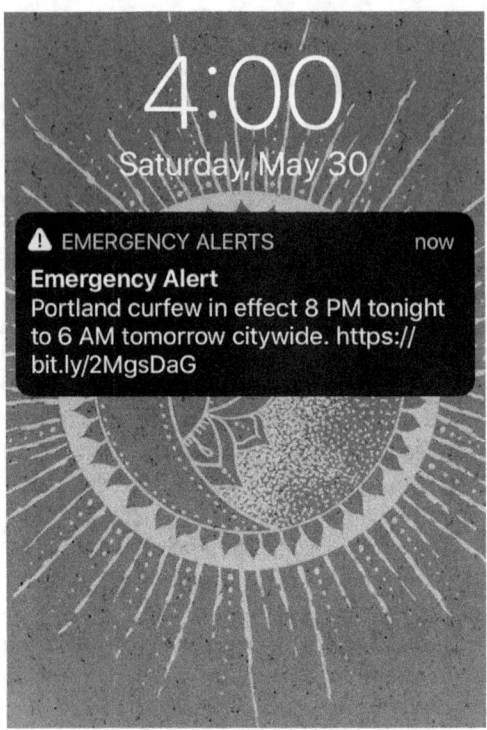

Figure 5.1 A Wireless Emergency Alert sent to Portland, Oregon, residents during the COVID-19 pandemic when the local government issued curfews.

Mexico, and South Carolina used WEAs to issue stay-at-home orders. In Portland, Oregon, a WEA was used to alert residents to a city-wide curfew (see Figure 5.1). The WEA system is an important tool for emergency risk communicators to consider as WEA messages can provide messages to people in a particular area on how to avoid becoming ill during an ongoing health emergency.

The corresponding tactic or communication product is the alert message template found within the WEA system. The alert message must include location, time frame, and health guidance information for those affected by the health emergency.

GovDelivery

GovDelivery is an electronic system that can be used to share information with citizens about health emergencies and other key government-related information.[24] Prior to GovDelivery, government agencies would send paper mailings.[25]

During COVID-19, Kitsap County in Washington state used GovDelivery to send out emails, texts, and social media messages about the outbreak and to counter misinformation.[26] Kitsap County had been using GovDelivery for 9 years, but during COVID-19 the county saw a double-digit percentage increase in subscribers to GovDelivery. Further, the county's COVID-19 daily bulletin included key information to answer citizen's questions received from call centers, media, and other channels.[26]

This consistent bulletin along with coordinated messaging shared via SMS and social media helped people identify Kitsap County as a trusted source of information during the health emergency. In addition to increased email subscribers, the county's Twitter (now known as X) and Facebook accounts saw a 10% growth, and its SMS messages reached over 830,000 recipients.[26]

The corresponding media tactics for GovDelivery are the newsletter, SMS text, and social media post templates that the system has set up. Leverage your agency's approved talking points and social media messages to create engaging newsletter content and social posts. Ensure message consistency when sending SMS messages about a health emergency and about the actions that the public can take to protect their health.

Town Halls

There are differences between media briefings and town halls or online forums. During a media briefing, the spokesperson is directly communicating with reporters. There's a set context, and everybody understands that there are reporters, a spokesperson, and set rules of engagement during press conferences. In contrast, in a town hall the spokesperson is communicating with everyone: the public *and* reporters. When a spokesperson is communicating with everyone including members of the public or those directly affected by the health emergency, the spokesperson must be prepared to interact and engage with the public's emotions. In a town hall, how the spokesperson communicates is vital.

Town halls can be more difficult for spokespeople than media briefings because town halls usually occur over a longer time frame. Media briefings are often about 30 minutes in length, whereas town halls can last for hours. Typically, the more speakers you have, the more interaction there will be between those attending the town hall.

During a town hall, the spokesperson will deal with multiple narratives and issues. In a media briefing, the spokesperson can control the narrative, but during a town hall, which encourages interaction with the public, multiple narratives will emerge. By conducting a stakeholder assessment prior to a town hall, the communication team will gain a good sense of the condition and emotions of the audience. Finally, there is potential for the spokesperson to be confronted with emotions, especially anger. Anger is not likely to be displayed during a media briefing, but it might very well be present in a town hall, and it is important to know how you can deescalate any such conflicts (see Chapter 11 for more information).

Town halls are created and organized by government agencies, organizations, and businesses to share information with a large group of people, engage in dialogue with the public and key stakeholders, and gather feedback on an issue affecting community. For emergency risk communicators, town halls provide a vital source of feedback for understanding public sentiment regarding the health agency's management of a health emergency. Like media briefings, most town halls were held in person before COVID-19, but with the rise of streaming technology online town halls are now more common.

When organizing a town hall, there are eight key steps to follow.

1 *Identify a location to host the town hall.* Most likely the health department will want to choose a neutral location or community-focused location to host the town hall. Town halls are not often held at the health agency but rather in a location that resonates with the community. When deciding on a physical location, consider the size of the room, the accessibility of the room, lighting, audio, electricity, and Wi-Fi availability. If the town hall is to be held are online, consider what platform (e.g., Zoom, WebEx, Teams) and what meeting style (e.g., webinar, live meeting) will be used. Next, consider the location where the town hall speakers will speak and consider matters regarding the camera

angle, lighting, and audio. Also consider how town hall attendees can ask questions. If the town hall is in person, ensure there are at least two microphones and mic runners who can make sure the questions are heard by all attendees.

2. *Identify partner agencies to cohost or speak at the town hall.* Including partner agencies to speak and present information to the community at the town hall demonstrates a partnership between the health agency and others to mitigate the health threat. Ensure partner agencies are included in any planning meetings to identify speaking topics, visuals, and other logistics related to the town hall.

3. *Identify team to support the event, including event moderator.* A town hall needs a formal facilitator or moderator to guide the flow of the event. The moderator will give a welcoming statement, introduce the speakers, and facilitate the question-and-answer session. The moderator monitors the audience, takes note of any drops in energy in the flow of dialogue, and supports conflict management actions if a confrontation escalates. In addition to the moderator who works the front of the room during the town hall, there also needs to be a back-of-room support team monitoring lights, audiovisual equipment, cameras, and other production-related items. For example, if the town hall is in person, it is important to have identified mic runners to ensure a microphone is provided to those asking questions. If the event is online, it is helpful to have a tech team supporting the online event. In addition to the moderator, it is a good idea to have an online host who will assist with any technological needs during the event such as muting and unmuting speakers and screen-sharing.

4. *Prepare backup plans and troubleshoot technology issues.* When hosting the media, it is good practice to ensure there is a backup plan and that you are ready to troubleshoot technology issues. Identify a second location in the event that your room or building is unavailable. Add signs and place greeters at the doors to ensure reporters get to the right location. For technology issues, meet with your tech team early and ensure you have tech support on the day of the event. Work with the spokesperson on a backup plan in the event that their power goes down or their Wi-Fi drops; a good backup plan is to have them call into the town hall instead of being on camera.

5. *Develop rollout and communications plans.* Develop a strategic communications plan to ensure the intended audiences are aware of the event and are able to attend. Develop a digital presence, including a dedicated web page and social media engagement, and alert the media via a press release.

6. *Day of town hall: Use a run-of-show document to organize team.* The moderator, speakers, and support team ought to use a run-of-show document to guide the production of the town hall. The run-of-show document includes the event agenda, timestamps, speaker information, and cues for key actions such as breaks or transitioning to the question-and-answer session. The run-of-show document helps guide and direct the moderator, speakers, and support team to stay on time and ensure each key action is completed to create a successful event.

7. *Gather feedback and continue dialogue.* Ensure the audience is given the opportunity to provide feedback after the town hall is complete. Provide QR codes to a feedback survey, but also identify a point of contact people can reach out to if they have more questions. Also share websites, email addresses, and phone numbers that people can use to provide feedback. Be sure to set up an email autoresponder so that people know that their emails have been received.

8. *Debrief afterwards.* After the town hall ends, it is good practice to hold an immediate debrief meeting to capture the successes and challenges of the event. Be sure to identify any action items that need to occur based on the event. Identify whether there were any issues that need to be corrected before any future town hall events.

The corresponding tactics for a town hall include talking points, slide decks, graphs, charts, and other visuals to support the speakers. Another key communication product is the run-of-show document for the production team – regardless of whether the event is online or in person. The run-of-show document will help orient everyone regarding the purpose of the event, outline speaker order and the roles and responsibilities of the production team, and indicate at what time the event will move to taking questions from the public.

Call Centers and Hotlines

In PHEP Capability 4: Emergency Public Information and Warning, establishing avenues for public interaction and information exchange includes the use of call centers and hotlines. Developing a call center doesn't have to be organized or managed solely by the public health agency. It is possible to leverage existing poison control centers, crisis hotlines, nurse advice lines, or community connection hotlines such as a 2-1-1 to support health emergency response activities and created a coordinated call center.[27] Calls centers are important because they provide another way for the information-seeking public to gather information about a health emergency. Further, when a call center is established, it can provide much-needed interaction with the public and build trust between the public and the health agency responding to the emergency.

It is good practice to ensure daily metrics about numbers of calls and the types or categories of calls that are being received, such as vaccination questions, symptoms of the illness, travel, or reporting illness, are shared with the communication team. These data can be used to inform and update communication strategies to ensure the agency is answering questions from the public and continuing to provide the most accurate and credible health information that is available.

The corresponding tactic or communication product for a call center is a prepared response. The prepared response is the official message and approved answered to a particular question. For example, if someone called about the symptoms of an illness, the prepared response would include the symptoms of that illness.

Digital and Social Media: Websites, Search Engine Optimization, Social Media, TikTok, Podcasts, and Chatbots

Digital channels are powerful external communications channels that ensure the provision of coordinated and consistent emergency risk information during a health emergency. Digital channels, including websites, GovDelivery newsletters, and social media, are large platforms that can reach many audience segments.

Websites

During COVID-19, state and federal health departments created COVID-19-dedicated websites with information about COVID-19 symptoms, health intervention and self-protection messages, dashboards with case counts by geographic location, testing information, and guidance.[28]

Websites are important channels for public health practitioners to use to share and disseminate important health and safety information. The key is to ensure that these channels are usable and accessible by all populations. When discussing websites, usability is formally defined as "the extent to which a system, product or service can be used by specified users to achieve specified goals with effectiveness, efficiency, and satisfaction in a specified context of use."[29] Accessibility is defined as the usability of a product, service, environment, or facility by people with the widest range of capabilities.[29]

Within the context of public health, usable and accessible websites need to communicate real-time and complex health and safety information to the public, partner agencies, community stakeholders, and the media through text, images, and other means to support those with language, hearing, eyesight, or other challenges that impact their ability to receive these materials.

A recent study of state health department COVID-19 websites used 148 evaluation criteria of website usability such as using images, optimizing for mobile device viewing, displaying information in a usable format, placing important information at the top and center, and options to view pages in a language other than English, and the researchers found that websites often were *not* usable or accessible.[28] In this study, the researchers found nine common issues that may have hindered emergency risk communication. These are listed in the following subsection, and they include but are not limited to: a lack of action messages, poor web page layout, issues with navigation menus, and a lack of content explanation for data dashboards.

Nine Recommendations to Improve Emergency Risk Communication on Websites

1 Ensure the web team, graphic designers, and communication specialists work with subject matter experts to design website graphics and data dashboards that convey the risk information to the public through the use of trend lines, warning signs, and different colors and icons signaling escalation and de-escalation of risk. Create interactive features for people to be able to select location information in order to understand the health risk by geographic area. Use "conventional urgency colors instead of non-standard color schemes (i.e., red, yellow, green, for high, moderate, and no urgency levels, respectively) so that the colors directly correspond to user mental models representing danger, moderate danger, and no danger. In addition to using colors, including patterned or textured areas could address accessibility concerns for color-blind users."[28]

2 Design for mobile viewing and ensure responsive designs and fluid layouts are implemented. Designers should design web pages to automatically adjust based on screen size and resolution. This is an important design consideration, particularly for web pages that include images or for dashboards containing tables and charts, where the content may not render and display properly and might not fit all screen sizes.

3 Provide a search function on the website. To ensure the public can find the information they need quickly, having a search function (i.e., site search) available on the website is key. This can take the form of a search box at the top of the website or a chatbot to assist the website visitor. Having a search function on the website can offset any website navigation issues or poorly laid-out pages that a website visitor might encounter.

4 Implement more language options. To ensure language accessibility, the study's authors recommended, at a minimum, embedding the freely available Google Translate or similar application programming interfaces to render pages in different languages for users. Additionally, ensure accessibility features are enabled for those with screen readers or who need large font sizes.

5 Clarity in website content. Website content needs to be organized in such a way that audience members can easily find the information they are looking for without excessive cognitive overload. At a minimum, the content should be organized to provide general

information about the situation, the risk factors, and how people can protect their health. Leverage the web page layout template to create pages with clear titles and subtitles, a logical sequence of information, and formatting features that highlight and define content pieces. Further, consider information density or the amount of information provided in a given space. During a health emergency, design web pages so that audience members are able to scan and quickly find pertinent health information without needing to invest a lot of effort.[28]

6. Use images and graphics to educate people on what actions to take to protect their health. Ensure these images complement the risk message so that the audience is able to take action without compromising their safety. Balance the amount and size of images so that page loading does not take too long, which might drive away web traffic. Make sure to include alternative text ("alt text") attributes to make the images accessible and inclusive.

7. Make sure to use a different color for visited links to distinguish these from unvisited links. This will help audience members to see what links they have already clicked on. When health departments update their websites and add more information, ensuring that previously visited links change color provides "a positive user experience when users need to navigate several pages of a public health website to find useful health information efficiently. Given the amount and mix of new and old links on these pages, if visited links are not distinguished, users may spend more time and feel frustrated clicking on and navigating through links that they may have already reviewed and did not intend to review again."[28]

8. Ensure websites support both online and print readability. The study's authors recommended not designing information that is only suitable for online reading. Since all web browsers have printing options, ensure that these pages are able to be printed.

9. Social media on websites. Make sure to include links to social media accounts such as X, Facebook, YouTube, and Instagram. Embed health department press conferences and tweets from health officials on the health department's website.

Search Engine Optimization

Search engine optimization (SEO) is often considered to be a tool that is relevant to marketing, but ensuring your agency's website includes metadata and alt text will help search engines find your agency's content during a health emergency. Search engines help people find information on the internet, and SEO helps place your website at the top of search results.[30] Due to the vast number of websites and web pages available, leveraging your site's metadata, which includes page titles, page text, site URLs, alt text for images, and graphics or images that constitute engaging content, will help make your agency's website more findable.[30]

Search engines use two basic algorithms when ranking websites. One algorithm ranks websites based on the quantity and quality of inbound and outbound web links. The other ranks websites according to relevance through search queries or keywords.[30] Google uses a combination of both of these algorithms.

For those maintaining your agency's website, there are two strategies to achieve SEO. One is using an on-page optimization strategy, which focuses on leveraging the page title, metadata, the titles of images, and anchor text. The other is off-page optimization, which focuses on web links that link to websites and web pages away from your agency's website and web links that are coming to your website from other websites (e.g., partners and stakeholders that provide links on their websites to your agency's website). Using these strategies will improve your agency's accessibility and findability on the internet. Doing so will also help those members of the public who are searching for credible and accurate health information to find official government sources and response information.

Key Tips for Emergency Risk Communicators to Improve SEO
Anchor Text
"Anchor text" refers to the visible characters and words that hyperlinks display when linking to a document or another web page. To optimize anchor text, ensure that the text is an exact match to a keyword you are targeting for an exact-match strategy or include a variation of the keyword on the page or document you are linking to for a partial-match strategy.[31]

- Make sure the anchor text is relevant to the page or document you are linking to.
- Keep the anchor text to as few words as possible instead of providing a long sentence.
- Keep the nature of the anchor text intact and do not stuff as many keywords as possible into the anchor text.

Keywords
Keywords are words that the public, partners, and stakeholders are using within search engines to find health information related to an emergency.

- Identifying keywords the public and others are using to locate health information can help you to strategize regarding your use of keywords on your agency's website in page titles and web page text. For example, during COVID-19, search terms included "coronavirus," "fever," "sore throat," "cough," "stay home," "facial masks," "social distancing," and "washing hands."[32]
- Understanding what terms the public is using to look for information is key when developing emergency risk communication content for your agency's website.

Page Titles
Page titles can be tailored for SEO purposes to support those who are searching for relevant health information and emergency risk information.

- Depending on how your agency's website is structured, there may be up to three page title options: the title of the web page, the page's SEO title, and a navigation web page title.
- Page titles can include keywords that you know the public and others are using to look for health information.
- It is helpful to keep page titles to 70 characters or fewer.[33]

Alt Text
Alt text is text added to images to make them more accessible.

- Alt text is also used by search engines to identify content on the web page and can also support an on-page SEO strategy.
- Alt text is also used by assistive screen readers or browsers with images disabled.
- If the browser cannot display the image for some reason, the alt text will be displayed instead. When creating alt text, use short, readable terms to describe the image.[34]

Inbound and Outbound Links

To maximize off-page optimization, including a combination of both inbound and outbound links will help increase the rank of your content on search engines and help those looking for health information to find your agency's content. Health departments are very good at including outbound links to federal and international health agencies such as CDC and WHO. Make sure to encourage your local partners and stakeholders to provide links from their websites to your agency's health emergency website.

Social Media

When engaging with social media channels, emergency risk communications need to review the health department's internal policies and ensure that resources are available to support social media platform management (e.g., Facebook, Instagram, X, YouTube, and LinkedIn). Social media accounts require daily maintenance even during nonemergency times. During an emergency, a health department may not want to add a new social media platform unless audience research indicates the agency is missing a key audience by not using a particular platform.

Social media platforms each have their own style, features, and norms of how to create and share content. Each platform will have its own unique way to convey information through text, images, video, use of emojis, hashtags, and @mentions. Each platform has a distinct way for people to follow or subscribe others for content updates. Some channels may allow for cross-posting, meaning that when the agency posts on Facebook, it will simultaneously cross-post on Instagram.

Due to the evolving nature of social media platforms and media technology, make sure to double-check each platform's guidance and training materials on how best to leverage its functions to disseminate the agency's key health messages.

The corresponding tactics or communication products for Facebook, Instagram, X, and LinkedIn include text, images, links, videos, hashtags, and @mentions. YouTube, by contrast, is a video-centered platform. To create social posts, review approved talking points and then tailor the talking points for each platform's unique audience. Setting up a photo or image library with approved images will help reduce the amount of time spent looking for appropriate images to match each social media post. Research on X messages revealed that, during health emergencies, tweets containing details regarding hazard impact, time, location, guidance, and source and that are delivered in a style that is clear, specific, certain, accurate, and consistent have a higher probability of positively impacting protective action-taking among persons at risk.[35]

Key Tips for Emergency Risk Communicators When Working with Social Media

1. Review organization policies about use of social media, including commenting, deleting, harassment/civil communication, and retention of posts.
2. Ensure there is team capacity to manage and monitor social media and address misinformation.
3. Engage in strategic planning of content creation by social media platform. Engage in continuing education regarding each of the social media platforms with reference to character limits, use of emojis, video content restrictions, hashtags, and @mentions.

4. Review processes regarding content review/clearance of materials. Ensure reviewers understand what feedback to provide regarding text, images, and video. Ensuring accessibility through language and Section 508 compliance guidelines.
5. Reuse content from previous media releases and press briefings to support social media engagement. Ensure content is tailored to each social media channel.
6. Embed social media into the web page. Ensure the health agency's social channels are featured on the health emergency web page, and embed video links for media briefings, interviews, and other key video content.
7. Repost or reshare partner content. Work with partner agencies to repost and reshare content related to the health emergency. Ensure reposting and resharing of information is outlined in the crisis communication plan.
8. Follow partners and influencers. Review current followers and accounts that the health agency is following. Consider adding new partners and influencers based on the type of health emergency. For example, particular influencers might resonate with an audience segment that is impacted by the health emergency.

TikTok

During COVID-19, a new platform rose to prominence: TikTok, a video-based platform. Some 62% of 18–29-year-old Americans say they use TikTok.[36] While many Americans use TikTok, the Chinese-owned company faced legal constraints prohibiting the use of the app on federal and state government phones based on national security risks regarding the Chinese government's ability to access American user data.[37]

Podcasts

Podcasts emerged in the early 2000s, but during COVID-19 the podcast industry shifted dramatically as telework became the de facto mode of work. Instead of listening to podcasts during the morning commute, listeners tuned in through their computers or mobile devices while multitasking, working out, cleaning, or working in their gardens.[38] Podcast types include traditional podcasts, enhanced podcasts, video podcasts, or vodcasting. Enhanced podcasts include slides, animations, or short videos to enhance the audio content. Vodcasting eschews the audio-only tradition of podcasting and includes video footage. According to the Pew Research Center, about half of Americans have listened to a podcast in the past year, and about 20% of Americans listen to podcasts a few times a week.[39] While people tune in to podcasts for entertainment or learning purposes, some listeners indicate that they listen to podcasts for news or to stay up to date on current events.[39]

Podcasts represent an important channel for emergency risk communications to leverage. While ensuring there are ample resources to maintain a regular podcast, health departments could host and manage their own podcasts. If the health agency does not have a podcast, working with partner agencies or landing an interview for a staff member on a well-known podcast can further spread health information regarding a health emergency. During COVID-19, CNN medical correspondent Sanjay Gupta was interviewed on the *Joe Rogan Experience* podcast to dispel misinformation about COVID-19.[40,41]

Chatbots

Chatbots – computer programs designed to simulate conversation with human users – were used during COVID-19 to help provide answers to questions about the outbreak. During COVID-19, chatbots were used to: disseminate health information and knowledge; aid in self-triage and personal risk assessment; monitor exposures and notifications; track COVID-19 symptoms and other health aspects; and combat misinformation and fake news.[42,43]

Chatbots can be programmed to ask and answer questions, create health records and histories of use, complete forms, and generate reports.[42]

The answers provided by these chatbots were based on information generated by WHO, CDC, and other health sources. Instead of having staff members engage with the public or having people call a hotline, chatbots on a health agency's website could provide information about COVID-19 symptoms, what people could do to protect their health, and personal risk assessments, as well as address misinformation.[42]

The two challenges of using chatbots during COVID-19 were the public's willingness to engage with a chatbot and the overall functionality of the chatbot. The public's willingness to engage with a chatbot is based upon whether they trust the technology to provide them with correct information and protect their privacy. Additionally, some people might not have had access to technology and therefore could not engage with chatbots. The overall functionality of the chatbot also impacts the adoption of this technology. Chatbots leverage existing databases (e.g., medical databases, information from WHO and CDC) and natural language capabilities to understand clinical terminology.[44,45] However, it can be hard to ensure that the chatbot has the latest and most accurate health information. Further, chatbots are not yet equipped to handle sensitive issues such as mental health concerns.

There may not be a corresponding tactic or communication product for a chatbot. Agencies ought to weigh the risks, benefits, and costs of deploying a chatbot on their website to determine whether this tool fits their communication and customer service needs.

Intersection of the 2018 California Camp Fire and CERC Principles
Madison Dulas, MSW, MS-DRL, LGSW

Introduction
The 2018 California Camp Fire is known as the deadliest wildfire in Californian history.[46] Significant and damaging health effects occurring during the Camp Fire, and lasting beyond the fire's containment, negatively impacted thousands. The utilization of CERC principles during this crisis will be explored, as will the lack of use of those CERC principles that would have been effective for conveying information to area residents. Upon analysis of the use of CERC principles, or lack thereof, implications for Butte County Public Health (BCPH) and other communicating entities will be presented for consideration regarding future disaster communications. Crisis communication by BCPH was sufficient, but it is vital to understand the intricacies of the Camp Fire and the resulting health-related impacts when analyzing such communications.

Overview of the Disaster

On November 8, 2018, the state of California was forever altered when the California Camp Fire began. The result of Pacific Gas and Energy's failure to maintain and replace components of its 50,000 electrical towers and 18,500 miles of transmission lines, the Camp Fire burned 153,000 acres, destroyed more than 18,000 structures, and caused 85 deaths before it was contained on November 25, 2018.[47,48] In the community of Paradise, California, over 85% of residential units were lost to the Camp Fire.[49] Devastating structural losses combined with ever-present, toxic smoke from the Camp Fire, which was harmful enough to warrant declaration of a public health emergency for the entire state of California by the US Secretary of Health and Human Services.[50] By 2023, the Camp Fire's immense destruction meant that the majority of burned areas were still in the recovery phase, and many residents remained impacted by the health-related effects they experienced during and after the Camp Fire.

Among the impacts of the Camp Fire were a variety of health-related effects that had the potential to cause severe long-term damage. These included the presence of significant amounts of toxic smoke, which contained dangerous levels of both metal contaminants and particulate matter (PM). Smoke containing elevated levels of lead and zinc, along with calcium, iron, and manganese, was found to have reached areas such as the Sacramento Valley and the San Francisco Bay Area, over 150 miles away from Paradise.[51] In nearby Chico, California, for instance, lead concentrations in the air were reported to reach 50 times average levels.[51] Such a degree of lead exposure can result in extremely harmful health effects including cancer, high blood pressure, difficulty reproducing, and behavioral changes and learning deficits in children.[51]

The toxicity generated by the Camp Fire was further compounded by the presence of PM, or minute particles in the smoke which represent as the largest health concern from wildfire smoke, as PM can reach the lungs' deepest recesses.[51] Throughout the Camp Fire's burn period, "... maximum PM levels increased across CA [California] by more than 300% compared to average levels seen during the same time period from 2010–2017."[51] Damaging health effects associated with inhaling PM include worsening of asthma, onset of various respiratory diseases, increases in infections and inflammation (e.g., pneumonia), and greater occurrences of hospital admissions.[51]

In addition to smoke-related impacts, poor water quality in the Camp Fire's burn area caused significant health concerns. Damage to water infrastructure and settling of ash and contaminants on lakes and water reservoirs led to contamination of drinking water.[52] Some 2,217 parts per billion (ppb) of the cancer-causing compound benzene, which has a federal limit of 5 ppb in drinking water, were found in water samples taken from the Camp Fire's burn area, along with elevated levels of aluminum and iron.[53] *E. coli* bacteria and polycyclic aromatic hydrocarbons, or chemicals stemming from burning wood, garbage, or gasoline, were also found in collected water samples.[54] As a result, BCPH issued a do-not-drink water advisory, lasting from January 2019 to August 2019, after which water customers were encouraged to continue engaging in water testing and treatment options for homes and businesses.[55]

Finally, hazardous fire debris also served as a health-related concern for those returning to their homes. Homeowners were confronted with debris and settled ash that contained toxic substances as a result of burned synthetic and hazardous materials, ranging from gasoline to household goods such as pesticides and cleaning products.[56] The toxic environment thus produced specific health threats to homeowners and response workers during cleanup, increasing the importance of these individuals properly equipping themselves with reentry health and safety protective equipment.[56]

While the immediate and long-term damages of the Camp Fire were severe and continued to be felt 5 years post-disaster, the nationally accredited BCPH played a significant role in providing crisis communication during the Camp Fire.[57] BCPH's phase-based and CERC-focused messaging was of benefit to all Paradise residents impacted by the many events associated with the Camp Fire.

Timeline of Key 2018 California Camp Fire Events
A timeline of key events in the 2018 California Camp Fire is provided in Table 5.2.

Table 5.2 Camp Fire Key Events Timeline

Date	Events
November 8, 2018	Camp Fire begins in remote stretch of canyon in Butte County, CA CA Governor Newsom declares State of Emergency in Butte County, CA, due to Camp Fire
November 9, 2018	Camp Fire spreads, burns entire town of Paradise, CA Toxic smoke from the Camp Fire begins to spread to Sacramento Valley and into the San Francisco Bay Area First press conference pertaining to the Camp Fire is held BCPH releases initial public statement on negative effects of wildfire smoke and promotes action items for residents via Facebook
November 10, 2018	Highest concentrations of lead detected in air in Chico, CA; lead concentrations reach 50 times average levels Second press conference pertaining to the Camp Fire is held; this is the first press conference in which public health-related information is shared by BCPH's PIO
November 12, 2018	President Trump makes a Federal Disaster Declaration for Camp Fire
November 13, 2018	US Secretary of Health and Human Services declares a Public Health Emergency for the state of California
November 14, 2018	BCPH releases health and action information related to returning to properties where hazardous fire debris remains
November 25, 2018	100% containment of Camp Fire is reached
Month of November 2018	PM levels are increased by more than 300% across California compared to November 2010–2017
December 1, 2018	California Air Resources Board notes substantial decrease in and return to safe level of PM in air
December 21, 2018	BCPH and Paradise Irrigation District await results of water sample testing for contaminants following the Camp Fire
January 18, 2019	California Water Boards issue a public warning not to drink or to cook with untreated surface water in Camp Fire burn areas due to the presence of contaminants in water
March 3, 2019	BCPH issues a water quality do-not-drink advisory for the majority of areas burned by the Camp Fire
August 6, 2019	BCPH issues a revised water quality advisory for residents in Camp Fire burn areas, lifting the do-not-drink advisory for some locations and encouraging individual home testing before resumption of water use

Overview of CERC Principles and Phase-Based Messaging

Effective communications during a public health emergency are necessary to ensure efficient responses are achieved. To meet this need, CDC created the CERC evidence-based framework, which utilizes psychological and communication sciences to develop six principles to assist organizations in communicating needed information to first responders and residents, allowing those on the receiving end of communications to take proactive steps to protect their health.[58] The six CERC principles that should be present in crisis communication responses are: Be First, Be Right, Be Credible, Express Empathy, Promote Action, and Show Respect.[58] Utilization of these six principles may vary based on the present communication phase, which tailors specific information to the current phase-based needs of the media, government, public and private entities, and those impacted by the disaster.[58] The following section will provide an overview of both the CERC principles and phase-based messaging.

CERC Principles

To begin with, *being first* focuses on the provision of information from an established and appointed communicating agency as quickly as possible. As disaster and crisis situations are time-sensitive, agencies should work diligently to be the first to provide incident-specific information.[58]

The incident-specific information that is released quickly must also meet the principle of *being right*. Communicating organizations and personnel should provide accurate, up-to-date information to audiences to help establish an organization's credibility.[58] This principle is achieved through the sharing of information and facts that are known in the moment, acknowledging details that are not known, and explaining what is being done to find missing information.[58]

In conjunction with being right, *being credible* is of the utmost importance when communicating in disaster situations. All communications and associated materials presented should honestly and truthfully convey the data, facts, and circumstances surrounding crisis situations.[58] This not only cements an organization as credible but can also grant a sense of peace to those receiving such accurate, reliable information in the midst of chaos.

While disseminating information, it is important that *empathy be expressed*. Times of crisis are often accompanied by harm and loss. Those communicating on behalf of an organization should be prepared to acknowledge the suffering being experienced by those receiving the communications and address common feelings and general challenges that are present.[58] Doing these things, while also being cognizant of the tone of any such messages, aids in building rapport and trust between a communicating organization and recipients of such information.[58]

As communication messages reach their end, the *promotion of action* should also be included. To help those receiving these messages regain a sense of control over current circumstances during crisis situations, to restore order, and to help calm fears, nerves, and anxiety, meaningful action items should be given to those impacted by disasters.[58] This is especially useful in terms of providing those impacted by crises with a sense of purpose, tasking them with significant items to carry out.

Finally, all communications, regardless of the present disaster or crisis, should embody the *showing of respect* to everyone receiving the message. During times when people feel particularly vulnerable, respectfully communicating through word choice and tone can help build rapport, garner trust, and promote cooperation between communicators and those on the receiving end of such communications.[58] When individuals feel respected, they may be more likely to acknowledge, respect, and follow the communication's warnings and shared information shared, regardless of the current disaster phase.

Phase-Based Messaging
Throughout crisis situations, a disaster event proceeds through different phases as the event changes and progresses; the same is true for crisis communications. Within crisis communications, three key communication phases exist: the initial, maintenance, and resolution or recovery phases of communication messaging.[58] As crisis situations evolve, so too do the "communication efforts and priorities that are to adapt and respond according" to the different needs of first responders, government entities, private and public organizations, the media, and those impacted by crises, resulting in phase-based messaging.[58]

During the initial phase of crisis communication, utilization of all six CERC principles should occur, with a particular focus on expressing empathy, providing accurate information that details risk explanations, promoting action, and establishing an organization's credibility.[58] This phase is often accompanied by sharing ways in which those receiving information can mitigate risk and what can be expected regarding the next steps of a crisis.

Transitioning to the maintenance phase, messaging during this phase is often more detailed, as ongoing risks are explained and background information pertaining to prior instances of similar events are shared.[58] During this phase, risk explanations for different audience segments (e.g., the elderly, those who are immunocompromised) are provided and misinformation or rumors are addressed, further supplemented by accurate, clarifying messaging.[58]

Lastly, resolution messaging serves as the final phase of crisis communication. Risk communications during this phase utilize empathy to motivate people to continue taking action so as to remain vigilant in protecting themselves from the current disaster.[58] This phase also capitalizes on the momentum of the focus placed on emergency preparedness and response and encourages communities to consider responses to future similar events, which may be revised or improved upon following evaluation of the current communication response.[58] In any crisis, utilization of the CERC principles and phase-based messaging can make a significant difference with respect to response and recovery efforts. Such utilization will be analyzed in the following section in terms of communications surrounding the Camp Fire.

Analysis of CERC Principles in Disaster
During the 2018 California Camp Fire, CERC principles were incorporated relatively well into BCPH's crisis communications. The following analysis highlights instances in which CERC principles were utilized fittingly, as well as instances in which such principles were not followed, the implementation of which may have resulted in more effective communication.

Example 1: Be Credible
During the initial phase of crisis communications, the CERC principle of *being credible* was first illustrated on the BCPH Facebook page. On November 9, 2018, details regarding the health effects of wildfire smoke were shared. This post also accurately detailed population groups who might be more sensitive to impacts from wildfire smoke, such as the elderly, children, or women who were pregnant.[59] Correct risk explanations were shared, as were honest action items that area residents could take that had "been proven to be most effective for protecting people from particles in smoke or ash."[59] Albeit a seemingly brief social media message, it provided simple risk explanations, including who was at risk and what were the health risks of the Camp Fire, along with promoting action, both of which are vital components of the initial phase of CERC phase-based crisis messaging.[58]

Example 2: Be Right
Moving on to the maintenance phase of crisis communications during the Camp Fire, the CERC principle of *being right* was apparent via another post to BCPH's Facebook page. Clarifying, accurate information was posted on BCPH's Facebook page on November 16, 2018, to address rumors and unclear facts, a key component of the maintenance-phase messaging.[58,59] The post's accurate information ultimately helped BCPH to establish credibility and reinforce the importance of mask wearing, given the known information about elevated levels of PM and metal contaminants in the air.[59]

Additionally, this post explained that while BCPH did not know how long it would be before the elevated levels of PM would decrease, an explanation regarding scheduled testing at air monitoring stations, with a commitment to provide updates regarding air quality levels, was provided in this Facebook post.[59] As a result, reinforcement of additional, accurate information related to the wearing of N95 masks, including not needing to change such masks every 8 hours and ensuring that they are tight-fitting, further guaranteed community members understood the ongoing risks and actions they could take to reduce related health risks. This is a key component of the maintenance phase of crisis communication.[58,59]

Example 3: Show Respect
The resolution phase of crisis communication during the Camp Fire also adequately followed CERC principles, specifically in relation to the importance of *showing respect*. Evidenced primarily by BCPH's PIO during many Camp Fire press conferences, this individual communicated up-to-date crisis information regarding public health threats with composure and body language that showed respect for the vulnerability of those listening.[58] Cognizant of the health-related threats and losses many had experienced, whether related to difficulty breathing or loss of life, the PIO frequently highlighted various ways in which listeners could receive health-related assistance for conditions stemming from the Camp Fire following the fire's containment.[58] Throughout the Camp Fire crisis communications by BCPH, the PIO was never once blamed others, used derogatory language, or dismissed audience or reporter questions related to health threats, further illustrating the respect shown by BCPH to all impacted by this disaster.

Example 4: Promote Action
In all of the crisis phases analyzed, BCPH can be credited with *promoting action* for area residents during and after the Camp Fire. During a November 13 press conference, BCPH's PIO relayed a variety of action items residents could undertake to further protect themselves from wildfire smoke impacts, as well as ways in which to protect against health threats when returning to burn sites and structures. The PIO encouraged area residents to continue wearing properly fitting N95 masks when outdoors, "utilize bottled drinking water, due to contaminated well water ... and obtain reentry health and safety kits or wear Tyvek suits/long pants, N95 masks, rubber gloves, and helmet protection" when reentering burn areas.[60] Discarding of any remaining food in residences, proper methods for cleaning food storage equipment, and replacing of in-home air filters were also discussed and presented by BCPH's PIO, all in an attempt to help those impacted by the Camp Fire restore some sense of order and control over their lives and so reduce feelings of unease.[58,60] Within each crisis communication phase, ranging from the initial phase to the resolution phase, BCPH frequently promoted actions for residents to take, facilitating effective responses to and recovery from the Camp Fire.[58]

Example 5: Be First
While BCPH utilized four of the six CERC principles well throughout its crisis communications, two CERC principles were not followed well. To begin with, the principle of *being first* was lacking during every phase of BCPH's crisis communications. With an understanding that crises are time-sensitive, quickly communicating information, particularly that related to health and safety, is crucial.[58] Cognizant that it is difficult to be the first to share information at a time when social and digital media are the main channels through which information is disseminated, allowing outside agencies or news media to claim the role of being the first to share such information, BCPH's inability to share pertinent information first is understandable. However, it was not until the second day of the Camp Fire – November 9, 2018 – that BCPH first shared risk information regarding the health threats associated with the impacts of the Camp Fire's smoke.[59] While the dissemination of this risk explanation on the second day of the Camp Fire was beneficial, sharing of health-related information on the day when the Camp Fire began would have provided residents – especially those living within the 20,000 acres that burned over the first 14 hours – with much-needed information, allowing them time to begin to protect themselves from the toxic smoke that would sit over California for days to come.[61] BCPH's delayed sharing of health-related information may have exacerbated the health effects experienced by some of those who were impacted by the Camp Fire.

Example 6: Express Empathy
Finally, *expressing empathy* was a CERC principle that was not followed in BCPH's crisis communication messaging, regardless of the messaging phase. Whether it be via BCPH's Facebook page, internet web page, or live communications from BCPH's PIO during press conferences, the suffering being experienced by thousands of individuals whose homes had burned or whose family members had died was unfortunately not acknowledged in any way.[58] Addressing of people's feelings – even those associated with the uncertainty regarding mask wearing, for example – was not done by BCPH. The building of trust and rapport between those impacted by the Camp Fire and BCPH did not occur in relation to the many challenges area residents faced.[58] Use of simple statements by BCPH – such as "We recognize your fears and concerns associated with the damaging health effects stemming from the Camp Fire" – during press conferences or in social media posts could have been extremely impactful, validating the feelings of those receiving these crisis communication messages, yet such statements were not delivered.

Discussion of Implications
Responding to and communicating during a disaster or crisis of any size and type are challenging yet necessary. BCPH did an adequate job overall of providing area residents, emergency personnel, government agencies, and private and public entities with needed information pertaining to threatening health effects from the 2018 California Camp Fire. Following analysis of the utilization of CERC principles throughout the phase-based messaging cycle, a few implications for those tasked with providing crisis communications in the future are presented.

First, although potentially difficult at a time when digital media is the norm, it is imperative that those providing crisis communications disseminate needed information as quickly as possible. While BCPH was unable to be the first agency to report on health-related impacts stemming from the Camp Fire, provision of information prior to the second day of a disaster should be expected from such agencies and organizations, especially those that have a duty to report and inform constituents of present dangers. Rapid crisis-related messaging from an established practitioner or agency such as BCPH, regardless of the crisis event, is vital to reducing the negative health effects such events may have on many people.

Another lesson learned from BCPH's dissemination of information relates to increasing access to communicated crisis information. Regardless of the speed at which information is released, such information should be made available on a variety of platforms and through various media to reach as broad of an audience as possible. Unfortunately, BCPH mainly utilized its social media channels in this event, making it difficult for those interested in revisiting crisis communications and action items on platforms such as BCPH's web page to find relevant, up-to-date information. While access to and the speed at which information is shared are vital, so too is how such information is presented to those listening.

Following a review of the crisis communication provided by BCPH during and after the Camp Fire, BCPH is encouraged to increase empathy in its future crisis messaging. No empathetic statements were present in any of BCPH's communications, whether spoken or via text. Simple adjustments (e.g., to tone of voice) could have conveyed some empathy to those listening. Instead, information was communicated in a straightforward and matter-of-fact way, which inhibited the building of rapport or trust between BCPH's PIO and those listening. Future crisis communications for any and all practitioners and organizations tasked with communicating crisis information should incorporate empathetic statements, even simple ones, which may take the form of acknowledging the fears and emotions of the audience.[58] Utilization of person-first language and acknowledgment of the challenges being experienced by those impacted by a disaster are likely to result in substantial buy-in and adherence to crisis information, as such an approach would involve being sensitive to the current, lived reality of many.

Finally, crisis communicators should look to BCPH's promotion of action within its crisis communication messaging as a model. BCPH did an excellent job of promoting action for area residents, emergency personnel, and public and private entities throughout the entirety of the response to the Camp Fire. Not only did BCPH's PIO provide action items that residents could follow during each messaging phase, but these actions were also realistic and effective, providing a sense of control to those experiencing immense instability.[58] The action items presented included accurate and credible accompanying information that helped rather than hindered area residents and emergency personnel. Those on the receiving end of BCPH's crisis communications were well-prepared to take micro-level actions that enabled their personal protection following each press conference involving BCPH's PIO. While analyses and revisions to crisis communications following a disaster are important, valuable lessons can be taken from BCPH's communications response to the 2018 Camp Fire and implemented in Butte County and other communications response agencies elsewhere.

Conclusion

Regarded as the deadliest wildfire in Californian history, the 2018 California Camp Fire has served as an invaluable case study pertaining to crisis communications. The Camp Fire incurred damaging health effects to thousands of individuals living and working in the areas burned. Fortunately, BCPH was able to utilize a majority of the CERC principles through a phase-based messaging system to accurately provide needed crisis communications to all impacted by the Camp Fire. Analysis of BCPH's inclusion of CERC principles – or lack thereof – has provided valuable lessons that other crisis communicators and organizations responding to disasters can use to convey pertinent information to area residents. While some aspects of BCPH's crisis communications were flawed, it ultimately played a significant role in mitigating the long-term, damaging health effects that could have severely impacted the lives of those thousands who had already become victims of the Camp Fire.

End-of-Chapter Reflection Questions

1 Identify a recent health emergency in which you successfully used at least five channels to communicate to your audiences, stakeholders, and partners. What channels did you use with each audience, stakeholder, or partner? How do you know that you used those channels successfully?
2 What types of metrics do you use to evaluate communication channels? How do you share these metrics during an emergency? How are these metrics used as inputs into your communication strategy?
3 If you had to identify a stretch goal (i.e., challenging target) for your agency regarding communication channels, what would it be and why? What support would you need to make this stretch goal a reality?
4 Field trip: Relationships are vital before and during health emergencies. Set up an in-person meeting with an emergency management staffer you haven't met yet or haven't seen in a while to discuss the current status of emergency risk communication in your agencies.

References

1 Daft RL, Lengel RH. Organizational Information Requirements, Media Richness, and Structural Design. *Manage Sci* 1986;**32**(5):554–71.
2 Ledford CJW. Changing Channels: A Theory-Based Guide to Selecting Traditional, New, and Social Media in Strategic Social Marketing. *Soc Mar Q* 2012;**18**(3):175–86.
3 CDC. *Crisis and Emergency Risk Communication October 2018*. Atlanta, GA, CDC, 2018.
4 CDC. *Crisis and Emergency Risk Communication October 2014*. Atlanta, GA, CDC, 2014.
5 Health Alert Network (HAN). *Centers for Disease Control and Prevention*. 2022. https://emergency.cdc.gov/han (Accessed April 10, 2024).
6 Epidemic Information Exchange (Epi-X). *Centers for Disease Control and Prevention*. 2018 https://emergency.cdc.gov/epix/index.asp (Accessed April 10, 2024).
7 Evanson AF. Epi-X: A Valueable Resource for Public Health. 2010. www.michigan.gov/-/media/Project/Websites/mdhhs/Folder2/Folder14/Folder1/Folder114/GLBHI2010Evanson.pdf?rev=343c36b5e9a04599b7a12d591d422671 (Accessed April 10, 2024).
8 Schwendinger J, Lahr E, Lynch J, McCollom M, Evanson AF. Use of CDC's Epidemic Information Exchange System as a Disease Surveillance Tool. *Emerg Threats J* 2011;**4**:11108.
9 Merkel MJ, Edwards R, Ness J, Eriksson C, Yoder S, Gilliam S, et al. Statewide Real-Time Tracking of Beds and Ventilators During Coronavirus Disease 2019 and Beyond. *Crit Care Explor* 2020;**2**(6):e0142.
10 About EMResource. *Texas Health and Human Services*. 2024. www.hhs.texas

.gov/providers/long-term-care-providers/long-term-care-provider-resources/regulatory-services-facility-surveyors-liaisons/about-emresource (Accessed April 10, 2024).

11 EMResource. *Indiana Department of Health.* 2024. www.in.gov/health/emergency-preparedness/emresource (Accessed April 10, 2024).

12 EMResource. *Wisconsin Department of Health Services.* n.d. www.dhs.wisconsin.gov/preparedness/systems/emresource.htm (Accessed April 10, 2024).

13 Mehta J, Yates T, Smith P, Henderson D, Winteringham G, Burns A. Rapid Implementation of Microsoft Teams in Response to COVID-19: One Acute Healthcare Organisation's Experience. *BMJ Health Care Inform* 2020;**27**(3):e100209.

14 Gupta R, Naik BN, Ganesh V, Singh A, Soni SL, Puri GD. Evaluation of Utility and Usefulness of Webinars on COVID-19 Management: A Questionnaire-Based Survey. *Ain-Shams J Anesthesiol* 2021;**13**(1):67.

15 Carvalho-Silva D, Garcia L, Morgan SL, Brooksbank C, Dunham I. Ten Simple Rules for Delivering Live Distance Training in Bioinformatics across the Globe Using Webinars. *PLoS Comput Biol* 2018;**14**(11):e1006419.

16 Aagaard J. On the Dynamics of Zoom Fatigue. *Convergence* 2022;**28**(6):1878–91.

17 Riedl R. On the Stress Potential of Videoconferencing: Definition and Root Causes of Zoom Fatigue. *Electron Mark* 2022;**32**(1):153–77.

18 McLuhan M. *Understanding Media.* London, Routledge, 1964.

19 Yap J, Chadhry C, Jha K, Mani S, Mitra S. Are Responses to the Pandemic Inclusive? A Rapid Virtual Audit of COVID-19 Press Briefings in LMICs. *World Dev* 2020;**136**:105122.

20 Allen WL, Bandola-Gill J, Grek S. Next Slide Please: The Politics of Visualization during COVID-19 Press Briefings. *J Eur Policy* 2024;**31**(3):729–55.

21 Writing Effective Talking Points. George Mason University Writing Center. 2014. https://writingcenter.gmu.edu/writing-resources/different-genres/writing-effective-talking-points (Accessed April 10, 2024).

22 Wireless Emergency Alerts (WEA). *Federal Communications Commission.* n.d. www.fcc.gov/consumers/guides/wireless-emergency-alerts-wea (Accessed April 10, 2024).

23 Bean H, Grevstad N, Meyer A, Koutsoukos A. Exploring Whether Wireless Emergency Alerts Can Help Impede the Spread of Covid-19. *J Contig Crisis Manage* 2021;**30**(2):185–203.

24 Granicus. *Digital Experiences for Government.* n.d. https://granicus.com (Accessed April 10, 2024).

25 Boerngen M. Effectiveness of Paperless Communication from the USDA Farm Service Agency. *J ASFMRA* 2019:27–32.

26 Granicus. Kitsay County, Washington. n.d. https://granicus.com/success-stories/kitsap-county-grew-audience-with-communications-during-covid-19 (Accessed April 10, 2024).

27 Public Health Emergency Preparedness and Response Capabilities: National Standards for State, Local, Tribal, and Territorial Public Health. *Centers for Disease Control and Prevention.* 2021. www.cdc.gov/orr/readiness/capabilities/index.htm (Accessed January 11, 2024).

28 Momenipour A, Rojas-Murillo S, Murphy B, Pennathur P, Pennathur A. Usability of State Public Health Department Websites for Communication during a Pandemic: A Heuristic Evaluation. *Int J Ind Ergon* 2021;**86**:103216.

29 ISO. Online Browsing Platform. *International Organization for Standardization.* 2018. www.iso.org/obp/ui/#iso:std:iso:9241:-11:ed-2:v1:en (Accessed April 10, 2024).

30 An S, Jung JJ. A Heuristic Approach on Metadata Recommendation for Search Engine Optimization. *Concurr Comput* 2019;**33**(3):e5407.

31. Burton W. Anchor Text: What Is It & How To Optimize It? 2022. www.searchenginejournal.com/how-to-optimize-anchor-text/466787/#:~:text=Anchor%20text%20is%20%E2%80%9Cexact%20match,a%20page%20about%20SEO%20services.&text=Anchor%20text%20that%20includes%20a,a%20page%20about%20Content%20Marketing (Accessed April 10, 2024).

32. Jimenez AJ, Estevez-Reboredo RM, Santed MA, Ramos V. COVID-19 Symptom-Related Google Searches and Local COVID-19 Incidence in Spain: Correlational Study. *J Med Internet Res* 2020;**22**(12):e23518.

33. Squarespace. Editing page titles. 2023. https://support.squarespace.com/hc/en-us/articles/206544147#toc-change-an-seo-title (Accessed April 10, 2024).

34. Squarespace. Adding alt text to images. 2023. https://support.squarespace.com/hc/en-us/articles/206542357-Adding-alt-text-to-images (Accessed April 10, 2024).

35. Sutton J, Spiro ES, Johnson B, Fitzhugh S, Gibson B, Butts CT. Warning Tweets: Serial Transmission of Messages during the Warning Phase of a Disaster Event. *Inf Commun Soc* 2014;**17**(6):765–87.

36. Gottfried J. Americans' Social Media Use. *Pew Research Center*. 2024. www.pewresearch.org/internet/2024/01/31/americans-social-media-use (Accessed April 10, 2024).

37. Bade G. Lawmakers shift gears on TikTok ban. *Politico*. 2023. www.politico.com/news/2023/10/09/what-happened-to-the-tiktok-ban-00120434 (Accessed April 10, 2024).

38. Bajaj S, Singh P. Analyzing Rise of Social Media: Podcasts During Covid-19 Pandemic. In: Manimekalai K, Poulpunitha S, editors. *Prevalence of Screen Addiction among College Students*. Tamil Nadu, Shanlax Publications, 2022; 134–52.

39. Shearer E, Liedke J, Matsa KE, Lipka M, Jurkowitz M. Podcasts as a Source of News and Information. *Pew Research Center*. 2023. www.pewresearch.org/journalism/2023/04/18/podcasts-as-a-source-of-news-and-information (Accessed April 10, 2024).

40. Rogan J. #1718 Dr. Sanjay Gupta. *The Joe Rogan Experience*. Spotify. 2021.

41. Gupta S. Dr. Sanjay Gupta: Why Joe Rogan and I sat down and talked – for more than 3 hours. *CNN*. 2021. www.cnn.com/2021/10/13/health/sanjay-gupta-joe-rogan-experience/index.html (Accessed April 10, 2024).

42. Almalki M, Azeez F. Health Chatbots for Fighting COVID-19: A Scoping Review. *Acta Inform Med* 2020;**28**(4):241–47.

43. Amiri P, Karahanna E. Chatbot Use Cases in the Covid-19 Public Health Response. *JAMIA Open* 2022;**29**(5):1000–10.

44. Health Bot. *Microsoft*. 2024. https://azure.microsoft.com/en-us/products/bot-services/health-bot (Accessed April 10, 2024).

45. Bitran H, Gabarra J. Delivering information and eliminating bottlenecks with CDC's COVID-19 assessment bot. *Microsoft*. 2020. https://blogs.microsoft.com/blog/2020/03/20/delivering-information-and-eliminating-bottlenecks-with-cdcs-covid-19-assessment-bot (Accessed April 10, 2024).

46. Gonzales R, Chappell B. California's Camp Fire becomes the deadliest wildfire in state history. *NPR*. 2018. www.npr.org/2018/11/13/667315613/californias-camp-fire-becomes-the-deadliest-in-state-history (Accessed April 23, 2023).

47. Brekke D. Report: PG&E knew high-voltage lines posed fire danger, but put off repairs. *KQED*. 2019. www.kqed.org/news/11760156/report-pge-knew-about-extensive-power-line (Accessed March 7, 2023).

48. National Institute of Standards and Technology. New timeline of deadliest California wildfire could guide Lifesaving Research and Action. 2021. www.nist.gov/news-events/news/2021/02/new-timeline-deadliest-california-wildfire-could-guide-lifesaving-research (Accessed March 10, 2023).

49. Economics & Planning Systems, Inc. Industrial Economics Incorporated. Camp Fire Regional Economic Impact Analysis. *3CORE*. 2021. https://3coreedc.org/wp-content/uploads/2021/03/Camp-Fire-Regional-Economic-Impact-Analysis-January-2021.pdf (Accessed March 10, 2023).

50. Hernandez L. Camp Fire, Woolsey fire prompt public health emergency declaration for California. *San Francisco Chronicle*. 2018. www.sfchronicle.com/california-wildfires/article/Camp-Fire-Woolsey-Fire-prompt-public-health-13390425.php (Accessed April 20, 2023).

51. California Air Resources Board. New analysis shows spikes of metal contaminants, including lead, in 2018 Camp Fire wildfire smoke. 2021. ww2.arb.ca.gov/news/new-analysis-shows-spikes-metal-contaminants-including-lead-2018-camp-fire-wildfire-smoke (Accessed April 20, 2023).

52. United States Environmental Protection Agency. Wildfires: How Do They Affect Our Water Supplies? *Environmental Protection Agency*. 2019. www.epa.gov/sciencematters/wildfires-how-do-they-affect-our-water-supplies (Accessed April 23, 2023).

53. Helmer J. Wildfires can spark widespread contamination of public water supplies. NRDC. 2020. www.nrdc.org/stories/wildfires-can-spark-widespread-contamination-public-water-supplies (Accessed April 20, 2023).

54. California Water Boards. Contamination found in streams following Camp Fire. *State of California*. 2019. www.waterboards.ca.gov/press_room/press_releases/2019/pr01182019_campfire_water_contaminants.pdf (Accessed April 20, 2023).

55. Proctor CR, Lee J, Yu D, Shah AD, Whelton AJ. Wildfire Caused Widespread Drinking Water Distribution Network Contamination. *AWWA Water Science*. 2020;2(4):e1183.

56. ABC10. Camp Fire Live Press Conference. *YouTube*. 2018. www.youtube.com/watch (Accessed April 20, 2023).

57. Butte County Public Health. Public health. *Butte County, California*. n.d. www.buttecounty.net/610/Public-Health (Accessed April 20, 2023).

58. Crisis & Emergency Risk Communication. *Centers for Disease Control and Prevention*. 2018. https://emergency.cdc.gov/cerc (Accessed April 20, 2023).

59. Butte County Public Health Facebook. *Facebook*. 2018. www.facebook.com/buttecountypublichealth (Accessed April 20, 2023).

60. KERO ABC News. Watch live: Press conference updating the condition of the camp fire. *YouTube*. 2018. www.youtube.com/watch?v=Pod0SyQ_GVM (Accessed April 20, 2023).

61. Sergent J, Petras G, Gelles K, Bacon J. 3 startling facts about California's Camp Fire. *Gannett Satellite Information Network*. 2018. www.usatoday.com/story/news/2018/11/20/camp-fire-3-startling-facts/2064758002 (Accessed April 20, 2023).

Part II **Communicating during a Health Emergency**

Chapter 6

Initial Messages during a Health Emergency
Addressing Uncertainty and Creating Trust with the Public

Chapter Objectives
- Describe the four components of an initial message.
- Explain how to include empathy in initial messages.
- Describe why it is important to address uncertainty during the early stages of an emergency.
- Identify initial messages by analyzing a real-world example.
- Be able to write communication objectives, identify audiences, develop key messages, identify channels, and identify communication products that are needed for initial messaging.
- Identify key tips for spokespeople, partner agencies, and call centers during the initial phase of a health emergency.
- Recall uncertainty reduction theory.

Overview of Phase-Based Messaging

As discussed in Chapter 1, development of emergency risk communication needs to consider the phase of the health emergency. Phase-based messaging comes from disaster sociology research on the distinct phases of an emergency and can be coupled with emergency risk communication messaging to understand what types of information audience members need during each phase of a health emergency.[1,2,3] Information needs will change, just like the emergency itself will change over time.

When a health emergency is first unfolding, this is the initial phase of the health emergency, and a health agency will want to move quickly to establish itself as a credible source of information and address uncertainty about the evolving health emergency.[4] If the health emergency has been going on for some time (e.g., in a foodborne illness outbreak) but now the outbreak has become larger and involves multiple counties or states, the health emergency is in what is known as the "maintenance phase."[4] In this phase, more information is known about the health emergency and about the virus or disease that is causing the health emergency. Messaging during the maintenance phase of a health emergency is different from messaging during the very beginning of a health emergency. And finally, when the health threat has been mitigated and the health emergency moves into the recovery phase, the communication messages again are different from the messages used in the initial or the maintenance phase.[4] This chapter and the following two chapters break down phase-based messaging into initial, maintenance, and recovery messaging and will look at the types of messages in each phase and how to write these messages with specific message characteristics that will resonate with audience members during each emergency phase.

Initial Messages: What They Are and How to Write Them

The initial phase of a health emergency is when some trigger event or catalyst has occurred that impacts public health.[4,5] Having responded to numerous health emergencies at the federal, state, and local level, I can confirm that the initial phase is short, typically only taking up the first 24–48 hours of the emergency, but it can last up to 1 week.[1,4] During these early hours of a health emergency, it is critical for the health agency to establish its authority and credibility as a responding agency, address uncertainty about the situation, promote actions people can take to protect their health, and offer empathetic communication.

During Hurricane Katrina, the US Centers for Disease Control and Prevention (CDC) used phase-based messaging to communicate health information during the initial, maintenance, and recovery phases of the hurricane.[1] Although natural disasters such as hurricanes, flooding, tornadoes, earthquakes, and wildfires are managed by emergency management agencies, there are often health impacts from these natural disasters. Communicating about health impacts during natural disasters should be based on the health expertise of public health officials and coordinated by the emergency management agency leading response efforts. In the initial phase CDC focused messaging on food and water safety, and in the maintenance and recovery phases it focused on injury prevention when reentering a home, carbon monoxide poisoning prevention, and mold cleanup.[1]

Initial Message Components

There are four key components of an initial message that will enable you to manage expectations, establish credibility, establish trust, and give people something to do to protect their health.[4] These initial message components are[4]:

- Addressing uncertainty
- Making a commitment
- Providing messages of self-efficacy
- Expressing empathy

The following subsections break down each of these message components and provide examples.

Address Uncertainty during the Early Stages of the Emergency

There are three message components that address uncertainty in an initial message:
- Explain what you know.
- Explain what you don't know.
- Explain what your agency is doing to find new information.

Addressing uncertainty will build and maintain trust and credibility with audiences and stakeholders by providing these key messages with openness and transparency.[6] Further, as the health agency addresses uncertainty, it is also managing expectations of the audiences by providing the information that the agency has about the health threat, by explaining what health information it does not have, and by stating that the health agency has a plan to find new information about the evolving health threat.

Addressing uncertainty will avoid the provision of overly reassuring statements that often backfire as new information emerges about the crisis.[7,8] An agency's credibility and the public's trust in that agency would be damaged if it was to say, in the immediate hours after a novel infectious disease outbreak is unfolding, "Not to worry. We've got this under control," but then, as more information is gathered about the novel infectious disease outbreak, the agency has to row back on these public words.

Let's break down these core message components.

What You Know

This message component looks at two key areas of what the health agency knows about the health threat: the risk or potential risk of the health threat and what people can do to protect their health. Even with novel infectious disease outbreaks, medical doctors and epidemiologists will have general information about the disease – for example, whether it is a respiratory or gastrointestinal illness. Depending on the general category of the virus or bug, medical subject matter experts can provide a general symptom profile and nonpharmaceutical actions people can take to protect their health, such as handwashing, physical distancing, and wearing a mask, among others.

Regarding risk explanations, there are key audiences – at-risk populations – that need to be addressed early during a crisis. Again, even if the outbreak is that of a novel infectious disease, medical subject matter experts know that people with underlying chronic health conditions, older adults, pregnant women, and children are generally at-risk populations. Regardless of the unfolding outbreak, groups will need to know if they are more at risk than others. If there are very limited data about who is at risk, focus on geographic area to help people understand if there is a risk in their community.

What You Don't Know

When the health agency states there are things it does not know, this represents a core function of accepting uncertainty about the current health crisis.[6] This is often one of the most difficult aspects of initial messages for leaders to convey during media briefings. Medical experts also tend toward waiting until more information is available before sharing information with the public and other key audiences. In the era of digital media, communicating early and often is key to establishing credibility and trust with a health department's audiences.

If the health department does not yet know the symptom profile or who is most at risk, explain this information to the public and other audiences. If this is a new virus, state that this is the case and offer comparisons to how this virus might be similar to other known viruses. Also state that the health department is waiting for new data to emerge in order to learn more.

As counterintuitive as it may seem, explaining what the health agency does not know will pay off in the long run during a crisis because doing so supports openness and transparency regarding the information that the health department has related to the health emergency.

What Your Agency Is Doing to Find New Information

The final aspect of addressing uncertainty is to inform the audience what the health agency is doing to find new information. Public health investigations and laboratory testing are agency activities that no one ever talked about prior to the COVID-19 pandemic. Now "contact tracing" and "confirmatory testing" are mainstream phrases.

In the initial phase of an emergency, explain what the health agency is doing to find information that the health department currently does not have. For example, perhaps the health agency is waiting on test results from a state laboratory, or the health agency might be monitoring the World Health Organization's (WHO) response might be in contact with multiple county health directors. It is vital to state the actions that the health agency is taking to address the crisis.

Example of Addressing Uncertainty Using These Three Message Components
- What we know: This is a novel virus. What we know today will likely change over time as we gather more information.
- What we don't know: We do not yet know who is most at risk, but we encourage people to monitor themselves for symptoms of a fever and to engage in frequent handwashing to avoid any potential spread.
- What the health department is doing to find new information: The health department is engaging in contact tracing and has sent laboratory samples to CDC for confirmatory testing.

Make a Commitment

Another component of an initial message is to make a commitment to those affected by the health emergency. Commitment statements have two parts. First, explain what the agency is doing to find new information about the emerging health crisis. This type of statement informs the audience that the agency has the responsibility for addressing this health threat and is taking action to manage and stop it. Providing this type of statement helps establish credibility in and the authority of the agency during a health response. The second part of a commitment message is letting the community know that the health agency will be there until the end of the health emergency. During the initial days and weeks of a health emergency, the agency can give a lot attention and resources to the response; however, over time, the agency's focus and amount of attention may change due to competing priorities. By establishing the health agency's commitment to ending the emergency, the agency can build and maintain trust with the community affected by the health emergency.

Message Example
- We are engaging in contact tracing. Contact tracing teams are talking to all people who are sick and identifying who they have come into contact with. This helps us find additional people who are ill and can help us build a symptom profile to better understand the virus.
- The health department is committed to finding the source of this outbreak and providing the necessary health interventions to protect the health of this community.

Self-Efficacy Statements

Another component of initial messages is a self-efficacy or self-protective health message. Essentially, these messages promote actions that those affected by the health emergency can take to protect their health. The term "self-efficacy" comes from research literature focused on one's personal efficacy or ability or capacity to carry out a particular action.[9,10] The term is used in emergency risk communication under the assumption that people have a level of efficacy or capacity to carry out simple actions to protect their health. Further, providing people with something to do during an emergency reduces anxiety.[11,12]

Message Example
- We do not yet know who is most at risk, but we encourage people to monitor themselves for symptoms of a fever and to engage in frequent handwashing to avoid any potential spread.
- Contact your health care provider immediately if you have a fever for more than 24 hours.

Empathy in Initial Messages

After COVID-19, there has been an emergence of research and interest in empathetic and compassionate communication during health emergencies and in how empathy might impact what self-protective measures people take.[13–19] In addition to empathy, the framework of mindfulness – nonjudgmental awareness – can also inform initial crisis messages (see Chapter 9).[20]

What Is Empathy?

Emotionally mature individuals are likely to be more empathetic, meaning they are more in touch with their own deep feelings and can imagine, or mentalize, the feelings of others.[21] For leaders and spokespeople engaging in emergency risk communication, being able to understand or at least imagine the feelings of others is critical during an emergency response. Further, empathetic individuals can deliver more authentic messages that resonate deeply with an audience. Psychologist Paul Ekman talked about empathy with the Dalai Lama, differentiating between different types of empathy and compassion. They argue that empathy isn't just knowing what the other feels, but also having the ability to feel with them.[22] Psychologist Daniel Goleman elucidates this further, offering that empathy can take on three different forms: cognitive, emotional, and compassionate[21]:

- *Cognitive:* Simply knowing how the other person feels and what they might be thinking.
- *Emotional:* When you feel physically along with the other person, as if their emotions were contagious.
- *Compassionate:* We not only understand a person's predicament and feel with them, but are spontaneously moved to help, if needed.

For emergency risk communication, emotional and compassionate empathy is most needed during press briefings and public speeches during a health emergency.

The following example of empathy is from the Governor of North Dakota, who delivered an emotional and compassionate empathetic message during COVID-19:

> In our state there are no requirements regarding masks, we're all in this together and there's only one battle we're fighting and that's the battle of the virus. I would really love to see in North Dakota that we could just skip this thing that other parts of the nation are going through where they're creating a divide – either it's ideological or political or something around mask versus no mask. This I would say is a senseless dividing line and I would ask people to try to dial up your empathy and your understanding.

If someone is wearing a mask they're not doing it to represent what political party, what candidates they support, they might be doing it because they've got a 5-year-old child who's been going through cancer treatments [pauses, speaking becomes more difficult due to emotional response], they might have [pauses, speaking becomes more difficult due to emotional response; tone of voice changes] vulnerable adults in their life who are currently of COVID and they're fighting. And so again I would just move to see our state is part of being North Dakota smart, also be North Dakota nice, North Dakota empathetic, North Dakota understanding to do this thing.

Because if somebody wants to wear a mask there should be no mask shaming. They should – you should look at them and say that person's wearing a mask because for them there's additional risk in their life. The first thing that somebody ought to assume is that they're doing it because they've got people in their life that they love and that they're trying to take care of and I think let's just start there.[23]

Mini-Case Study: Richard Besser and H1N1 Initial Crisis Message

When reading the following message, look for the four components of an initial message highlighted earlier. Write down examples of each.

> Our hearts go out to the people in Mexico and the people in the United States who've been impacted by this outbreak. People around the country and around the globe are concerned with the situation we're seeing and we're concerned as well. As we look for cases of swine flu we are seeing more cases of swine flu. We expect to see more cases of swine flu. We're responding and we're responding aggressively to try and learn more about this outbreak and to implement measures to control this outbreak. Let me provide for you an update in terms of where we are today and what kinds of public health actions are being taken here as well as abroad.
>
> Today we can confirm that there are 20 cases of swine flu in the United States. We have five affected states. There are eight cases confirmed in New York City. There's one case confirmed in Ohio; two in Kansas; two in Texas; and seven in California. And again as we continue to look for cases I expect that we're going to find them. We've ramped up our surveillance around the country to try and understand better what is the scope, what is the magnitude of this outbreak.
>
> The good news is all of the individuals in this country who have been identified as cases have recovered, only one individual had to be hospitalized; but I expect as we continue to look for cases we are going to see a broader spectrum of disease, and what we know about this virus is it looks to be the same virus as is causing the situation in Mexico, and given the reports out of Mexico I would expect that over time we're going to see more severe disease in this country.
>
> There's some things that it's important people understand. Flu viruses are extremely unpredictable, and variable outbreaks of infectious diseases are extremely unpredictable and variable, and so over time what we say about this and what we learn will change.
>
> Expect changes in terms of the number of cases. We're going to try and give you consistent information and have it on our website once a day so that we don't get into the situation where you're hearing different numbers of cases throughout the day. We're going to report that daily.
>
> We expect that we're going to be changing our recommendations over time based on what we learned and that's an important thing. You'll start to see different activities taking place in different parts of the country depending on the local outbreak picture and that's good.

You want people to respond based on what the situation is in their community, based on what situations are in particular countries. Because of the speed at which things are progressing, you will at times find inconsistent information, and we're going to work really hard to make sure that that doesn't stay up for long, but as we're updating recommendations and they're going out through various sources you may find some inconsistency. And we will work to minimize that.

This is moving fast, but I want you to understand that we view this more as a marathon. We do think that this will continue to spread, but we are taking aggressive actions to minimize the impact on people's health. It's important that people understand that there is a role for everyone to play when there's an outbreak going on.

There are things that individuals do, there are things that families do, communities do, to try and reduce the impact at the individual level. It's important people understand how they can prevent respiratory infections with very frequent handwashing.[24]

Quick Response Communication Planning: Identify Communication Objectives, Audiences, Key Messages, and Channels and Develop Communication Products/Materials

When engaging in emergency risk communication, it is always important to think through your communication strategy and ensure your agency has a plan to specifically address the health emergency. It is also important to identify a communication objective, key audiences, key messages, and channels to disseminate the information and develop any communication products that need to be released. This information will be used to draw up the crisis and emergency risk strategy, and it will inform the communication plan for the health emergency response.

In this chapter and Chapters 7 and 9, quick response communication planning will be included to deepen learning regarding the development of initial, maintenance, and recovery messages. The same examples will be used in each chapter so the reader can compare and contrast how quick response planning and key messages change throughout the life cycle of a crisis.

Communication Objectives

A communication objective is a measurable, time-bound, and audience-focused action.[25] Often communication strategies and objectives are designed to create awareness, educate, or persuade the audience.[25]

Example 1

Measles: The county health department will communicate with school district officials and affected individuals to increase awareness about a suspected measles outbreak over the next 3 days.

Example 2

Foodborne illness: The county health department will work with local fair organizers, ill individuals, and food truck vendors to identify the source of a suspected foodborne illness outbreak over the next 3 days.

Example 3
Unknown novel infection: The county health department will alert the media to share the latest information about an emerging infectious disease over the next 24 hours.

Audiences

As outlined in Chapters 3 and 4, identify your audiences and audience segments and their information needs. Understanding *which* audience needs *what* type of information will help you to organize and strategize on key messaging. Using the audience segment variables outlined in Chapter 3, the following examples develop audience segments that will receive emergency risk communication messages during the initial phase of an emergency.

Example 1 Measles
Audiences include schoolchildren and their parents, adults who have not received the measles, mumps, and rubella (MMR) immunization, school districts officials, and health care providers. See Table 6.1 for audience segments for this example.

Table 6.1 Audience segments by risk variable for a measles outbreak

Variable	Definition	Audience segment
Risk level	Who is most at risk based on current health threat?	Schoolchildren (plus parents as children are minors) Adults who have not received the MMR immunization
Location or proximity	Who is closest to the risk or health threat?	Schoolchildren by vaccination status (plus parents as children are minors)
Employment	Is there a particular industry that is affected by the health crisis?	School district officials and health care providers

Example 2 Foodborne illness
Audiences include but are not limited to fair attendees, fair organizers, food vendors, and health care providers. See Table 6.2 for audience segments for this example.

Table 6.2 Audience segments by risk variable for a foodborne illness outbreak

Variable	Definition	Audience segment
Risk level	Who is most at risk based on current health threat?	Fair attendees who ate at food carts
Employment	Is there a particular industry that is affected by the health crisis?	Fair organizers Food vendors Health care providers

Example 3 Unknown novel infection
Audiences include but are not limited to individuals who live in a particular county and who have underlying health conditions. See Table 6.3 for audience segments for this example.

Table 6.3 Audience segment by risk variable for an unknown novel infection

Variable	Definition	Audience segment
Risk level	Who is most at risk based on current health threat?	Individuals who live in a particular county
Location or proximity	Who is closest to the risk or health threat?	Individuals who live in a particular county
Health condition	Who has current health conditions that may be at a heightened risk (e.g., age, underlying medical conditions, pregnant)?	Individuals who live in a particular county and who have specific underlying medical conditions
Employment	Is there a particular industry that is affected by the health crisis?	Health care providers

Key Messages

Communication objectives will guide emergency risk communicators about the audience and the information that the health agency will provide. Key messages are the specific messages that the agency wants to communicate that are aligned with the communication objectives. For example, if the communication objective is creating awareness about an infectious disease, there are specific key messages that need to be created. During the initial phase of the emergency, the key messages will need to address uncertainty, make a commitment to those affected by the health emergency, provide messages of self-efficacy, and express empathy. For emergency risk communicators, key messages are grounded in Crisis and Emergency Risk Communication (CERC) principles and initial message components. The following examples provide high-level key messages that emergency risk communicators might use to guide the development of talking points, web page copy, and social media messages.

Example 1 Measles

Key Message 1: Express empathy and make a commitment.

- It can be unnerving when our little ones are ill or when our friends' children are ill. Dealing with a measles outbreak can test even our most patient parents.
- Here at the county health department, we want you to know we hear the fear and frustration from you about this outbreak and we are working with you, the school district, and our local hospitals to quickly resolve this situation and get our little ones on the road to good health.

Key Message 2: Address uncertainty.

- I'd like to share what we know, what we don't know, and what we are doing to learn more about this measles outbreak.
- The county health department has been working with local school districts since Tuesday when the first case was diagnosed.
- The case is an unvaccinated young child, and we encourage everyone to respect the privacy of this child and their family.

- Through contact tracing, we are identifying those who have been exposed to the ill individual, and we will continue to engage in contact tracing over the next 2 days.
- We do not yet know how big this outbreak could get, so I'd like to share with you what people can do to protect their health.

Key Message 3: Provide a self-efficacy message.

- Measles is a serious, potentially life-threatening disease that can make people very ill, especially young children. Children with measles usually start with a fever, cough, runny nose, and red eyes. This is often followed by a rash inside the child's mouth, followed a few days later by flat round spots on the face and hairline that spread down the trunk. Complications include pneumonia, encephalitis, miscarriage, preterm birth, hospitalization, and death.[26]
- Per CDC's vaccine schedule, in general all children should receive the first MMR dose by 12–15 months of age and the second dose between 4 and 6 years.[26]
- Those who aren't sure about their immunization status should call their local health department or health care provider. Those who were born before 1957 have likely already been exposed to the virus and are immune. Those born between 1957 and 1971 should check with a doctor to ensure they've been properly immunized as vaccines administered during that time may not have been reliable.[26]

Example 2 Foodborne illness

Key Message 1: Express empathy and make a commitment.

- So many of us come out to the local county fair each year to visit the exhibits and support our community. It is unfortunate when such a fun and carefree event can turn into a very unpleasant experience. The county health department is working quickly with the fair organizers and food vendors to identify the source of what is making so many people ill.

Key Message 2: Address uncertainty.

- I'd like to share what we know, what we don't know, and what we are doing to learn more about this outbreak.
- The county health department has been working with the fair organizers, food vendors, and health care providers to look at the symptom profile and identify the source of the outbreak.
- We do not yet know the particular food or virus that is causing the illness. Specimens are being collected, and once the test results return, we will make those available.

Key Message 3: Provide a self-efficacy message.

- We'd like to encourage people who ate at the county fair to monitor for symptoms including:
  - Diarrhea, which may be bloody
  - Nausea
  - Abdominal pain
  - Vomiting
  - Dehydration
  - Low-grade fever (sometimes)[27]

- Please contact the county health department at 123-567-8899 to report your symptoms and to provide additional information to our contact tracers.
- Seek emergency medical assistance if you have severe symptoms such as severe abdominal pain or watery diarrhea that turns very bloody within 24 hours.[27]

Example 3 Unknown novel infection

Key Message 1: Address uncertainty.

- I'd like to share what we know, what we don't know, and what we are doing to learn more about this emerging outbreak.
- Here's what we know: An emerging virus has been found in our state, and it looks to be related to the emerging virus of avian influenza that is going on in the eastern part of the United States. About 50 people in County Black have become ill with the virus, and 10 of them are currently in the intensive care unit receiving treatment.
- Here's what we don't know: We do not yet know if it is the avian influenza virus that is causing the illness. Specimens are being collected, and once the test results return, we will make those available.

Key Message 2: Express empathy and make a commitment.

- We all remember the devastating effects of COVID-19, and it feels unfair for our county to be impacted by yet another major health emergency. Since 2023, the county health department has been working diligently to improve our syndromic surveillance systems, improve our internal emergency protocols, and improve our risk communication messaging so that if we have another novel health threat, we are ready to respond. The county health department is ready to respond, and we are working with the state health department to monitor the situation. We will be here to support our community through this outbreak whether it is a short or long emergency response.

Key Message 3: Provide a self-efficacy message.

- As we gather more information about the virus, there are things everyone can do to protect their personal health and those in their community:
  - Frequent handwashing or use of hand sanitizer.
  - Wear a mask in public and in indoor spaces where physical distancing is different.
  - Please monitor county.health.gov for the latest updates.

Channels

As outlined in Chapter 5, think about what channels are available to you for sharing information and what audiences use which channels.

Example 1 Measles

Consider which channels are available and what would be the best way to communicate health information to reach the audiences segments that have been identified. See Table 6.4 for channel identification for this example.

Table 6.4 Communication channels for each audience segment during a measles outbreak

Audience	Communication channel
Schoolchildren (plus parents as children are minors) Adults who have not received the MMR immunization	Email to parents Email to school workers School website Health department website Media relations Health department social media channels
Schoolchildren by vaccination status (plus parents as children are minors)	Email to parents
School district officials and health care providers	Conference calls or virtual meetings with school officials Health Alert Network message for clinicians

Example 2 Foodborne illness

Consider which channels are available and what would be the best way to communicate health information to reach the audiences segments that have been identified. See Table 6.5 for channel identification for this example.

Table 6.5 Communication channels for each audience segment for a foodborne illness outbreak

Audience segment	Communication channel
Fair attendees who ate at food carts	Media relations Fair social media channels
Fair organizers Food cart vendors Health care providers	Face-to-face meetings Emails Health Alert Network message for clinicians

Example 3 Unknown novel infection

Consider which channels are available and what would be the best way to communicate health information to reach the audiences segments that have been identified. See Table 6.6 for channel identification for this example.

Table 6.6 Communication channels for each audience segment for an unknown novel infection

Audience segment	Communication channel
Individuals who live in a particular county	Media relations Health agency website Health agency social media channels
Individuals who live in a particular county and who have specific underlying medical conditions	Media relations Health department website Health department social media channels
Health care providers	Health Alert Network message

Communication Products

As outlined in Chapter 5, think through what communication materials need to be developed based on channel selection.

Example 1 Measles

Table 6.7 outlines the types of communication products that would need to be created for each communication channel.

Table 6.7 Communication products that can be sent on communication channels for a measles outbreak

Communication channel	Communication product
Email to parents Email to school workers School website Health department website Health department social media channels Media Relations	Letter and email copy about outbreak Web page copy Social media messages (including visuals, hashtags, and web URLs for more information Talking points
Email to parents Conference calls or virtual meetings with school officials Health Alert Network message for clinicians	Letter and email copy about outbreak Talking points Health Alert Network message copy

Example 2 Foodborne illness

Table 6.8 outlines the types of communication products that would need to be created for each communication channel.

Table 6.8 Communication products that can be sent on communication channels for a foodborne illness outbreak

Communication channel	Communication product
Media relations Fair social media channels	Talking points Social media messages (include visuals, hashtags, and web URLs for more information)
Face-to-face meetings Emails Health Alert Network message for clinicians	Talking points Email copy Health Alert Network message copy

Example 3 Unknown novel infection

Table 6.9 outlines the types of communication products that would need to be created for each communication channel.

Table 6.9 Communication products that can be sent on communication channels for an unknown novel infection

Communication channel	Communication product
Media relations Health department website Health department social media channels	Talking points Web page copy Social media messages (include visuals, hashtags, and web URLs for more information)

Table 6.9 (cont.)

Communication channel	Communication product
Media relations Health department website Health department social media channels	Talking points Web page copy Social media messages (include visuals, hashtags, and web URLs for more information)
Media relations Health department website Health department social media channels	Talking points Web page copy Social media messages (include visuals, hashtags, and web URLs for more information)
Health Alert Network message	Health Alert Network message copy

Key Tips for Spokespeople, Partners Agencies, and Call Centers

During every phase of a health emergency, spokespeople, partner agencies, and call centers need to receive consistent and coordinated information from the health agency. Here are some key tips for those who are spokespeople or who work at partner agencies or call centers:

Spokespeople: As a spokesperson, educate yourself about the agency's communication policies and ensure you have a working relationship with your emergency risk communication agency. Get a briefing from lead subject matter expert or incident management team to gain situational awareness regarding the health emergency. Reach out to other leaders within your agency and in partner agencies to discuss health emergencies and engage in active listening. Engage in mock presentations and practice talking points before your first media briefing.

Partner agencies: Identify key points of contact for the health emergency, including the incident manager, public information officer, chief medical officer, and other key roles according to the Incident Command Structure. Ensure you have received directions on meeting frequency and have received meeting information and been given access to any shared project management systems.

Call centers: Ensure there is a working relationship between the public information officer and crisis communication team, that the call center is able to receive key information to create prepared responses, and that the call center is able to provide key metrics to the health agency to inform the communication strategy.

Theory Callout: Uncertainty Reduction Theory

Interpersonal researchers Berger and Calabrese developed uncertainty reduction theory to understand how people reduce uncertainty about each other when meeting for the first time.[28] Uncertainty can also occur in intimate relationships when people break their partner's trust or violate a set boundary, or when engaging with people from a culture that is different from one's own. Uncertainty reduction theory offers eight axioms or propositions of what occurs in uncertainty reduction[28]:

1. As verbal communication increases, uncertainty decreases.
2. Increases in nonverbal expression cause decreases in uncertainty. As uncertainty decreases, nonverbal expressions increase.
3. Information-seeking behavior increases with increased uncertainty and decreases with decreased uncertainty.
4. Intimacy of communication increases as uncertainty decreases.
5. High levels of uncertainty produce high levels of reciprocity.
6. Personal similarities reduce uncertainty.
7. Liking decreases when uncertainty increases, and it increases as uncertainty decreases.
8. Having shared networks/mutual friends decreases uncertainty.

While this theory was established for interpersonal communication, emergency risk communicators can use the theory to understand how an audience might seek out and process information from a health agency during the initial phases of a health emergency. Further, the principles of the theory suggest that when a health agency communicates early and often about a health threat, the uncertainty of an audience is likely to decrease as it receives such health information.

Analysis of the CERC Framework during the Flint Water Crisis
Mae M. Brooks, MPH

Overview of the Crisis
Flint, Michigan, formerly known as "Vehicle City," is in Genesee County and sits in eastern Michigan, comprising approximately 80,000 residents. Established in 1819, Flint quickly rose to glory when it became the home of Durant-Dort Carriage Company, a manufacturer of horse-drawn vehicles, and then General Motors, an automotive manufacturer.[29] The glory days of the 1960s were short-lived, however; as quickly as the city thrived, it then began to decline just as fast in the 1980s, with factories closing, thousands losing their jobs, rising crime rates, and increasing poverty.[29] A public health crisis would be the worst possible situation for a struggling city already in economic duress; however, in 2014, the Flint Water Crisis began.

In April 2014, as a cost-saving measure, Flint changed its water supply from the Detroit Water and Sewage Department to the Flint River as a temporary measure until a new water pipeline could be developed.[29] The river water was already considered corrosive, but corrosion control agents were not used to treat the water before public use.[30] Subsequently, aging pipes throughout homes, businesses, and schools began to corrode, releasing lead into the water. The Flint Water Crisis began in May 2014, immediately after the water supply switched and appropriate efforts were not implemented to provide clean water to the public. However, actions to rectify the problem did not begin until 2015. For approximately 15 months, the citizens of Flint complained, pleading for a solution to their water that tasted, smelled, and looked different.[29]

Throughout those months, *E. coli* and total coliform bacteria, trihalomethanes (THMs), and high lead levels were detected in the water.[29] Exposure to lead was the primary health concern, as lead is a toxin that can cause various effects such as developmental delays, learning difficulties, weight loss, high blood pressure, memory problems, reduced sperm count, and risk of miscarriage/stillbirth.[31] In addition, health problems such as Legionnaires' disease began to rise. Legionnaires' disease is a respiratory illness that can appear similar to pneumonia, with symptoms of headaches, muscle aches, shortness of breath, and chest pain.[32] In December 2015, months after the crisis began, the newly elected mayor, Karen Weaver, declared a state of emergency.[30] In the following months, the governor, Rick Synder, and President Barack Obama declared a state of emergency.[30]

Many federal, state, and local agencies such as the Michigan Department of Environmental Quality (MDEQ), the Michigan Department of Health and Human Services (MDHHS), the Genesee County Health Department (GCHD), the US Environmental Protection Agency (EPA), and CDC played a role in the response; however, this analysis will only address the communication and crisis responses from MDHSS to the public.[33] The primary goal of MDHHS is to address public health concerns for the entire state, providing effective communication with the public and active collaboration with federal, state, and local partners.[34] As it is a leading public health agency in Michigan, we want to examine the response and communication of MDHHS using the evidence-based framework of CERC principles throughout the Flint Water Crisis.

Timeline of Key Crisis Events
- On April 25, 2014, Flint officials switched the water supply from the Detroit Water and Sewerage Department to the Flint River.
- In May 2014, immediately after the switch, Flint residents complained about the water's taste, smell, and color.
- Over the following months, *E. coli*, coliform bacteria, THMs, and lead were detected in the water, and boil water advisories were issued in the city.
- In October 2014, MDHHS was made aware of a rise in cases of Legionnaires' disease by the local health department.
- In May 2015, MDHHS noted in a surveillance report that the Legionnaires' disease outbreak was over.
- In July 2015, MDHHS noted high lead levels in the water; however, this was deemed "seasonal but not related to the water supply."
- In August 2015, a Virginia Tech team of researchers and students determined that corrosive water from the Flint River was causing pipes to leak lead into the water.
- In September 2015, clinician and researcher Dr. Mona Hanna-Attisha, at Hurley Medical Center, released data from her research study indicating high lead levels in children's blood due to this water.
- On September 29, 2015, the local health department issued a health advisory not to drink the water. A few days later, MDHHS declared an emergency. Soon after, President Barack Obama issued a state of emergency.
- On October 16, 2015, Flint switched its water supply back to the Detroit Water and Sewerage Department as the city's drinking water source.
- During 2016–2018, lawsuits were filed against various agencies and indictments were issued to several employees, including four MDHHS employees.

Overview of CERC Principles and Phase-Based Messaging
CDC developed the CERC framework to facilitate efficient and effective communication with the public during an emergency.[35] The framework includes six core principles: Be First, Be Right, Be Credible, Express Empathy, Promote Action, and Show Respect. The CERC principles emphasize effective communication in providing timely, honest, relatable, and

respectful messages to the public.[35] *Be First* is the first principle, and it outlines the importance of being the first source to provide information on emergencies in a time-sensitive manner.[35] The second principle of *Be Right* requires the provision of accurate and credible information, which lead to the subsequent principle of *Be Credible*.[35] Credibility is essential during a crisis, as communicators must establish openness and trust with the public.[35] *Empress Empathy* is the next principle, emphasizing the importance of understanding the public's challenges and showing genuine compassion.[35] *Promote Action* is essential in terms of providing the public with ways to be engaged while staying safe and contributing to the response.[35] Lastly, *Show Respect* is an accumulation of all the previous principles, as when communicators provide prompt, accurate, genuine, compassionate, and cooperative messaging, this yields the principle of *Show Respect*.[35]

In every crisis, there are four phases. The CERC manual defines the phases as Precrisis, Initial, Maintenance, and Resolution.[36] In each phase, different CERC principles can be applied, along with additional messages, components, and concepts that the spokesperson or risk communicator should emphasize.[35] As the crisis evolves, the messaging also changes, and applicable CERC principles can be used to tailor correspondence to the community and different audience segments within it.[29]

Analysis of CERC Principles during the Crisis

Be First

On MDHHS's website, within the "News" tab, the first mention of lead exposure was posted on October 5, 2015. (MDHHS's YouTube channel and X account [formerly Twitter] over the past 10 years were also reviewed, and this posting was identified as the first such news release to be archived and made publicly available. Other released information may have been removed or not have been archived.)

The following are excerpts from the first press release:

Free water filters will be available to current Michigan Department of Health and Human Services clients and Flint residents at four locations beginning Tuesday, October 6, at 9 a.m. through a partnership between the MDHHS and the Genesee County Community Action Resource Department. Free National Sanitation Foundation certified water filters are being provided to Flint residents as part of the administration's comprehensive approach to addressing water concerns in the area.[37]

Although blood lead levels throughout the city of Flint have remained steady, last week, MDHHS data was found to be consistent with a recent Hurley Children's Hospital study indicating increased blood lead levels in children residing in two Flint ZIP codes after a 2014 change in water source. While lead paint remains the number one cause of lead poisoning in Michigan, the recent data prompted MDHHS to take action to reduce potential lead exposures through water sources.[37]

MDHHS is urging parents in Flint and throughout the state to do their part in preventing elevated blood lead levels in children. For more information about steps you can take now, visit www.michigan.gov/lead, or contact your local health department. For updates on Flint water and available resources, visit www.michigan.gov/flintwater.[37]

Although this was the first news release we can identify on MDHHS's website and other social media channels, it does not sufficiently meet the CERC principle of Be First. The messaging states:

Although blood lead levels throughout the city of Flint have remained steady, last week, MDHHS data was found to be consistent with a recent Hurley Children's Hospital study indicating increased blood lead levels in children residing in two Flint ZIP codes after a 2014 change in water source.[37]

This message is referring to a separate press conference conducted on Thursday, September 24, 2015, by Dr. Mona Hanna-Attisha, an independent researcher and clinician at Hurley Medical Center, in which she released data indicating the increase in blood lead levels in children since the change in water supply in 2014.[33] In the message, MDHHS stated that "last week" it had found Hurley study's data to be consistent with the state's data regarding lead levels; however, it stated that prior to this point, these data had not aligned.[37] MDHHS was not the first source to release information regarding the elevated lead levels of water in people's homes; Dr. Hanna-Attisha was. A week after Dr. Hanna-Attisha's press conference, the local health department released a health advisory regarding the water quality in Flint.[33] On October 1, 2015, MDHHS publicly agreed with the health advisory and with the findings from the Hurley research study.[33]

This message was released in the initial phase of the crisis. Although the message did not adhere to the Be First CERC principle, it did include some initial key message components of self-efficacy and commitment.[35] MDHHS displayed its commitment by providing free water filters to the public and arranging access to these resources at various locations.[37] In addition, the message provided self-efficacy messaging by encouraging the public to access information about preventing elevated blood levels of lead and utilizing filters to obtain safer drinking water.[37] Message components of uncertainty and empathy were absent from this initial messaging.

Be Right
In MDHHS's news media release in January 2016, it noted that MDHHS could not conclude that the Legionnaires' outbreak in Genessee County was related to the corrosive water from the Flint River.[38] From June 2014 to October 2015, approximately 86 individuals contracted Legionnaires' disease, and 12 died due to the condition.[29] MDHHS noted that they knew of the Legionnaires' disease outbreak in Genesee County; however, no action was taken or information was presented to the public.[33] In 2016, when MDHHS began to report on the outbreak, it persistently stated that it could not conclude with certainty that the outbreak was due to the contaminated and untreated water:

> While the MDHHS cannot conclude that the increase is related to the water emergency in Flint, the State of Michigan is treating this situation with the same urgency and transparency as the lead response in the city of Flint.[38]

In May 2018, MDHHS further concluded that the only source of the outbreak was linked to McLaren Flint Hospital, not the Flint water system.[39] Cases of Legionnaires' disease were identified at McLaren Flint Hospital in 2016; however, many experts conclusively confirmed that the outbreak began with the change in water supply in 2014.[40] Not only was MDHHS again late in notifying the public, but it also failed to provide truthful and accurate information to the public regarding the Legionnaires' disease outbreak.[33]

Regarding lead exposure, communications from MDHHS's website or X or YouTube feeds only could be found after October 2015. However, a congressional hearing transcript was available and did note inaccuracies in the information MDHHS employees shared with the public in 2014.[41] In the congressional hearing on April 13, 2016, a Texas representative questioned the former director of MDHHS, Nike Lyons, regarding inaccurate information from officials stating that the spike in lead levels in the water was "seasonal and not related to the water supply."[41] The initial report on lead exposure was incorrect and dismissed the potential risk, as there is no safe blood lead level in children according to the CDC.[42]

MDHHS did not meet the CERC principle of Be Right during various phases of the crisis. The inaccurate messaging regarding the spike in lead levels occurred during the initial stage, and the denial of the source of the Legionnaires' disease outbreak occurred during the maintenance stage. Maintenance message components such as providing a deeper risk explanation, making a commitment to the public, and addressing rumors and inaccurate information were absent.[43] MDHHS's inability to deliver accurate information contributed to rumors developing and increased the amount of misinformation being presented to the citizens of Flint.

Be Credible

From the onset of the crisis, the public was continuously presented with inaccurate information. The public's outcries were disregarded, and they were told that their water supply concerns were unjustified.[30] The mothers, fathers, children, and elders were all ignored and poisoned for approximately 15 months before MDHHS could no longer deny their claims and concerns. In 2016, after the truth about the lead poisoning and the rise of Legionnaires' disease became public, media attention was heightened, and the crisis was then discussed by the 2016 presidential candidates, senators, and media outlets nationally.[44] Accusations of blame and demands for accountability were rising as it became known that many local, state, and federal agencies had failed to protect the citizens of Flint. MDHHS responded to the rumors and criticism regarding its lack of action by stating that it had acted and would release its emails indicating as much.[45] MDHHS was on the defensive and wanted to reiterate its mission and commitment to Flint's citizens.[45] Even with MDHHS's "proof" of it releasing emails and acknowledging the public's concerns, its credibility had been compromised.

The following are examples of MDHHS messages from this time:

> Recent comments in the media are inconsistent with the collaboration that has taken place between the Michigan Department of Health and Human Services and the Genesee County Health Department. MDHHS is releasing some of its earliest email conversations between its epidemiologists and the Genesee County Health Department regarding legionella cases.[45]

> When it comes to health, our team and the partners we turn to for support have not lost sight of our mission: protect the health of our residents by bridging the gaps to promote more and better opportunities for success in Flint.[45]

> We know that the Legionnaires outbreaks have added to public concerns. We want Flint to know we take these concerns seriously – that we have investigated these cases and committed our staff to support and guide the local investigations.[45]

Due to MDHHS's inability to provide accurate information to the public, the CERC principle of Be Right was not met. Subsequently, its credibility was diminished, and this lack of the timely provision of information persisted throughout the crisis.[43] When these emails were released, the public didn't have a reason to trust in or believe that MDHHS could protect them or provide accurate news about the crisis. In this maintenance message, we can see attempts to address misinformation and to make a commitment to the community to mitigate their risk and concerns regarding Legionnaires' disease; however, these attempts to provide credible information and make a commitment to the community come too late in the emergency. Throughout this emergency response, the agency would struggle to maintain trust with the community.[43]

Express Empathy
Throughout the crisis, we can observe communications from the state health department mentioning its focus on the safety of the public, but none of the messaging showed genuine compassion.[20] Compassion and empathy are complex characteristics to emote or evaluate, but they do not appear to be present in the messaging regarding the Flint crisis. In the messaging, MDHHS noted referred to "families" and that "lead exposure is our top priority"; however, this is a minimal effort.[46] The messaging did not reflect the fears and suffering that the public experienced in not being able to meet their basic need for clean water.[43] The messaging did not address the health department's delays in discovering or rectifying the crisis sooner. The communication from the state health department lacked messages that empathetically related to what the public had experienced and suffered throughout the past year.

The following are examples of MDHHS messaging from this period:

As testing continues, our focus remains on helping families reduce all potential exposures to lead.[29]

Free water filters and replacement cartridges are still available to Flint residents.[29]

We have made progress in testing and identifying those with elevated blood lead levels, and the department will continue to work closely with the Genesee County Health Department to reach these families.[46]

Ensuring that families in the Flint area have access to resources that will help reduce the potential for lead exposure is our top priority.[46]

To help residents properly install water filters, and to demonstrate how to replace the original when it expires, MDHHS has created an instructional video on its YouTube channel. For this and other updates, visit www.michigan.gov/flintwater.[46]

The communications were released in the maintenance phase of the crisis. They did not meet the CERC principle of Express Empathy. Nevertheless, they did provide a deeper risk explanation of the effects of lead in minors. They indicated a commitment to the community, as free water filters were being provided and video resources were available to show citizens how to install these filters.[46]

Promote Action
The following messages were provided during the maintenance phase of the crisis. Each of them demonstrates the CERC Principle of Promote Action appropriately.

Avoiding smoking is the single most important thing you can do to lower your risk of infection. Smoking increases the chances that you'll develop LD [Legionnaires' disease] if exposed to *Legionella* bacteria.[47]

People can get Legionnaires' disease by breathing in small droplets of water (mist) that contain *Legionella* bacteria. In general, *Legionella* does not spread from one person to another. People also don't get Legionnaires' disease from drinking water but may be exposed if water goes down the airway.[48]

Making sure that hot tubs and warm pools have the right disinfectant (i.e., chlorine) levels is important for killing *Legionella* bacteria. These disinfectant levels can be hard to maintain when water temperature is high. You do not need a special filter to remove *Legionella* bacteria in your drinking water.[47]

Showers: Because they remain damp, shower heads could hold *Legionella* bacteria. Removing the shower head, manually cleaning it to remove scale and sediment, and soaking it in a mixture of 1 tablespoon of household bleach to 1 gallon of water for about 2 hours will disinfect the shower head.[47]

After MDHHS stopped denying the existence of the crisis and started to accept the truth, they began to provide the public with many self-efficacy messages to protect themselves and their families. The messaging included proactive steps to "avoid smoking" and ensuring pools and hot tubs have the "right disinfectant" to kill bacteria such as *Legionella*.[47] Maintenance message components of interventions, deeper risk explanations, and committing to the community were present.[43] The communications included risk explanations, as details regarding how the bacteria spreads and symptoms of the disease were provided in straightforward language.[48] In addition, interventions for families to treat and clean bodies of water such as showers, humidifiers, and water heaters were included.[47]

Show Respect
In the initial and maintenance phases of messaging, the CERC principle of Show Respect was not followed, as dishonesty and a lack of respect for the public were prevalent. However, MDHHS demonstrated this CERC principle during the resolution phase. Here are examples of MDHHS's messaging:

Flint families with children who qualify for food assistance benefits will receive an additional $30 per child monthly beginning in March.[49]

The Legislature appropriated $7 million in federal Temporary Assistance for Needy Families block grant dollars for emergency food assistance for Flint children, with half going to the Michigan Department of Health and Human Services and half going to the Michigan Department of Education. The two departments pooled the money to provide the additional food assistance benefits for children in Flint.[49]

Eating nutritious foods is crucial to mitigating the impact of lead exposure on the health of Flint residents – including children who are particularly at risk. That's why this additional food assistance is so important. The state of Michigan is committed to helping the residents of Flint in coordination with our partners, including the federal government and Michigan State University.[49]

After lead consumption was no longer a concern, efforts and initiatives were implemented to help assist those affected and exposed to high lead levels.[49] Mobile food banks were opened at 14 locations across the city to provide citizens with nutritious ingredients and vitamins to combat lead exposure.[49] This initiative provided the city with an extra 7 million dollars for Flint victims.[49] MDHHS demonstrated here respect and cooperation with partners and stakeholders to establish the initiative in order to serve the community.[36]

Conclusion
After evaluating MDHHS's response and emergency risk communication during the Flint Water Crisis, the following lessons should be learned.

Transparency and Honesty
MDHHS consistently provided delayed and inaccurate information to the public while jeopardizing the health of all citizens of Flint. Due to the amount of misinformation, poor timing, and lack of promptness in the initial and maintenance phases of the crisis, MDHHS was unable to establish credibility and trust, which set the precedent for the crisis and further compromised the effectiveness of the department's response. Openness,

transparency, and honesty must not be compromised during a crisis as the public always has the right to know.[43] New information can surface and inaccuracies can occur; however, MDHHS must be able to prioritize relaying the truth promptly while acknowledging uncertainty and maintaining trust and credibility.[43]

Collaboration
Throughout the crisis, many mixed messages from local, state, and federal agencies existed.[33] Conflicting messages can breed confusion and increase fear among the public.[36] Attempts to discredit and refute data from external partners such as the Hurley medical staff or the Virginia Tech team were unnecessary and further discredit damaged MDHHS's credibility and integrity.[33] As the leading health department in Michigan, it is MDHHS's responsibility to promote collaborative efforts with partners and stakeholders and utilize its resources to verify, review, and provide accurate information to the public rapidly.

Adherence to the CERC Principles and Phase-Based Messaging
The six core CERC principles were not applied or used when communicating with the public during the Flint Water Crisis. The CERC principles of Be First, Be Right, Be Credible, and Express Empathy were absent from all the stages of the crisis, which is unacceptable. Each of these core principles should be heavily utilized at the onset of a crisis to establish trust with the public during such tumultuous times.[29] The CERC principles of Promote Action and Show Respect appeared in the later stages of the crisis. Additional work is needed to incorporate these principles into all stages of crisis responses in order to provide more effective communication.

Adherence to the phase-based messaging of the CERC framework was skewed, as is shown in the following example: In January 2016, MDHHS posted a news release regarding the increase in Legionnaires' disease in Flint. This messaging appeared during the maintenance phase of the crisis. Since the Legionnaires' disease outbreak was urgent and unexpected, this messaging should have occurred during the initial phase of the crisis. MDHHS lacked promptness in its messaging, which detrimentally impacted the public.[40] These actions also resulted in multiple criminal charges of involuntary manslaughter related to Legionnaires' disease deaths and willful neglect of duty regarding concealing and later misrepresenting the lead data.[40] These charges were made against four MDHHS employees.[40]

I encourage MDHHS to accept accountability for its deficiencies in upholding its mission statement to protect the public and for its ineffectiveness in providing efficient emergency risk communication throughout the Flint Water Crisis. Adopting the CERC principles in the future will be vital to rebuilding trust in the department's ability to provide effective emergency communication not only to Flint's citizens, but to all Michiganders.

End-of-Chapter Reflection Questions

1. Write your own initial messages for an infectious disease outbreak and identify the key message components: address uncertainty, make a commitment, provide empathy, and provide a self-efficacy message.
2. Review previous health department messages from a recent outbreak. Did the messaging address uncertainty? If not, how could it be improved based on the information provided in this chapter?

3 Review previous health department messages from a recent outbreak. Did the messaging include empathy? If not, how could it be improved based on the information provided in this chapter?

4 Consider how you would disseminate your initial message through different channels. Which three channels would you use and why?

5 Discuss your agency's policies and procedures about releasing information to the media before sharing it with partner agencies. What are the benefits and drawbacks of these policies and procedures?

References

1 Vanderford ML, Nastoff T, Telfer JL, Bonzo SE. Emergency Communication Challenges in Response to Hurricane Katrina: Lessons from the Centers for Disease Control and Prevention. *J Appl Commun Res* 2007;**35**(1): 9–25.

2 *Facing Hazards and Disasters: Understanding Human Dimensions.* Washington, DC, The National Academies Press, 2006.

3 *Facing the Unexpected: Disaster Preparedness and Response in the United States.* Washington, DC, The National Academies Press, 2001.

4 CDC. *Crisis and Emergency Risk Communication October 2018.* Atlanta, GA, CDC, 2018.

5 Seeger M, Sellnow T, Ulmer R. *Communication and Organizational Crisis.* London, Bloomsbury Academic, 2003.

6 Communicating risk in public health emergencies: A WHO guideline for emergency risk communication (ERC) policy and practice. *World Health Organization*, 2017. www.ncbi.nlm.nih.gov/books/NBK540733 (Accessed April 10, 2024).

7 Seeger M. Best Practices in Crisis Communication: An Expert Panel Process. *J Appl Commun Res* 2006;**34**(3): 232–44.

8 CDC. *Crisis and Emergency Risk Communication October 2014.* Atlanta, GA, CDC, 2014.

9 Bandura A. Self-Efficacy: Toward a Unifying Theory of Behavioral Change. *Psychol Rev* 1977;**84**:191–215.

10 Bandura A. Social Cognitive Theory of Mass Communication. In: Bryant J, Zillmann D, editors. *Media Effects: Advances in Theory and Research*, 2nd edition. Mahwah, NJ, Lawrence Erlbaum Associates, 2002; pp. 121–53.

11 Burns KM. *Emergency Preparedness Self-Efficacy and the Ongoing Threat of Disasters.* Unpublished dissertation, George Washington University, 2014.

12 Wirtz P, Rohrbeck C, Burns KM. Anxiety Effects on Disaster Precautionary Behaviors: A Multi-Path Cognitive Model. *J Health Pyschol* 2017;**24**(10): 1–11.

13 Baiano C, Raimo G, Zappullo I, Marra M, Cecere R, Trojano L, et al. Empathy through the Pandemic: Changes of Different Emphatic Dimensions during the COVID-19 Outbreak. *Int J Environ Res Public Health* 2022;**19**(4):2435.

14 Franke VC, Elliott CN. Optimism and Social Resilience: Social Isolation, Meaninglessness, Trust, and Empathy in Times of COVID-19. *Societies* 2021; **11**(2):35.

15 Grignoli N, Petrocchi S, Bernardi S, Massari I, Traber R, Malacrida R, et al. Influence of Empathy Disposition and Risk Perception on the Psychological Impact of Lockdown During the Coronavirus Disease Pandemic Outbreak. *Front Pub Health* 2021;**8**:567337.

16 Karnaze M, Bellettiere J, Bloss C. Association of Compassion and Empathy

with Prosocial Health Behaviors and Attitudes in a Pandemic. *PLoS One* 2022;**17**(7):e0271829.

17 Petrocchi S, Bernardi S, Malacrida R, Traber R, Gabutti L, Grignoli N. Affective Empathy Predicts Self-Isolation Behaviour Acceptance during Coronavirus Risk Exposure. *Sci Rep* 2021;**11**(1):10153.

18 Morstead T, Zheng J, Sin N, King D, DeLongis A. Adherence to Recommended Preventive Behaviors during the COVID-19 Pandemic: The Role of Empathy and Perceived Health Threat. *Ann Behav Med* 2022;**56**(4):381–92.

19 Zahry NR, McCluskey M, Ling JY. Risk Governance during the COVID-19 Pandemic: A Quantitative Content Analysis of Governors' Narratives on Twitter. *J Contin Crisis Manage* 2023;**31**(1):77–91.

20 Kabat-Zinn J. *Mindfulness-Based Interventions in Context: Past, Present, and Future*. Washington, DC, American Psychological Association, 2003.

21 Goleman D. *Emotional Intelligence*. New York, Bantam Book, 1995.

22 Dalai Lama TG, Ekman P. *Emotional Awareness: Overcoming the Obstacles to Psychological Balance and Compassion: A Conversation between the Dalai Lama and Paul Ekman*. New York, St. Martin's Essentials, 2008.

23 North Dakota governor in tears at split over face mask use in the US. *Guardian News*. 2020. www.youtube.com/watch?v=UBdpkgfJH9w (Accessesd April 10, 2024).

24 Besser R. Media briefing on H1N1 [MP4]. 2009.

25 *Study Guide for the Examination for Accreditation in Public Relations*. Wilmington, DE, Universal Accreditation Board/Public Relations Society of America, 2021.

26 New York State Department of Health Provides Updates On Nassau County Measles Case. *New York State Department of Health*. 2024. www.health.ny.gov/press/releases/2024/2024-03-23_measles.htm (Accessed April 10, 2024).

27 First aid: Foodborne illness. *Mayo Clinic*. 2024. www.mayoclinic.org/first-aid/first-aid-food-borne-illness/basics/art-20056689#:~:text=Seek%20emergency%20medical%20assistance%20if,You%20suspect%20botulism%20poisoning (Accessed April 10, 2024).

28 Berger CR, Calabrese RJ. Some Explorations in Initial Interaction and Beyond: Toward a Developmental Theory of Interpersonal Communication. *Hum Commun Res* 1975;**1**(2):99–112.

29 Denchak M. Flint Water Crisis: Everything you need to know. *NRDC*. 2018. www.nrdc.org/stories/flint-water-crisis-everything-you-need-know (Accessed July 1, 2023).

30 Kennedy M. Lead-Laced Water in Flint: A Step-By-Step Look at the Makings of a Crisis. NPR. 2016. www.npr.org/sections/thetwo-way/2016/04/20/465545378/lead-laced-water-in-flint-a-step-by-step-look-at-the-makings-of-a-crisis (Accessed July 1, 2023).

31 Mayo Clinic. Lead Poisoning – Symptoms and Causes. 2022. www.mayoclinic.org/diseases-conditions/lead-poisoning/symptoms-causes/syc-20354717 (Accessed July 1, 2023).

32 Mayo Clinic. Legionnaires' disease – Symptoms and causes. 2021. www.mayoclinic.org/diseases-conditions/legionnaires-disease/symptoms-causes/syc-20351747 (Accessed July 1, 2023).

33 Flint Water Advisory Task Force. Commissioned by the Office of Governor Rick Snyder State of Michigan. 2016. www.michigan.gov/-/media/Project/Websites/formergovernors/Folder6/FWATF_FINAL_REPORT_21March2016.pdf?rev=284b9e42c7c840019109eb73aaeedb68 (Accessed July 1, 2023).

34 About MDHHS. *Michigan.gov*. 2019. www.michigan.gov/mdhhs/contact-mdhhs (Accessed April 29, 2024).

35 CDC. *Crisis and Emergency Risk Communication October 2018*. Atlanta, GA, CDC, 2018.

36 CDC. CERC: Psychology of a Crisis. Crisis & Emergency Risk Communication

(CERC) Manual. 2018. https://emergency.cdc.gov/cerc/ppt/CERC_Psychology_of_a_Crisis.pdf (Accessed July 1, 2023).

37. Water filters available for MDHHS clients in Flint beginning Tuesday. *Michigan.gov.* 2019. www.michigan.gov/mdhhs/inside-mdhhs/newsroom/2015/10/05/water-filters-available-for-mdhhs-clients-in-flint-beginning-tuesday (Accessed April 29, 2024).

38. Increased Cases of Legionnaires Disease Investigated in Genesee County. *Michigan.gov.* 2019. www.michigan.gov/mdhhs/inside-mdhhs/newsroom/2016/01/13/increased-cases-of-legionnaires-disease-investigated-in-genesee-county (Accessed July 1, 2023).

39. MDHHS completes Genesee County Legionnaires' Disease case review, finds only one common source. *Michigan.gov.* 2019. www.michigan.gov/mdhhs/inside-mdhhs/newsroom/2018/05/29/mdhhs-completes-genesee-county-legionnaires-disease-case-review-finds-only-one-common-source (Accessed April 29, 2024).

40. Fleming LN. Ex-health director Lyon gets emergency Supreme Court hearing on Flint case. *The Detroit News.* 2022. www.detroitnews.com/story/news/michigan/flint-water-crisis/2022/03/23/ex-health-director-lyon-gets-emergency-supreme-court-hearing-flint-case/7146777001 (Accessed July 1, 2023).

41. Flint Water Crisis: Impacts and Lessons Learned [Internet]. *Govinfo.gov.* 2017. www.govinfo.gov/content/pkg/CHRG-114hhrg20534/html/CHRG-114hhrg20534.htm (Accessed July 1, 2023).

42. CDC. NBP – Factsheet – Lead. 2013. www.cdc.gov/biomonitoring/lead_factsheet.html#:~:text=No%20safe%20blood%20lead%20leve (Accessed April 29, 2024).

43. CDC. CERC: Crisis Communication Plans. Crisis & Emergency Risk Communication (CERC) Manual. 2018. https://emergency.cdc.gov/cerc/ppt/CERC_Crisis_Communication_Plans.pdf (Accessed July 1, 2023).

44. Quinn A. What the Flint water scandal says about US politics in 2016. *The Conversation.* 2016. https://theconversation.com/what-the-flint-water-scandal-says-about-us-politics-in-2016-55789 (Accessed July 1, 2023).

45. MDHHS releases emails related to the Genesee County Legionnaires Disease investigations. *Michigan.gov.* 2019 www.michigan.gov/mdhhs/inside-mdhhs/newsroom/2016/02/09/mdhhs-releases-emails-related-to-the-genesee-county-legionnaires-disease-investigations (Accessed April 29, 2024).

46. MDHHS releases latest data outlining blood lead levels in Flint; follow-up care, case management resources continue for families. *Michigan.gov.* 2019 www.michigan.gov/mdhhs/inside-mdhhs/newsroom/2015/12/03/mdhhs-releases-latest-data-outlining-blood-lead-levels-in-flint-follow-up-care-case-management-reso (Accessed April 29, 2024).

47. Michigan Urges Continued Legionella Precaution. *Michigan.gov.* 2019. www.michigan.gov/mdhhs/inside-mdhhs/newsroom/2016/05/27/michigan-urges-continued-legionella-precaution (Accessed April 29, 2024).

48. Genesee County has its first confirmed case of Legionnaires' disease in 2016. *Michigan.gov.* 2016. www.michigan.gov/mdhhs/inside-mdhhs/newsroom/2016/07/06/genesee-county-has-its-first-confirmed-case-of-legionnaires-disease-in-2016 (Accessed April 29, 2024).

49. Flint families will receive $7 million in additional food assistance. *Michigan.gov.* 2019. www.michigan.gov/mdhhs/inside-mdhhs/newsroom/2017/02/16/flint-families-will-receive-7-million-in-additional-food-assistance (Accessed April 29, 2024).

Part II Communicating during a Health Emergency

Chapter 7

Maintenance Messages during a Health Emergency
How to Protect the Public's Health and Debunking Misinformation

Chapter Objectives
- Describe the four components of a maintenance message.
- Explain why it is important to provide health risk information by audience segment.
- Compare and contrast messaging for nonpharmaceutical and pharmaceutical interventions.
- List three ways to debunk rumors and misinformation.
- Be able to write communication objectives, identify audiences, develop key messages, identify channels, and identify communication products that are needed.
- Identify key tips for spokespeople, partner agencies, and call centers during the initial phase of a health emergency.
- Recall the rumor management framework.

In Chapter 6, we studied initial messages that typically occur during the first 24–48 hours of a health emergency and can last until 3–7 days into an emergency. Often the transition from the initial phase to the maintenance phase is based upon new information coming from laboratory test results. It is common that a health emergency such as a foodborne illness outbreak or an infectious disease outbreak is initially managed solely by the program or division that oversees disease or foodborne illness surveillance. However, if the outbreak becomes larger or gathers media attention or a fatality occurs, emergency risk communication will become a forefront issue, often requiring more communication expertise from the health department's media and external relations office. As the health emergency escalates, requiring more department resources, it moves from the initial phase into the maintenance phase. Often the maintenance phase can be one of the longest phases of a health emergency. For example, look at the COVID-19 pandemic: The virus emerged in the fall of 2019, and the World Health Organization (WHO) declared the emerging coronavirus cases a Public Health Emergency of International Concern on January 30, 2020, and named the evolving outbreak as a pandemic on March 11, 2020.[1] The maintenance phase ran from March 2020 to about May 2023, although COVID-19 is still a health threat today.[2]

For many health emergency responses, emergency risk communicators may find themselves already in the midst of the maintenance phase instead of starting messaging during the initial phase. This can be due to the health threat (e.g., infectious disease) having already been transmitted in the community before the health department has been alerted to its existence.

The Crisis and Emergency Risk Communication (CERC) framework has been developed to guide the development of emergency risk messaging, but the framework seems to be missing guidance for long-term outbreaks or outbreaks that last for several months or even years, as many people witnessed during the COVID-19 pandemic response. In Chapter 8, we will look at long outbreaks and how to incorporate health communication campaign principles into the maintenance phase for such outbreaks.

Maintenance Messages: What They Are and How to Write Them

There are four key message components of a maintenance message that will support the CERC principles of Be Right, Be Credible, Promote Action, and Show Respect.[3]

Maintenance message components include the following[3]:

- Providing deeper risk explanations
- Providing interventions
- Making a commitment to the community
- Addressing rumors and misinformation

The following subsections break down each of these message components and provide examples.

Providing Deeper Risk Explanations

As the health emergency moves into the maintenance phase, laboratory tests are likely to confirm the nature of the causative virus. If lab results confirm the specific virus or disease causing the health emergency, then you have more information to share about the health risk. By understanding what the health risk is, emergency risk communicators and epidemiologists can work together to communicate to the public, stakeholders, and partners about who is most at risk.

There are two different ways to approach risk explanations and communicating them to the public. One way is to identify which groups in the community are at risk. Since public health is focused on population health or community health, health threats are likely to impact different members of the community in different ways. For example, common at-risk or vulnerable populations include those over the age of 65, people with chronic health conditions, pregnant women, children, individuals with limited hearing or eyesight, individuals with limited mobility, and those who are not able to access and use standard health care resources.[4,5,6]

For example, in the fall of 2023, respiratory syncytial virus (RSV) emerged in the United States, affecting older adults and some other high-risk adults. The American Lung Association released a risk explanation about who was at risk by identifying three high-risk groups for severe RSV: adults with chronic lung or heart disease; adults with weakened immune systems; and all older adults, especially those aged 65 years and older.[7]

The second way to approach risk explanations is to identify potential risk exposure by situation. For example, during the 2022 Mpox outbreak, emergency risk communication messages focused on activities that could put a person at risk of contracting Mpox. Mpox can be transmitted human to human through contact with body fluids, through prolonged face-to-face contact, or through contact with clothing used by an individual who has Mpox.[8] The Centers for Disease Control and Prevention (CDC) messaging highlighted the risk of exposure to Mpox as a result of the following situations or activities (see Figure 7.1):

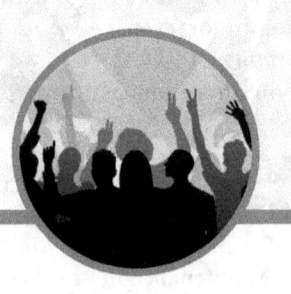

 Get the vaccine if you
- Are a gay, bisexual, or other same-gender loving man who has sex with men or are transgender, gender non-binary, or gender-diverse.
- Have had sexual or intimate contact with someone who may have mpox. Get vaccinated as soon as possible after exposure, regardless of your sexual or gender identity.

AND if you, in the last 6 months, have had or expect to have

- One or more sexually transmitted infections
- A weakened immune system because of another illness, like HIV
- Sexual or intimate contact with a person who is at risk of mpox
- Anonymous sexual or intimate contact, or more than one sexual partner

 ✗ Get both doses unless
You had a severe allergic reaction (such as anaphylaxis) after getting your first dose of the JYNNEOS vaccine.

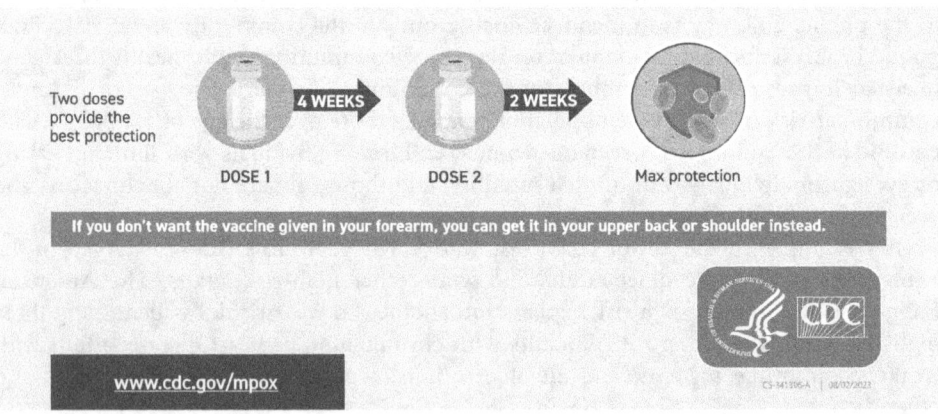

Figure 7.1 CDC infographic explaining the risk of exposure to Mpox based on activity
Source: CDC. The use of this material does not imply endorsement by CDC, Agency for Toxic Substances and Disease Registry, US Department of Health and Human Services, or the United States Government of the author. This material is available on the CDC website free of charge: www.cdc.gov/poxvirus/mpox/collections/pages/get-mpox-vaccines.html

- Are a gay, bisexual, or other same-gender-loving man who has sex with men or are transgender, gender nonbinary, or gender-diverse.
- Have had sexual or intimate contact with someone who may have Mpox.
- In the last 6 months, have had or expect to have

- One or more sexually transmitted infections (STIs).
- A weakened immune system because of another illness, like HIV.
- Sexual or intimate contact with a person who is at risk of Mpox.
- Anonymous sexual or intimate contact or more than one sexual partner.

Providing Interventions

The next component of a maintenance-phase message is providing pharmaceutical and nonpharmaceutical interventions and message components that align with the CERC principle of Promote Action.[3] "Nonpharmaceutical interventions" means that there are no medicines involved. Nonpharmaceutical interventions include handwashing, covering coughs, isolation and quarantine for ill or exposed individuals, and social or physical distancing.

Pharmaceutical interventions are used if and when they're available. Examples of pharmaceutical interventions include vaccines, prophylaxis, or antivirals. Vaccines are given to prevent the occurrence of illness. Prophylaxis is given to people who have been exposed early on in the infectious stage of an outbreak. Antivirals are mediations that help the body fight the infection, ease symptoms, and shorten the length of the infection.

The New York City Health Department provided the following pharmaceutical and nonpharmaceutical intervention information on its website regarding RSV[9]:

Prevention
There are new vaccines and medicines to help prevent RSV in people ages 60 and older and to infants and young children.

Everyone can decrease the risk of getting and spreading RSV and other respiratory viruses:
- Cover your cough and sneeze with a tissue or your arm.
- Wash your hands often. Use hand sanitizer when soap and water are not available. Remind and help children to wash their hands.
- Stay home when sick and keep children who are sick home from school and day care. Avoid close contact with people at increased risk for severe infection when you are sick.
- Clean frequently touched surfaces, especially if someone in the household is sick.
- Avoid close contact with people who are sick, especially if you are at increased risk for severe infection.
- Get tested for flu, COVID-19 and RSV, as appropriate.
- Wear a face mask.
- Get an annual flu shot and stay up to date with your COVID-19 vaccinations.
- Parents of young children should be careful to wash their own hands and their children's hands often and avoid close contact with people who are sick. Keep children who are sick home from school.

Adults 60 and Over
- There are two new RSV vaccines available (Arexvy and Abrysvo) for adults ages 60 years and older. Talk to your health care provider about whether RSV vaccination is right for you.

Infants and Young Children
- Two monoclonal antibody products are available to protect infants and young children from severe RSV infection.
- Nirsevimab (Beyfortus) – a new product recommended for all infants less than 8 months old during their first RSV season. Nirsevimab is also recommended for

infants 8–19 months old who are at increased risk of severe RSV infection and entering their second RSV season.
- Palivizumab (Synagis) – available for infants and young children with certain underlying health conditions who are at high risk of severe RSV infection and who have not or cannot receive nirsevimab.
- In addition, the new Abrysvo RSV vaccine is recommended for pregnant people during weeks 32 to 36 of pregnancy to protect the infant. If vaccine is not given during pregnancy, it is recommended that the newborn receive nirsevimab. In most cases, only one option (vaccination of the pregnant parent or nirsevimab given to the infant) is needed to protect the infant. Expecting parents should discuss with their provider which option is right for them.

Making a Commitment to the Community

Making a commitment to the community is also an initial message component, and it is important to continue commitment messaging throughout the health response.[3] Expressing commitment will support your agency's credibility as long as the agency continues to follow through on what it committed itself to do in the first place.

As discussed in Chapter 6, making a commitment to those affected by the health emergency, stakeholders, and partner agencies supporting the response is made up of two components. First, explain what the agency is doing to find new information about the emerging health crisis. This informs the audience that the agency has the responsibility for addressing this health threat and is taking action to manage and stop this health threat. Providing this type of information helps establish credibility and authority for your agency during the health response. The second part of a commitment message is letting the community know you will be there until the end of the health emergency. During the initial days and weeks of a health emergency, the agency can give a lot of attention and resources to the response; however, over time, the agency's focus and amount of attention may change due to competing priorities. By establishing the health agency's commitment to ending the emergency, the agency can build and maintain trust with the community affected by the health emergency.

During the maintenance phase, commitment messaging needs to include key actions that the health department has been taking to address the health threat, acknowledging any challenges, frustrations, or issues that have arisen.

The following is a statement from former US Vice President Mike Pence on March 17, 2020, demonstrating a commitment to the public regarding the COVID-19 response[10]:

> As I said, the President has continued to push our task force to bring a whole-of-government, a whole-of-America approach. And we continue to be inspired by the way our nation's governors, the nation's businesses are responding.
>
> We spoke just yesterday with the leaders of every broadcast network in America that will soon be unveiling a public service campaign using CDC guidelines. And specifically, as we work on the issue of supplies – meetings yesterday with Department of Defense officials about excess supplies; the President and I will be meeting today to speak about the supply chain for hospitals – we would make one specific request, and that is: We would urge construction companies to donate their inventory of N95 masks to your local hospital and forego additional orders of those industrial masks.
>
> . . .

At the President's direction, we will – we will continue to do whatever it takes. We'll continue to marshal the best of the American people, the best of all the people behind me, the people behind them, our state and local officials. And we will get through this, and we will get through this together.

Addressing Rumors

During the maintenance phase of an emergency, rumors and misinformation will emerge. Rumors emerge where there isn't enough information *or* some part of correct information gets told and retold, introducing slight changes to the information with each retelling. Each time we repeat and retell a story, we might inadvertently change it by inserting what we thought we heard based on how that information get filtered through our frame of reference, which is made up of our belief systems, knowledge, and previous experience.

The following subsections provide three tactics for addressing rumors and misinformation:
- Develop and maintain a facts/myths web page.
- Address misinformation in media briefings and statements.
- Ask other organizations for help.

Develop and Maintain a Facts/Myths Web Page

When rumors or myths begin to emerge, a health agency needs to provide correct and accurate information to the public about the health threat. One tactical way to address rumors and myths is to develop a dedicated web page addressing these myths and providing the facts. Previous research recommends stating the fact first and then stating the myth. By stating the information in this order it is possible to recalibrate the individual to accept this information as accurate rather than reinforcing the incorrect information by stating it first.[11]

The facts/myth web page information can also be shared on social channels and with partners to help amplify the correct and accurate information. WHO's website addressing myths and facts only states the facts about COVID-19 and includes infographics with more information.[12] The web page's title is "Coronavirus disease (COVID-19) advice for the public: Mythbusters," and the web page's content includes hyperlinked subheadings on a variety of topics that have been associated with false information such as but not limited to alcohol-based sanitizers, bleach, masks/CO_2 intoxication, and supplements.[12]

Address Misinformation in Media Briefings and Statements

Another way by which emergency risk communications can address rumors is by having a spokesperson speak on these matters directly during media briefings or by including a relevant quote within a health agency media statement.[13,14] Leveraging media briefings is a great way for spokespeople to directly address rumors or false information and provide accurate information. Additionally, an agency can issue an official media statement as a written document providing the same information. Using the media to combat rumors or false information can ensure the broad reach of a message. Further, it can bolster the credibility of a health agency by ensuring that the most accurate health information is available for the public.

The following is an example from the US Virgin Islands Governor Albert Bryan Jr. addressing a rumor that residents of the US Virgin Islands had been test subjects for the new COVID-19 vaccine.[15] The rumors emerged after the television show *60 Minutes* ran a segment about the logistics of delivering vaccines across the United States, including the US Virgin Islands. The US Virgin Islands Department of Health issued a formal statement and included a link to the *60 Minutes* transcript to verify the information that the television show had issued.[16]

> "There is no basis for these false statements being propagated on social media platforms, and, in fact, they are harmful to the health and well-being of our community in that they instill unnecessary fear and doubt among residents and could potentially cause some Virgin Islanders to forgo using a safe vaccine that could protect them against the virus," Governor Bryan said.
>
> "I am as anxious and hopeful as anyone that an effective vaccine be developed as quickly as possible to protect all Americans against COVID-19," Governor Bryan said. "However, I will not put the public health of our community at risk, and I will not approve distribution of a vaccine that has not been thoroughly vetted and approved by the Food and Drug Administration and that has not been meticulously tested."
>
> The Governor urges USVI [US Virgin Islands] residents to get accurate and authentic information from legitimate sources, such as the Virgin Islands Department of Health, the Centers for Disease Control and Prevention or Government House and to dismiss baseless misinformation from social media platforms.[15]

Ask Other Organizations for Help

To address rumors and misinformation, it can be helpful to enlist other organizations to help debunk misinformation and amplify scientifically accurate information. Working with stakeholders who are advocates of the health agency is beneficial for addressing rumors in the following two ways:

1. Doing so extends the exposure and reach of the message. Leverage additional organizations and subject matter experts outside of the health agency. Empowering others to share accurate health information increases the reach of messaging, and leveraging peer-to-peer outreach provides an opportunity for medical and health care professionals to share such information throughout their personal and professional networks.
2. Medical providers are trusted sources of information. Research continues to demonstrate the power of trusted messengers, especially those from within the medical community.[17] Providing health care providers with accurate health information represents an important channel for providing members of the public with the right information to protect their health based on information from someone they already trust.

For example, the grassroots campaign "This Is Our Shot" and the sister campaign in Spanish language "VacunateYa" was supported by the California Department of Health, the Public Health Institute, the California Medical Association, and dozens of other stakeholders and partners.[17]

The intention of the campaign was to leverage members of the health care industry to share accurate and credible information about the COVID-19 vaccine through stories, photos, and videos. Specifically, this campaign was focused on those who have been subjected to structural inequality and who are mistrustful of traditional institutions and so are likely to be hesitant to receive a vaccine.[18]

"This Is Our Shot" offered tools and resources for advocates who were willing to share accurate health information with others. The tools included a Covid Vaccine Conversation Guide, a MixInfoRx Toolkit, and educational videos that could be reshared on social media. "VacunateYa" focused on educating and empowering the Latino/x community to get vaccinated, as statistics revealed that this community was particularly vulnerable to COVID-19.[19] The three key pillars of this effort included engagement, empowerment, and education, again leveraging health care workers to share and amplify accurate health information about COVID-19 vaccines.

> **Mini-Case Study: University of Oregon Meningitis Outbreak**
>
> In early January 2015, the University of Oregon confirmed a case of meningitis in a student who lived off campus. The laboratory testing revealed the particular type of meningitis as serogroup B. Through contact tracing, close contacts of the case were identified and given prophylaxis, which means that they were given a type of medical treatment that would help prevent the spreading of that infection within their own bodies.
>
> In late January, a second case of meningitis serogroup B was laboratory confirmed in a student who lived on campus.[20] Contact tracing revealed close contacts, and those individuals were given prophylaxis to make sure they would not get sick. The epidemiological investigation revealed that there was no link between the two cases, meaning that there was no way to say whether these two cases were at all involved with each other or had been around each other to spread the disease.
>
> Two days after the second case fell ill, another case of meningitis serogroup B was reported.[21,22] Through epidemiological investigation it was discovered that there was a link between case 2 and case 3.[23] About 2.5 weeks after case 3 was reported, a fourth case, named Lauren Jones, died from meningitis. This young woman lived in the dorms on campus and was a member of the acrobatics team.[24] In terms of the crisis communication life cycle, the death of a case could be identified as a trigger event that starts the initial life cycle of a health emergency.[25] Although three cases were occurring prior to this death, a fatality in an outbreak triggers the need for emergency risk communication messaging.[3]
>
> CDC recommends that broader community vaccination be considered when there have been more than three cases of infection by a single meningococcal serogroup within a 3-month period *without a direct epidemiological link between the cases* and yielding an attack rate of greater than 10 cases per 1,000 in the community at risk.[23]
>
> The University of Oregon was working with Lane County Public Health officials on the situation, but when the death of the student occurred, Lane County Public Health requested epidemiological and risk communication assistance from the Oregon Health Authority, the state public health department.[26] Through collaboration, the health officers and emergency risk communicators from Lane County Public Health and Oregon Health Authority began to develop an intervention strategy to mitigate the health threat and think strategically about emergency risk communication messaging. Through research, health officials discovered that there were other universities (Princeton and the University of California, Santa Barbara) that had also faced serogroup B outbreaks, and the Food and Drug Administration (FDA) granted emergency authorization to use a vaccine to prevent serogroup B.[26] At the time of the University of Oregon outbreak, CDC's Advisory Committee on Immunization Practices had recently approved the vaccine for limited groups.[23]

There were two major challenges that health officials had to face: the cost of the vaccine and timing, as spring break was just a few weeks away. To ensure the $300 vaccine was not cost-prohibitive for anyone at risk seeking vaccination, the University of Oregon worked with health insurance companies, Oregon Health Plan/Medicaid, and others to ensure that the costs of vaccines were covered.[26,27,28] To address timing, two actions were taken: First, the University of Oregon worked with health officials to set up mass vaccination clinics, putting to the test point-of-dispensing plans outlined in public health emergency response plans; and second, state health officials developed a letter to be sent to parents explaining the health risk and informing them to encourage their children to get vaccinated while at home during spring break.

In collaboration with the University of Oregon, a mass vaccination campaign was planned for March 2–6, 2015, at the university's basketball arena. During the mass vaccination event about 9,000 students were immunized.[23] The university's spring break occurred during March 21–29, 2015, meaning that many students returned to their homes away from Eugene, Oregon, where the university is located. Health officials in concert with the university sent letters to parents explaining the risks of the health situation and encouraged students to get vaccinated at their local pharmacies.[23]

The following subsections break down the key emergency messages that were sent during this health emergency by CERC life cycle phase.

Initial-Phase Messages

Empathy
Messages of empathy were present in the response after the death of Lauren Jones. Most notable are the heartfelt sentiments provided by coaches and staff at the University of Oregon who directly knew Lauren. The following are examples of those empathetic messages:

> "This is a terrible and sudden loss for our whole Oregon community, as well as our acrobatics and tumbling team family. Lauren was such a positive and bright spirit every day, and her smile was contagious. She will be greatly missed, and our prayers and deepest condolences go out to her whole family, friends, previous teammates and anyone else who had the opportunity to know Lauren." University of Oregon, acrobatics and tumbling coach Chelsea Shaw.[24]

> "All of us in the UO [University of Oregon] family are deeply saddened by Lauren's sudden passing and extend our sympathies to her family and friends. As we honor Lauren's spirit, we are providing comfort and support to her coaches, teammates and fellow student-athletes as they go through the grieving process." University of Oregon athletic director Rob Mullens.[24]

Commitment
During early February, the University of Oregon and Lane County Public Health provided messages of commitment regarding the actions that were being taken to mitigate the health threat and the collaboration between the two agencies:

> "There was one student who was examined and referred for additional screening. This was done out of an abundance of caution due to increased exposure risk by nature of proximity," said Dr. Pat Luedtke of Lane County Public Health. "At this time all exposed community members have been identified and contacted."

> "We are extremely pleased with the level of collaboration and coordination between the UO and public health," said Mike Eyster, executive director of the University Health

Center. "Our folks acted quickly, worked with medical professionals to identify areas of risk and provided prophylaxis those who needed it."

The UO distributed notices to approximately 1,200 students Tuesday evening. "The large number of notifications should not be perceived as 1,200 individuals are at the same level of potential exposure. Procedurally, it is more important for us to reach the individuals so they can begin self-monitoring for symptoms and come speak to medical staff to assess their individual risk," Eyster said.[20]

Maintenance-Phase Messages

The death of Lauren Jones was covered by the media in mid-February, and the focus of messaging then changed from empathy and commitment to deeper risk explanations and interventions. As discussed in Chapter 6, initial messaging typically lasts from 24 to 28 hours after a trigger event but can last up to 3–7 days after a trigger event.[3,29] The pivot from initial phase to maintenance phase occurred as health emergency response operations began to ramp up activity for the mass vaccination clinic, and so messaging shifted to deeper risk explanations and interventions. The following subsections provide examples of maintenance-phase message components of providing deeper risk explanations and interventions.

Providing Deeper Risk Explanations
Laboratory tests confirmed *Neisseria meningitidis*, serogroup B.[23] Based on the available information, health officials followed protocols to identify close contacts and provide prophylaxis. With the death of Lauren Jones and the lack of a direct link between all of the cases, health officials began to understand that the disease had moved beyond the prophylaxis ring of close contacts and that there was a health risk to a broader group of individuals. The following question therefore arose: Who was most at risk?

As we discussed in Chapter 6, determining who is at risk will determine audience segments for messaging. For this outbreak, the University of Oregon wanted to know who exactly was at risk. Based on the epidemiological investigation and the physical location of the cases, Oregon Health Authority identified the following three groups as most at risk and recommended these groups for vaccination:

- All University of Oregon undergraduates
- Undergraduates from other colleges who live in the "13th & Olive" apartment complex in Eugene
- Graduate students and faculty who either live on campus or have a medical condition (asplenia, sickle cell disease, or complement deficiency) that puts them at increased risk for meningococcal disease[23]

Providing Interventions
The University of Oregon meningitis outbreak required emergency risk communication messaging regarding both nonpharmaceutical interventions and pharmaceutical interventions. The following two subsections provide overviews of this key messaging.

Nonpharmaceutical Interventions
After the identification of the third case and prior to the mass vaccination clinic, the University of Oregon delivered messages promoting actions and nonpharmaceutical interventions. Campus-wide emails were sent to all students, faculty, and staff explaining the signs and symptoms of meningitis and the actions to take to prevent the spread of the

infection.[26] These actions included handwashing; not sharing eating utensils, straws, toothbrushes, lip balm, or cosmetics; seeking medical attention if ill; and updating vaccination records with the university health center. Similar information was shared with parents through the Parents' Association.[26]

Pharmaceutical Interventions

The pharmaceutical intervention for this outbreak was a series of mass vaccination clinics that occurred over 13 months after the initial case was identified.[26] The vaccination strategy focused on students opting in instead of mandating the vaccine.[26,30]

Emergency risk communication activities for the mass vaccination clinics were twofold. One part was a media relations push, with public health medical experts explaining the risk of the health threat and the importance of vaccination.[31] The second part was the health communication campaign to encourage students to get vaccinated. The University of Oregon led efforts to create communication products designed for college students to encourage them to get vaccinated. The following section provides examples of both.

Media Relations

Dr. Paul Cieslak, Oregon Health Authority, and Dr. Patrick Luedtke, Lane County Health Officer, were the spokespeople for their respective health agencies.[32] Media interviews on television, college radio, broadcast radio, and in newspapers were scheduled throughout the first day of the mass vaccination campaign.

Health Communication Campaign Messaging

Communication Objective

- The measurable communication objective was to vaccinate 22,000 undergraduate students through multiple vaccination clinics leading up to spring break.[26] The mass vaccination clinics were organized to handle up to 5,000 students per day. By March 19, 2015, 9,000 of the 22,000 students had been vaccinated.[33]

Audience

- The main audience was University of Oregon undergraduate students.
- Additional audiences included faculty, staff, and parents of students.

Key Messages and Communication Products

- The mass vaccination communication campaign was led by the University of Oregon and the main key message was to get vaccinated.
- The campaign materials leveraged the school colors of the university – bright green and gold. The tagline – "Get the Vax" – was displayed on posters, stickers, sidewalk corners, table tents, the university website, and social media.[34] Posters included images of student leaders and student athletes with their shirt sleeves rolled up and displaying a bandage with the university logo and the tagline "Get the Vax."[26]
- After a student received the vaccination, they could take their photo in a photo booth that featured the tagline "I Got the Vax." They could also get a bracelet or a tote bag branded with the same message. One online poster featured adhesive bandages in the school's green and gold colors with its "O" symbol at the center.[34]

Communication Channels

- Faculty received a PowerPoint presentation for display at the beginning of classes to inform students of the various clinic locations and hours of operation.

- The same slides were used for digital displays in several buildings across campus.
- Notifications of immunization clinics were posted in the university's class registration system, ensuring students viewed clinic details when logging into the system.
- Advertisements were also placed in the student newspaper.[26]

Making a Commitment to the Community
The maintenance message component of commitment was demonstrated by state health officials after the on-campus vaccination clinics. A sixth case was confirmed in an off-campus student, and state health officials focused messaging on the importance of vaccination. They soon realized that dealing with this health threat would take months.[27]

"We need parents to help us get the word out to students about this dangerous, potentially deadline disease, and why it's crucial for students to get the meningitis B shot right now. No one should be complacent about this disease. University of Oregon undergraduates who have not been vaccinated are at risk of infections, serious illness, and death." Paul Cieslak, MD, medical director of infectious disease and immunization programs.[27]

"The meningococcal outbreak is not over. We won't be at all surprised if we see more cases. That's why undergrads and those with high-risk medical conditions should get vaccinated right away. It's the best way to reduce your risk of being infected." Paul Cieslak, MD, medical director of infectious disease and immunization programs.[27]

Addressing Rumors
For this particular outbreak, no rumors emerged that needed to be addressed. Not every health emergency will see the emergence of rumors.

Misinformation, Disinformation, and Infodemics

"Misinformation," "disinformation," and "infodemics" are terms that were commonly used throughout the COVID-19 health emergency response. *Misinformation* is information that is not correct and is being spread without knowing that the information is incorrect.[35] Misinformation is different from rumor because misinformation can be created by content generators who believe that this information is correct.[36] *Disinformation* is a form of misinformation or inaccurate information that is being purposefully shared in an effort to malign political, social, or health situations due to underlying interests of power and corruption.[35,36,37] An *infodemic* is "an overabundance of information" – some accurate, some not – that makes it hard for people to find trustworthy sources and reliable guidance when they need it.[38] Infodemics are related to the volume of information that is available.[36,38]

COVID-19 Infodemic

WHO's director general Tedros Adhanom Ghebreyesus said, "We're not just fighting a pandemic; we're fighting an infodemic."[39] The prevalence of rumors and conspiracy theories was so great on social media during the COVID-19 pandemic that WHO developed a framework to address misinformation.[40] As emergency risk communicators face the issue of managing an infodemic, it is important to pause and look at the core issues of an infodemic:

1. The emergence of incorrect or potentially incorrect information
2. Trust in government
3. The amount of uncertainty about the health emergency
4. The great availability of information sources

The COVID-19 pandemic revealed particular challenge for emergency risk communicators: the advancements of technology to create and manipulate digital media and the speed and scale at which information can be shared globally.[36] The core issues of an infodemic are rumors or misinformation, trust in government, uncertainty in a crisis, and the great availability of information sources. These can be addressed using CERC and phase-based maintenance messaging. This section outlines how CERC provides strategies to address the challenges of an infodemic.

Rumors and misinformation are not new phenomena to emergency risk communicators. Rumors and misinformation have been around since World War II and occurred during the 1918 influenza pandemic, the 1980s HIV/AIDS epidemic, and the 2003 SARS outbreak.[36,41]

As outlined in CERC phase-based maintenance messaging, addressing rumors is a critical component of emergency risk communication. The three strategies to address misinformation include developing and maintaining facts/myths web pages, addressing misinformation in media briefings, and asking other organizations for help. These strategies align with interventions that COVID-19 misinformation researchers recommend: amplifying accurate information, filling information voids, and debunking false information.[36,42]

Another issue that CERC can address in regard to an infodemic is trust in the government. COVID-19 revealed that people in the United States had little to no trust in the government, especially when they felt health recommendations were politically influenced.[43] Trust in the government must be addressed regardless of the health emergency phase. For emergency risk communicators who find themselves working on a health emergency in the throes of the maintenance phase, establishing trust and credibility can be challenging, but doing so is not necessarily impossible. Strategies to promote trust through emergency risk communication include: making a commitment to those affected by the emergency that the agency will work to address and mitigate the health threat; expressing empathy and listening to the concerns of stakeholders; releasing aggregate datasets so research institutions and independent researchers can analyze the data; and communicating transparently about the risks that are known regarding the health threat.

Addressing uncertainty is a critical component during an infodemic. As outlined in Chapter 6, uncertainty is inherent during a health emergency, especially during the initial phase of such an emergency. Through the multiyear global pandemic of COVID-19, uncertainty was present in both the initial and maintenance phases. Specifically, uncertainty surrounded the identification of the virus, the symptoms and transmissibility of the virus, the severity of the illness, its long-term effects, and the source of the virus. Uncertainty also arose regarding the pharmaceutical interventions, including the development of the vaccines using a new technology and the risks and benefits associated with these vaccines.

Starbird and fellow researchers have explained that people engage in a process called "sensemaking" as a way to make sense of a situation and the information they are receiving.[44] Through this process, it is possible for people to misunderstand something and so create their own form of information. In this regard, researchers at the University of Washington have expressed hesitancy at labeling such information as "misinformation" because doing so ultimately labels the information as objectively false and incorrect.[36] From an emergency risk communication standpoint, when health officials deem something as misinformation and label it as incorrect, trust between the health agency and the audience engaging in the rumor or misinformation is reduced due to the establishment of a polarizing "us versus them" or "right versus wrong" narrative. To alleviate this potential polarization, one strategy to address trust and create a dialogue regarding potential misinformation is to offer opportunities for dialogue and listening through virtual webinars with question-and-answer sessions, virtual or in-person town halls, or community-based listening sessions. The goal of these sessions would be to focus on long-term trust development through a series of dialogue and listening sessions over a course of months instead of an annual or biannual town hall meeting.

CERC advises a media monitoring strategy to ensure the media is reporting the agency's messages accurately.[45] If the information is not reported correctly, follow up with the reporter to provide a correction. During the 2001 anthrax attacks in the United States, media monitoring was used as a proxy for audience feedback. Due to the heightened media attention and fast-evolving nature of health emergencies, news media stories can be grouped together and analyzed by theme. This data analysis then can be used by emergency risk communicators to inform the development of a communication strategy or to identify potential gaps in health agency messaging.[46] Social monitoring and listening technologies have evolved to allow us to understand audience sentiments, overall trends on social media, and information-seeking behavior, with the aim of helping businesses monitor their digital presence and customer opinions.[47,48] Social monitoring and social listening tools can be designed and developed for a health agency, or an agency can contract with a public relations or marketing firm to monitor and listen on their behalf. Monitoring and listening to social media during an infodemic can help identify whether there are information gaps, rumors, or misinformation that are arising, as well as providing details regarding emerging topics or trends that the health agency needs to consider in its future messaging.[46]

The New York City Department of Health and Hygiene used a social media monitoring team during a 2013 full-scale Ebola exercise in 2013 and a Legionnaires' disease outbreak response in 2015.[49] The key functions of this social media monitoring included situational awareness, assessing the success or failure of public messaging, and identifying rumors and misinformation. The social media monitoring reports were shared with the Planning Section and the Public Information Officer. The reports helped to support decision-making regarding crisis management and to inform communication strategy, especially when rumors had been identified.

What Is Government Censorship?

Researchers have analyzed the strategies used by governments across the world took to address COVID-19 misinformation.[50] Some governments prioritized disseminating accurate information, while other governments arrested citizens and journalists who discussed the virus or the governments' handling of the pandemic response.[50] Some strategies to address misinformation have landed US health officials and researchers in legal trouble, with allegations of suppressing free speech and potentially violating the First Amendment.[51,52,53]

In the United States, a legal case called *Murthy v. Missouri* involved five social media users and two state governments claiming that their free speech was suppressed after social media companies were pressured by US government agencies (i.e., the White House, CDC, the Federal Bureau of Investigation [FBI], and Department of Homeland Security) to remove or downgrade their posts.[54] The debate raged between legal, public health, and medical experts as to where the line was to be drawn between ensuring protection of free speech under the First Amendment and ensuring that the government is able to prevent harm to the public.[55] Allowing the government to adjudicate on health information could have negative consequences relating to the government potentially being unable to distinguish accurate from false information, especially with scientific knowledge as to what is "true" and what is "false" continuing to evolve, and the potential for the suppression of accurate information that proves to be scientifically true later.[55]

In June 2024, the US Supreme Court released its opinion on *Murthy v. Missouri*. In short, the Court ruled that the five social media users and two state governments who had brought the claim of suppressed free speech could not fully demonstrate that a harm or injury had occurred or could occur, nor that the government fully controlled the social media platform's decision-making processes to restrict or censor user messages.[56] The Court's decision is based upon a "doctrine of standing" (i.e., Article III of the Constitution) that requires that the people filing the suit must have "suffered (or risk imminently suffering) a concrete and particularized injury that is traceable to the opposing party's alleged wrong doing and that the court can redress."[57] By invoking Article III, the Supreme Court is essentially stating it has no jurisdiction to officially decide on whether the First Amendment had been violated because those bringing the case could not demonstrate that harm or injury had occurred or that the government fully controlled the social media platform's decision-making process.[57]

In light of the Supreme Court's ruling, big questions still remain for emergency risk communicators to consider when developing a communication strategy:

- How can emergency risk communicators ensure accurate health information is made available to the public to educate them about health risks?
- What constitutes appropriate (and legal) action to correct false health information during a health emergency?

Quick Response Communications Planning: Identify Communication Objectives, Audiences, Key Messages, and Channels and Develop Communication Products/Materials

During the maintenance phase of a health emergency, it is important to review and update communication objectives, key audiences, key messages, channels, and communication materials and products and update the communications strategy from what was established in the initial phase of the health emergency. Below includes descriptions of each of these topics and examples that are related to the maintenance phase of a health emergency.

In this chapter and Chapters 6 and 9, quick response communication planning will be included to deepen learning regarding the development of initial, maintenance, and recovery messages. The same examples will be used in each chapter so the reader can compare and contrast how quick response planning and key messages change throughout the life cycle of a crisis.

Communication Objectives

A communication objective is a measurable, time-bound, and audience-focused action.[58] Often communication strategies and objectives are designed to create awareness, educate, or persuade the audience.[58]

The following communication objective examples have been updated to reflect objectives that could be aimed for during the maintenance phase. These objectives have been updated from Chapter 6, which focused on objectives for the initial phase of the health emergency.

Example 1

Measles: The county health department will coordinate with school districts and health care provides regarding vaccination interventions and continue to monitor the outbreak throughout the incubation period.

Example 2

Foodborne illness: The county health department will continue to engage in contact tracing and provide updates to the public and partner agencies with new information.

Example 3

Unknown novel infection: The county health department will provide health intervention information and highlight vaccine priority groups.

Audiences

As outlined in Chapters 3 and 4, identify your audiences and audience segments and their information needs. Understanding *which* audience needs *what* type of information will help you to organize and strategize on key messaging. Using the audience segment variables outlined in Chapter 3, the following examples develop audience segments that will receive emergency risk communication messages during the maintenance phase of an emergency.

Example 1 Measles

Audiences continue to include schoolchildren and their parents, adults who have not received the measles, mumps, and rubella (MMR) immunization, school districts officials, and health care providers. For the maintenance phase, as the emergency evolves, two new audiences were added: community-based advocacy groups and elected officials. See Table 7.1 for audience segments for this example.

Table 7.1 Audience segments by risk variable for a measles outbreak

Variable	Definition	Audience segment
Risk level	Who is most at risk based on current health threat?	Schoolchildren (plus parents as children are minors) Adults who have not received the MMR immunization
Location or proximity	Who is closest to the risk or health threat?	Schoolchildren by vaccination status (plus parents as children are minors)
Employment	Is there a particular industry that is affected by the health crisis?	School district officials and health care providers
Values	What does the audience segment value, believe in, and support?	Informed Consent Action Network (group does not support vaccination) Vaccinate Your Family (group does support vaccination)
Organizational affiliations	What organizations do individuals in this segment belong to or associate with?	Local elected officials

Example 2 Foodborne illness

Audiences continue to include but are not limited to fair attendees, fair organizers, food cart vendors, and health care providers. For the maintenance phase, as the emergency evolves, two new audiences were added: fair attendees from other counties in the state and food suppliers who gave products to food vendors. See Table 7.2 for audience segments for this example.

Table 7.2 Audience segments by risk variable for a foodborne illness outbreak

Variable	Definition	Audience segment
Risk level	Who is most at risk based on current health threat?	Fair attendees who ate at food carts
Employment	Is there a particular industry that is affected by the health crisis?	Fair organizers Food cart vendors Health care providers
Location or proximity	Who is closest to the risk or health threat?	Fair attendees from other counties in the state
Employment	Is there a particular industry that is affected by the health crisis?	Food suppliers who gave products to food vendors

Example 3 Unknown novel infection

Audiences still include but are not limited to individuals who live in a particular county and who have underlying health conditions. For the maintenance phase, as the emergency evolves, four new audiences were added: incident management teams from other government agencies, the media, elected officials, and advocacy groups. See Table 7.3 for audience segments for this example.

Table 7.3 Audience segments by risk variable for an unknown novel infection

Variable	Definition	Audience Segment
Risk level	Who is most at risk based on current health threat?	Individuals who live in a particular county
Location or proximity	Who is closest to the risk or health threat?	Individuals who live in a particular county
Health condition	Who has current health conditions that may be at a heightened risk (e.g., age, underlying medical conditions, pregnant)?	Individuals who live in a particular county and who have specific underlying medical conditions
Employment	Is there a particular industry that is affected by the health crisis?	Health care providers
Organizational affiliations	What organizations do individuals in this segment belong to or associate with?	Incident management teams from other government agencies The media Elected officials
Values	What does the audience segment value, believe in, and support?	Anti-Mask League (group does not support wearing masks)

Key Messages

Communication objectives will provide you with a broad strategy about who you want to communicate with and the information that you'd like to provide. Key messages are the specific messages that the agency wants to communicate that are aligned with the communication objectives. For example, if the communication objective is to create awareness about an infectious disease, there are specific key messages that need to be created. During the maintenance phase of an emergency, the key messages include providing deeper risk explanations, providing interventions, making a commitment to the community, and addressing misinformation and rumors.

Example 1 Measles

Key Message 1: Providing deeper risk explanations and health interventions.

- The county health department continues to recommend measles vaccination for those have been exposed and are unsure if they have been vaccinated.
- Vaccinations are available through local health care providers.

Key Message 2: Making a commitment to the community.

- The county health department continues to monitor the situation and will continue to do so for the next 3 weeks.
- At that time the health department and school districts will assess the number of new cases and any potential risks to the community.
- We will continue to keep the public up to date if any guidance changes.

Key Message 3: Addressing rumors and misinformation.

- We have become aware of several rumors regarding vaccines. I'd like to address some of those today.

- o Rumor 1: Patient 0 is an already-vaccinated child or illegal immigrant. Let me clarify that none of the epidemiological evidence we have supports this claim. As we know, there has been a lag in childhood vaccinations due to the pandemic. There has also been a lag in childhood vaccinations due to religious and lifestyle choices. Here at the county health department, we advocate for our community to vaccinate their children to prevent measles.
  - o Rumor 2: The county health department has been hosting measles parties to support community immunity. This is 100% false. The county health department works hard to prevent infectious diseases from spreading in our community through promoting vaccinations. We very much advocate for our community to vaccinate their children to prevent measles.
- Finally, I'd like to close today by offering our measles facts and myths website: countyhealthmeaslesfacts.gov.
- We will continue to update this page and provide the most accurate information as it becomes available.

Example 2 Foodborne illness

Key Message 1: Providing deeper risk explanations and health interventions.

- The county health department has been in contact with neighboring counties and is learning about how this outbreak has grown. It was initially thought that one of our food vendors was the source of the outbreak.
- We have now learned that our outbreak is linked to a larger outbreak at CDC.
- Due to the increase in numbers, including in other counties, and being a part of the national outbreak, we have established an Incident Command Structure to coordinate our efforts.
- We'd like to encourage people who ate at the county fair to monitor for symptoms including:
  - o Diarrhea, which may be bloody
  - o Nausea
  - o Abdominal pain
  - o Vomiting
  - o Dehydration
  - o Low-grade fever (sometimes)[59]
- Please contact the county health department at 123-567-8899 to report your symptoms and to provide additional information to our contact tracers.
- Seek emergency medical assistance if you have severe symptoms, such as severe abdominal pain or watery diarrhea that turns very bloody within 24 hours.[59]

Key Message 2: Making a commitment to the community.

- We are working with our neighboring counties to continue to identify ill individuals in our community and understand how our outbreak is linked to the national outbreak.
- We are in contact with CDC, and CDC will be sending support to help us quickly identify the source of this outbreak.

- We will continue to work to find the source of the outbreak and work with our food vendors to ensure proper food handling procedures are followed.

Key Message 3: Addressing rumors and misinformation.

- We have become aware of a rumor regarding potentially tainted local tomatoes. I'd like to address that rumor today.
  - Rumor: The source of the outbreak is a local supplier of tomatoes. Let me clarify that none of the epidemiological evidence we have supports this claim. As we know, our outbreak is linked to a larger national outbreak. One of the local farms that does supply tomatoes to the food cart vendors does not have a national distribution. So, at this time, based on the epidemiological data we have, our local tomato farmers are not considered the source of the outbreak.

Example 3   Unknown novel infection

Key Message 1: Providing deeper risk explanations and health interventions.

- Today we'd like to confirm that the emerging virus in our state is linked to the avian influenza virus that first started in the eastern part of the United States.
- We are in contact with CDC, and CDC is monitoring this situation very closely.
- It appears that the virus is mutating and is able to spread from human to human through close, prolonged, and unmasked contact with an ill individual.
- Symptoms include fever, pink eye, sore throat, and coughing.
- We'd like to recommend individuals with underlying medical conditions and pregnant women wash their hands frequently, maintain a 6-foot distance when out in public areas with others, and wear masks when in public spaces.
- There is no vaccine available for this particular virus. CDC, FDA, and the White House are looking into vaccine development for this influenza virus. The seasonal influenza vaccine will not provide protection against this virus.

Key Message 2: Making a commitment to the community.

- This outbreak comes so soon after COVID-19, so many of us are feeling shocked that we could be here again.
- The county health department pledges to be here with our community throughout this outbreak. As the Greek historian Thucydides wrote, "The bravest are surely those who have the clearest vision of what is before them, glory and danger alike, and yet notwithstanding, go out to meet it."
- We have been here before, we made it through, and we will make it through again.

Key Message 3: Addressing rumors and misinformation.

- We have become aware of a rumor regarding vaccinations. I'd like to address that rumor today.
  - Rumor: The seasonal influenza vaccine will work against this virus. Let me clarify that the regular seasonal influenza vaccine we get every year will not work against this virus. This current outbreak is a new and mutated strain. This is similar to what happened during COVID-19. CDC, FDA, and the White House are looking into creating a new vaccine that will offer protection against this virus.

Channels

As outlined in Chapter 5, think about what channels are available to you for sharing information and what audiences use which channels.

Example 1 Measles

Consider what channels are available and what would be the best way to communicate health information so as to reach the audiences segments that have been identified. See Table 7.4 for channel identification for this example.

Table 7.4 Communication channels for each audience segment for a measles outbreak

Audience segment	Communication channel
Schoolchildren (plus parents as children are minors) Adults who have not received the MMR immunization	Email to parents Email to school workers School website Health department website Health department social media channels Media relations
Schoolchildren by vaccination status (plus parents as children are minors)	Email to parents
School district officials and health care providers	Conference calls or virtual meetings with school officials Health Alert Network message for clinicians

Example 2 Foodborne illness

Consider what channels are available and what would be the best way to communicate health information so as to reach the audiences segments that have been identified. See Table 7.5 for channel identification for this example.

Table 7.5 Communication channels for each audience segment for a foodborne illness outbreak

Audience segment	Communication channel
Fair attendees who ate at food carts	Media relations Fair social media channels
Fair organizers Food cart vendors Health care providers	Face-to-face meetings Emails Health Alert Network message for clinicians

Example 3 Unknown novel infection

Consider what channels are available and what would be the best way to communicate health information so as to reach the audiences segments that have been identified. See Table 7.6 for channel identification for this example.

Table 7.6 Communication channels for each audience segment for an unknown novel infection

Audience segment	Communication channel
Individuals who live in a particular county	Media relations Health department website Health department social media channels

Table 7.6 (cont.)

Audience segment	Communication channel
Individuals who live in a particular county	Media relations Health department website Health department social media channels
Individuals who live in a particular county and who have specific underlying medical conditions	Media relations Health department website Health department social media channels
Health care providers	Health Alert Network message

Communication Products

As outlined in Chapter 5, think about what communication materials need to be developed, such as talking points, web page copy, and visuals such as charts and graphs.

Example 1 Measles

Table 7.7 outlines the types of communication products that would need to be created for each communication channel.

Table 7.7 Communication products that can be sent on communication channels for a measles outbreak

Communication channel	Communication product
Email to parents Email to school workers School website Health department website Health department social media channels Media relations	Letter and email copy about outbreak Web page copy Social media messages (including visuals, hashtags, and web URLs for more information) Talking points
Email to parents Conference calls or virtual meetings with school officials Health Alert Network message for clinicians	Letter and email copy about outbreak Talking points Health Alert Network message copy

Example 2 Foodborne illness

Table 7.8 outlines the types of communication products that would need to be created for each communication channel.

Table 7.8 Communication products that can be sent on communication channels for a foodborne illness outbreak

Communication channel	Communication product
Media relations Fair social media channels	Talking points Social media messages (including visuals, hashtags, and web URLs for more information)
Face-to-face meetings Emails Health Alert Network message for clinicians	Talking points Email copy Health Alert Network message copy

Example 3 Unknown novel infection

Table 7.9 outlines the types of communication products that would need to be created for each communication channel.

Table 7.9 Communication products that can be sent on communication channels for an unknown novel infection

Communication channel	Communication product
Media relations Health department website Health department social media channels	Talking points Web page copy Social media messages (including visuals, hashtags, and web URLs for more information)
Media relations Health department website Health department social media channels	Talking points Web page copy Social media messages (including visuals, hashtags, and web URLs for more information)
Media relations Health department website Health department social media channels	Talking points Web page copy Social media messages (including visuals, hashtags, and web URLs for more information)
Health Alert Network message	Health Alert Network message copy

Key Tips for Spokespeople, Partner Agencies, and Call Centers

During every phase of a health emergency, spokespeople, partner agencies, and call centers need to receive consistent and coordinated information from the health agency. Here is some key tips for those who are the spokespeople or who work at partner agencies call centers during the maintenance phase of a health emergency:

Spokespeople: Ask the communications team to send you a copy of the media monitoring report. Stay on top of media trends, thought leader conversations, and public sentiment. Be mindful of public activities and ensure that, as a public figure, you follow any health guidance that is recommended for the public. During the COVID-19 response, many spokespeople and local leaders became news stories when they did not adhere to local public health guidance, including not hosting parties of six or more individuals or not wearing masks in public.

Partner agencies: Continue to participate in Incident Command System meetings and webinars. Obtain a copy of the communication plan and understand what messages your agency could be amplifying.

Call centers: Provide a metrics report about the amount and type of calls received by the call center. Work with the communications team if there are gaps in messaging. For example, if you are receiving many calls about the health intervention, check whether the public messaging about the health intervention is adequate. If not, bolster the public messaging and update the call center's prepared responses.

Theory Callout: Rumor Management Framework

The rumor management framework is not a specific theory as such, but Kate Starbird and her colleagues at the University of Washington's Center for an Informed Public have been studying rumors in digital environments for decades.[44,60] Starbird's work is important to emergency risk communicators because she looks at rumors specifically within the context of crises and emergencies, providing a unique perspective on how uncertainty or a government's lack of openness in public messaging can create and fuel rumors.

Spiro and Starbird created a framework to help assess whether a rumor will go viral (see Table 7.10). The framework looks at three high-level categories: information and event conditions; contextual features; and systems effects. Within information and event conditions, there are two dimensions to consider: uncertainty regarding the evolving emergency and whether there is diminished trust in official information providers. Emergency risk communicators can review messaging and see whether key messages have addressed the uncertainty regarding the evolving health emergency by sharing what the agency knows, what the agency does not know, and what the agency is doing to find more information to mitigate the health impact. If key messages have addressed uncertainty, consider whether the agency's reputation or trust with the community has been diminished. If lack of trust is a factor, consider how to leverage partner agencies to share key information and make small steps toward repairing trust in the agency. For example, ensure that the agency follows through on each of the commitments made to the public to address health emergencies.

The second category of contextual features includes significance/impact, familiarity/repetition, novelty, emotional valence, compelling-ness of evidence, and participatory potential. Each of these dimensions looks at the context of the health emergency. The key takeaways here are how impactful the rumor is on a particular group of people, how familiar the information is relating to the rumor, what level of novelty the rumor has, whether the rumor invokes strong reactions, whether there is compelling evidence (e.g., videos and pictures), and what the participatory nature of the rumor is. All of these factors play into how the rumor is spread. This information is important for emergency risk communicators to consider when correcting false information and providing scientifically accurate information.

Finally, the third category of systems effects looks at the position of the rumor within the social network and algorithmic or network manipulation. Looking at the position of the rumor spreader within the social network will provide a sense of how many followers this individual has and the potential research of their message. The algorithms underlying social media platforms might then allow a rumor to go viral if the system is set up to spread the post based on how many people interact with it.

This framework can help emergency risk communicators to understand why rumors emerge, providing them with an opportunity to respond to and correct false information.

Table 7.10 Rumor threat framework, which helps us to assess whether an event will generate viral rumors and which rumors will spread

GROUP	DIMENSIONS	DESCRIPTION
INFORMATION AND EVENT CONDITIONS	Uncertainty	As events (infections, train wrecks, elections) unfold, uncertainty powers both generation and spread of rumors. For specific rumors, ambiguous evidence will lead to more spread.
	Diminished Trust	Diminished trust in "official" information providers (government, media, etc.) pushes people toward more informal communication channels, catalyzing rumoring.
CONTEXTUAL FEATURES	Significance / Impact	The strength of a specific rumor is proportional to its importance in the lives of those spreading it. Events with greater potential impact on people's lives will catalyze more, and more viral, rumors.
	Familiarity / Repetition	A common set of building blocks underlie many rumors, which may make them resonate with familiarity. This, plus repetition, can enhance plausibility and boost spread.
	Novelty	People spread rumors to inform and entertain. Crises and other emergent events provide novel content that can be assembled into rumors.
	Emotional Valence	Rumors that stimulate strong emotions – including anger, fear, and outrage – will be more likely to spread. Events that stimulate strong emotions may catalyze the creation of viral rumors.
	Compelling-ness of Evidence	Evidence that piques interest and adds tangibility – e.g., first-person accounts, photos, and videos – will catalyze the creation and enhance virality of rumors.
	Participatory Potential	Rumors that allow people to participate – to add evidence or share their experiences and interpretations – are likely to spread further.
SYSTEM EFFECTS	Position within the Social Network	Social networks shape the spread of rumors. Rumors will spread further if they reach central or high-audience nodes in a network or move from one network to another (e.g., a rumor in an anti-vaccine network jumps into ethnonationalist networks).
	Algorithmic or Network Manipulation	In online environments, rumors can be intentionally seeded or spread for strategic gain. Often those efforts game underlying networks and recommendation systems.

Source: Kate Starbird and Emma S. Spiro. Reproduced with permission from *Issues in Science and Technology*, 2023.

2022 Mpox Outbreak in Louisiana
Emma Caroli de la Rosa, MPH

Overview
Monkeypox, later abbreviated as Mpox, is a virus in the same family as smallpox with similar but more mild symptoms and a lower mortality rate. The most identifiable symptoms of Mpox are a rash that can appear on a person's hands, feet, face, or genitals, with the appearance of pimples that scab over. Individuals with the Mpox virus may also experience symptoms such as fever, chills, swollen lymph nodes, exhaustion, headaches, and other flu-like effects.[61] Mpox is spread through skin-to-skin contact with an individual who has the virus. It is not an STI, but sexual contact was how the disease was most often transmitted during the 2022 outbreak. The best way to prevent transmission is to avoid close contact with people who have the virus and to get the two-dose vaccination.

The vaccination for Mpox – JYNNEOS – was originally approved in 2019. It is administered through two subcutaneous injections over 4 weeks to adults (18 years and old) who are at risk for Mpox transmission.[62] CDC found that in the United States individuals who received two doses of the JYNNEOS vaccine had an 86% vaccine effectiveness rate in terms of preventing against Mpox, and individuals who received one dose had a 75% vaccine effectiveness rate. Getting just one dose of the vaccination is associated with a 7.4-fold decrease in likelihood of infection.[63]

The 2022, a US outbreak of Mpox began with a case reported in Boston on May 17, after an individual traveled to the United States from Nigeria.[64] The outbreak reached its peak in July, with 2,891 cases reported in the country. Almost all of the cases were males (99%), disproportionately affecting men who have sex with men (MSM), with 94% of the transmissions associated with sexual contact between MSM.[64] Mpox was declared a public health emergency by the US Health and Human Services Department on August 4, 2022.[64]

The most at-risk population for the virus was gay and bisexual men, as well as any other MSM. Louisiana has high rates of new HIV incidence and STI incidence: the third highest in the country for chlamydia and gonorrhea diagnoses and sixth highest in the country for HIV.[65] Mpox is not often deadly, but it has worse impacts on people who are immunocompromised. Half of all people living with HIV in Louisiana have an AIDS diagnosis.[65] Given the trends of STIs and HIV in Louisiana, the demographics, and the known information about the Mpox outbreak, it was of extreme importance for public health officials in Louisiana to rapidly address this emerging health concern.

There was a focus on the two highly populous cities of Baton Rouge and New Orleans by the Louisiana Department of Health (LDH) to get at-risk individuals vaccinated. These two cities are the most densely populated in Louisiana, and they also have the highest concentrations of STI and HIV cases.[65] In New Orleans there is an annual gathering in early September for the LGBTQ community called Southern Decadence. People come from all over the Southern United States to celebrate the Southern Decadence festival, which is similar to a Pride-type festival, in the historic French Quarter. LDH and local agencies targeted New Orleans to prevent the spread of Mpox before and during the event. Free vaccination events were held in major LGBTQ hotspots in New Orleans on August 30 and in Baton Rouge on August 27.[65] In total, there were 307 Mpox cases reported in Louisiana during this outbreak, with the main concentration of them (103 cases) reported from the greater New Orleans area.[65]

Timeline of Key Events
- May 12, 2022: Outbreak begins in the United States with first case reported.
- May 23 2022: CDC launches emergency response, expanding testing and prevention.

- July 7, 2022: First case identified in Louisiana.
- August 2022: US Department of Health and Human Services declares Mpox a public health emergency.
- August 9, 2022: JYNNEOS vaccine is approved for emergency authorization for adults determined at risk for Mpox.
- August 24, 2022: Vaxxtravaganza, a free vaccination event, is held in the French Quarter of New Orleans.
- August 27, 2022: LDH holds first vaccination event in Baton Rouge.
- August 30, 2022: Southern Decadence Health Hub begins providing free Mpox vaccines in New Orleans.
- August 30, 2022: LDH expands vaccination inclusion criteria.
- August–September 2022: 13,000 vaccination doses given in Louisiana.
- September 1–5, 2022: Southern Decadence festival held in New Orleans.
- January 2023: Outbreak totals are reported as 307 in Louisiana and 30,400 in the whole of the United States.
- February 22, 2023: LDH Mpox dashboard on its website is paused.

CERC Principles and Phases

CDC provides agencies with guidance on how to communicate effectively through its CERC manual and guidelines. The six core principles of CERC are Be First, Be Right, Be Credible, Express Empathy, Promote Action, and Show Respect.[66] Be First means that an agency must address a crisis as soon as possible. There may not be a full picture available in the initial phase when this principle is demonstrated, so the agency should provide what information is available and indicate what information they are trying to find. To Be Right, an agency must explain that what any information it provides is proven to be true. It is acceptable to say that there are no answers on certain aspects of a crisis. To adhere to this principle, the agency should explain what is being done to find out more about unknowns. An agency can Be Credible by telling only the truth of what is known. Even if the truth might cause a reaction of fear or panic, it is best practice to get ahead of the information and not hide it from the public. The principle of Express Empathy is important especially at the beginning of a crisis. It helps to build trust and acknowledges the reactions that community members are having. To help with the difficult feelings people are experiencing during such times, it is helpful to Promote Action. This involves giving the community a task to complete to help them stay safe. This can be as simple as providing reminders regarding proper handwashing techniques, or it can be more complex, such as advice on evacuating the safety of a location. Following the principle of Show Respect enables an audience to trust that the agency is working for them.

The different CERC principles have varying levels of importance at different times during a crisis. The phases of a crisis identified by CDC are the precrisis, initial, maintenance, resolution, and evaluation phases.[66] In the precrisis phase an agency is preparing plans, strengthening and maintaining connections with community partners and stakeholders, and developing systems and recommendations for a crisis. In the initial phase the crisis has just been identified. All of the six CERC principals are to be demonstrated in an agency's initial crisis response message. The message should give as much risk information as is available at the time, recommend any known actions to protect community members, and commit to being with the community throughout the crisis. In the maintenance phase messages can focus on segments of higher-risk populations and be tailored accordingly. There will be more information available at this stage, and the agency should be showing support in their responses to the crisis. The important CERC principles during this phase are Be Right, Be Credible, Show Respect, and Promote Action. In the resolution phase the crisis has been mitigated or resolved, and so it is time to acknowledge what the agency and community did well and what they can do better next time. This may involve passing new legislation, celebrating achievements, evaluating the agency's long-term impact on the community, and moving toward the new normal. Be First and Express Empathy are less important during this stage than the other four CERC principles. The evaluation phase is often occurs within in the recovery phase. The agency can conduct a hotwash or after-action review, in which the response team reviews the actions it took during the crisis and how well these actions worked, as well as what could be done better next time. Stakeholders should be invited to give feedback and be given the information gathered during this evaluation.[66]

Analysis of the CERC Principles

Initial Message
The first time LDH acknowledged Mpox was in a media release on July 7, 2022, when the first case was identified in the state.[67] This communication can be found as an announcement on LDH's website and Instagram and Facebook feeds, and it was briefed to the media on the same day. The live delivery of the message was uploaded and can still be found on YouTube.[68] The statement acknowledges what LDH knows and what it is working to find out. It gives information on what Mpox is, how it spreads, its symptoms, and how to prevent its transmission. Included on the web page announcement is a link to the situation summary and facts for sexually active persons who are identified as being at risk. There is no contact information given on the web page, but such information is communicated at the end of the live briefing. The following is an extract from this initial message:

> The Louisiana Department of Health (LDH) is reporting the first detected case of monkeypox infection in a Louisiana resident. This individual is from LDH Region 1 (Orleans, Plaquemines, Jefferson, St. Bernard). In addition, an out-of-state resident visiting Louisiana also tested positive for monkeypox. No further information will be shared about these cases to protect the patients' privacy. LDH WILL HOLD A TECHNICAL BRIEFING FOR MEDIA THIS AFTERNOON TO DISCUSS MONKEYPOX IN LOUISIANA. ADDITIONAL DETAILS ARE FORTHCOMING. There are likely more undiagnosed human cases of monkeypox existing in Louisiana than have been formally tested and identified to date.
>
> LDH is working closely with the U.S. Centers for Disease Control and Prevention (CDC) and the patients' healthcare providers to identify and notify individuals in Louisiana who may have been in contact with the patients while they were infectious. LDH has kept providers in Louisiana up to date, urged providers to be on the lookout for symptoms in patients, and shared specific monkeypox reporting and specimen submission guidance. Since May 2022, 605 monkeypox cases have been identified in 36 states. Globally, more than 7,200 cases have been reported from 54 countries; the case count continues to rise daily. Information about international cases is available from the WORLD HEALTH ORGANIZATION and information about U.S. cases is available from the CDC. There have been no deaths in the U.S. to date.[67]

While LDH was successful in reporting the first case of Mpox in the state in a timely manner, there are no announcements accessible showing that it had addressed the Mpox outbreak before it reached Louisiana. The outbreak disproportionality affected gay and bisexual men and other MSM and was mostly spread through intimate contact. Since Louisiana ranks in the top three states in the United States for chlamydia and gonorrhea infections and ranks sixth highest in terms of new HIV diagnoses,[69] LDH could have addressed the outbreak before it reached Louisiana given its similarity to STIs in terms of its potential transmission. In a media release on June 28, 2022, CDC advised public health agencies to prioritize gay and bisexual men and all other MSM to engage in Mpox testing and vigilance.[70] LDH could have messaged this community about engaging in such vigilance once the virus was confirmed to have entered the United States but before it had been identified in Louisiana.

Therefore, while the message did not necessarily achieve the CERC principle of Be First, it does demonstrate the principles of Be Right and Be Credible by identifying the first case in Louisiana, and it also demonstrates Promote Action by advising providers to be on the lookout for Mpox symptoms. The recorded live briefing of the announcement demonstrates that Dr. Joseph Kanter, who delivered the risk message, showed respect and empathy. He reassured the audience in this message that this virus would not be as serious as the COVID-19 pandemic. He also spoke about the population that was at highest risk and what they should look for regarding the symptoms of Mpox, which promoted action in the target population. The full message demonstrated LDH's commitment to continuing to update community members on Mpox, as LDH expected to identify more cases in the state.[67]

Maintenance Messages

LDH ramped up its maintenance message response once the JYNNEOS vaccine was approved for use for preventing Mpox in August. FDA approved the vaccine for those aged 18 years and older who were at high risk for Mpox on August 9, 2022. The social media accounts for LDH show at least weekly postings about Mpox vaccine events and risk communication messages that were occurring as early as August 27, less than 3 weeks after FDA approved the vaccine for emergency use. The first vaccine event documented at which the Mpox vaccine was distributed was on August 27 at three LGBTQ-centered bars in the Baton Rouge area. These events were held at night in places where the priority population was likely to be, showing respect for the community by meeting them where they were at. They also demonstrated LDH's commitment to the community and to promoting action. The announcement of this trio of events was accompanied by a risk description explaining the potential for contracting Mpox through different behaviors (see Figure 7.3). For example, the most risky behaviors are described as "direct contact with infectious rash, scabs, or body fluids; intimate contact; all forms of sexual contact."[71] The least risky behaviors listed include but are not limited to "dancing at a party outside with mostly clothed people; co-worker to co-worker transmission; trying on clothing at a store; or touching a doorknob."[71] This chart also used a color-coding system to categorize the behavior by risk level. For example, the riskiest behaviors are color-coded red, then risky behaviors are color-coded orange, behaviors that have a possible risk are color-coded yellow, and the least risky behaviors are color-coded green.

This post conveys the CERC principles of Be Right and Be Credible by providing information on how Mpox is transmitted, specifically regarding what activities represent the lowest to highest risk of transmission. It promotes action by encouraging individuals to participate in less risky activities, by promoting the Southern Decadence Health Hub, and by giving multiple forms of contact to get further information. The post shows respect to the community by trusting them to make decisions for themselves regarding what activities they will or will not participate in. Instead of simply telling people not to do an activity because it is a high-risk one, this graphic acknowledges that people might still choose to engage in risky behaviors and entrusts them with the knowledge to make their own decisions. This hits the CERC maintenance message points of "ensure community understands ongoing risks and actions they can take to reduce risk or harm."[66]

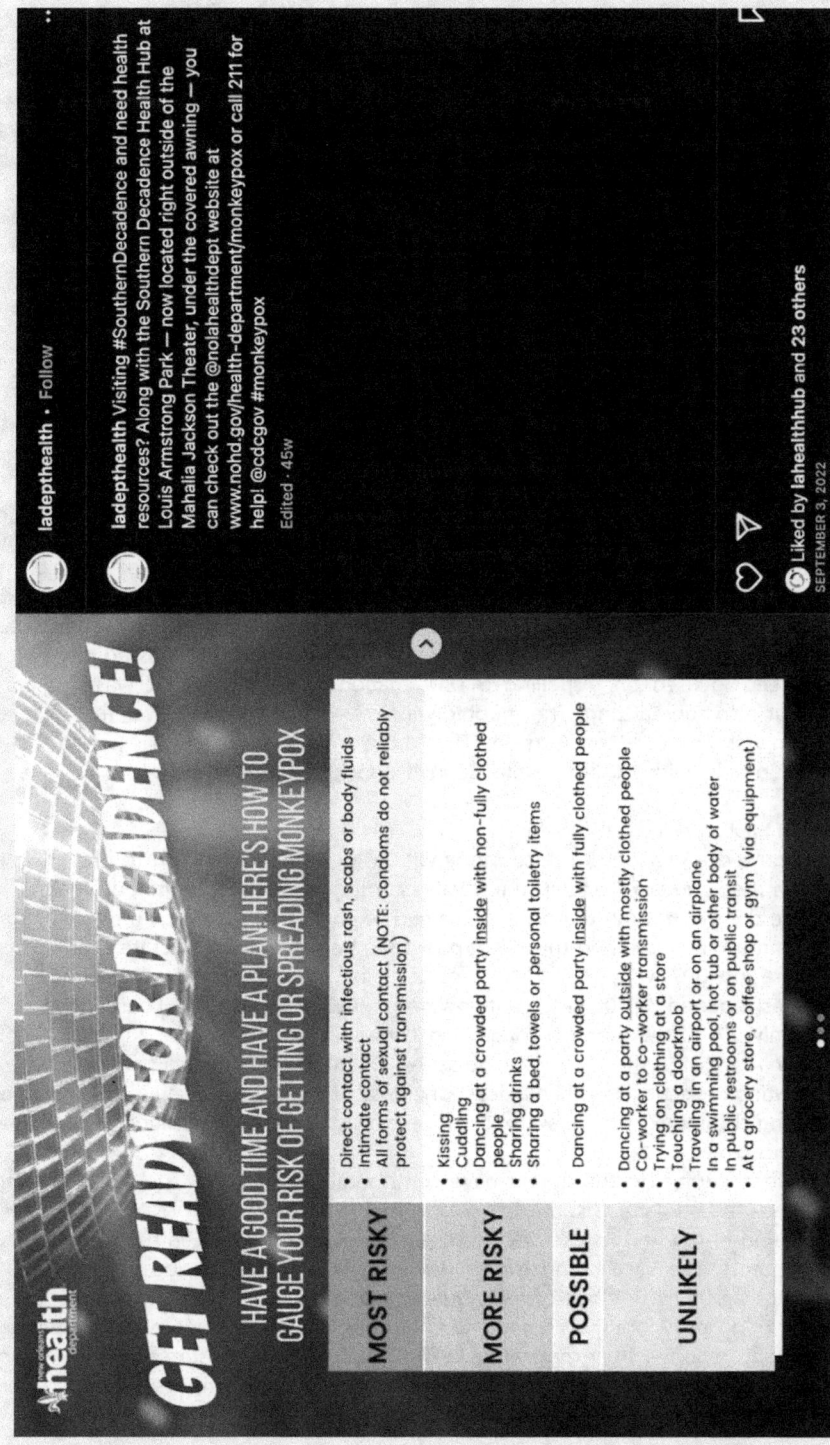

Figure 7.2 New Orleans Department of Health social media graphic that explains the health risk of getting or spreading Mpox at the Decadence event. Reproduced with permission from the Louisiana Department of Health.

The highlighting of the Southern Decadence Health Hub by LDH was a timely and targeted response to the outbreak. In the city of New Orleans specifically, the Mpox outbreak came just before Southern Decadence, a large in-person event for the LGBTQ community. Since this event would involve a large gathering of individuals who were most at risk for Mpox, LDH quickly put together vaccination events for the Decadence crowd (Figure 7.2). On August 30, LDH announced that the Southern Decadence Health Hub would begin its partnership with CDC, and vaccination events would begin on September 1 in the French Quarter where the festival events would be occurring.[72] This presence at the event during the Mpox outbreak was crucial to showing commitment to the community and promoting action to prevent the spread of the virus.[73]

These vaccine events showed respect for the at-risk community, helping to build their trust in the agency. They were held in locations where this population was already going for the festivities. The services were free and included other health services that the population might need, representing a further showing of respect. Health units and community clinics in each parish were made available for testing and vaccination, including for people with no insurance.[73] The branding was inviting and nonstigmatizing.

A "Vaxxtravaganza" event was held in the week leading up to Decadence in the same location, providing free Mpox vaccinations. The staff present for this event also tested for STIs and HIV.[72,73] This event was announced to local press publications, thereby helping to reach those audiences who might not look at LDH's website or social media pages. The number of events and their availability demonstrated a commitment to promoting action.

A further way in which LDH showed the CERC principles Be Right and Be Credible was by attempting to dispel any myths surrounding Mpox. An image posted on LDH's Instagram feed focused on dispelling misinformation about Mpox that was not only incorrect but also stigmatizing. The graphic was in a question-and-answer format, and the question was whether Mpox was an STI, and the answer – "No, Mpox is not an STI" – was written in bold, with a longer explanation also included.[74]

Discussion of Implications

Louisiana showed a swift response to Mpox with a focus on vaccination to prevent the spread. With the Southern Decadence festival occurring at the peak of the outbreak, LDH chose to see the event as an opportunity instead of panicking. The focus on vaccination and risk communication around this event proved to be successful. The state's total cases in 2022 were just 307, with 103 of these cases being reported in New Orleans.[65] The United States reported 34,400 cases nationwide in 2022, meaning that Louisiana's cases made up only 1% of the national total.[64] In Louisiana, as of February 20, 2023, 9,448 individuals had initiated the Mpox vaccine series. The Mpox vaccine is a two-dose series. People initiating the series have had at least one dose of the two-dose series. A majority of those seeking the Mpox vaccine were in the southeast region of Louisiana, where New Orleans is located.[75]

There are a few factors that might have contributed to the LDH's success in limiting cases of Mpox in Louisiana, a state that was at high risk for this outbreak. LDH's timely communication of risk and its vaccination response seem to have been the most significant contributors. The vaccination events were wildly successful; a local news station reported lines around the block of individuals waiting for vaccination, with the events running out of doses before their scheduled end times. The reporter interviewed queuing individuals who reported their motivation to limit their risk of exposure to Mpox, which, despite being a fairly novel virus, seemed to be familiar to the attendees already.[76] This shows the success of LDH's risk communication campaign.

LDH emphasized the CERC principles of Be Credible, Be Right, and, most of all, Promote Action. The messages were focused on proven credible actions that the at-risk population could take to prevent Mpox transmission. The communication was respectful to the community in that is engaged in nonstigmatizing messaging and met the priority population where they were at. Having vaccinations available for free and advertising for people who were uninsured to come to a parish or community clinic also showed respect. However, there was not very much empathy expressed in this messaging, and the initial message could have been sent out sooner. Nevertheless, it appears that LDH's approach worked well. It could improve its responses even further by putting more emphasis on these two CERC principles of Be First and Express Empathy.

End-of-Chapter Reflection Questions

1. Write your own maintenance messages for an infectious disease outbreak and identify core maintenance message components. Compare and contrast your message to one created by a local health agency.
2. Consider how these maintenance messages address risks by audience segment. What additional information do you need from your epidemiologists? How would you share and explain risk information on a dashboard on your agency's website?
3. Consider how you would use community stakeholders and partners to help get these messages out.
4. Consider how you would disseminate your maintenance messages on different channels. Which three channels would you use and why? Are these the same as the initial message channels? Why or why not?
5. Rumors and misinformation are major challenges during health emergencies. Review how your agency has dealt with rumors and misinformation in the past. What are the strengths and weaknesses of those previous activities?
6. Consider hosting a series of internal listening sessions with public health staff on infodemics and misinformation. Discuss the challenges of rumors and misinformation during health emergencies. Discuss potential opportunities for the health agency to help it successfully navigate rumors and misinformation moving forward.

References

1. Coronavirus disease (COVID-19) pandemic: Overview. *World Health Organization*. 2024. www.who.int/europe/emergencies/situations/covid-19 (Accessed April 21, 2024).
2. Cubanski J, Kates J, Tolbert J, Guth M, Pollitz K, Freed M. What Happens When COVID-19 Emergency Declarations End? Implications for Coverage, Costs, and Access. *Kaiser Family Foundation*. 2023. www.kff.org/coronavirus-covid-19/issue-brief/what-happens-when-covid-19-emergency-declarations-end-implications-for-coverage-costs-and-access/#:~:text=May%2011%2C%202023.-,On%20Jan.,to%20the%20COVID%2D19%20pandemic (Accessed April 21, 2024).
3. CDC. *Crisis and Emergency Risk Communication October 2018*. Atlanta, GA, CDC, 2018.
4. Populations and Vulnerabilities. *Centers for Disease Control and Prevention*. n.d. www.cdc.gov/nceh/tracking/topics/PopulationsVulnerabilities.htm (Accessed April 21, 2024).

5. Wingate MS, Perry EC, Campbell PH, David P, Weist EM. Identifying and Protecting Vulnerable Populations in Public Health Emergencies: Addressing Gaps in Education and Training. *Pub Health Rep* 2007;**122**(3):422–26.

6. Chin M. Populations at Risk: A Critical Need for Research, Funding, and Action. *J Gen Intern Med* 2005;**20**(5):448–49.

7. RSV in Adults. *American Lung Association*. 2024. www.lung.org/lung-health-diseases/lung-disease-lookup/rsv/rsv-in-adults (Accessed April 21, 2024).

8. Amer F, Khalil HES, Elahmady M, ElBadawy NE, Zahran WA, Abdelnasser M, et al. Mpox: Risks and Approaches to Prevention. *J Infect Public Health* 2023;**16**(6):901–10.

9. Respiratory Syncytial Virus (RSV). *New York City Health*. n.d. www.nyc.gov/site/doh/health/health-topics/respiratory-syncytial-virus.page (Accessed April 21, 2024).

10. Remarks by President Trump, Vice President Pence, and Members of the Coronavirus Task Force in Press Briefing. *Trump White House*. 2020. https://trumpwhitehouse.archives.gov/briefings-statements/remarks-president-trump-vice-president-pence-members-coronavirus-task-force-press-briefing-4 (Accessed April 14, 2024).

11. Yeh M, Jewell R, Hu MY. Stereotype Processing's Effect on the Impact of the Myth/Fact Message Format and the Role of Personal Relevance. *Psychol Market* 2013;**30**(1):36–45.

12. Coronavirus disease (COVID-19) advice for the public: Mythbusters. *World Health Organization*. 2022. www.who.int/emergencies/diseases/novel-coronavirus-2019/advice-for-public/myth-busters (Accessed April 14, 2024).

13. Managing Misinformation in the Media. *Centers for Disease Control and Prevention*. 2017. https://emergency.cdc.gov/cerc/cerccorner/article_121616.asp (Accessed April 14, 2024).

14. Responding to Rumors and Misinformation. *Centers for Disease Control and Prevention*. 2017. https://emergency.cdc.gov/cerc/cerccorner/article_072216.asp (Accessed April 14, 2024).

15. Governor Bryan Addresses False Rumors Regarding USVI and COVID-19 Vaccine. *Government of the Virgin Islands*. n.d. https://doh.vi.gov/governor-bryan-addresses-false-rumors-regarding-usvi-and-covid-19-vaccine (Accessed April 14, 2024).

16. Martin D. Inside the Operation Warp Speed effort to get Americans a COVID-19 vaccine. *CBS News*. 2020. www.cbsnews.com/news/covid-19-vaccine-distribution-60-minutes-2020-11-08 (Accessed April 14, 2024).

17. Lalani H, DiResta R, Baron R, Scales C. Addressing Viral Medical Rumors and False or Misleading Information. *Ann Intern Med* 2023;**176**(8):1113–20.

18. About Us. *This Is Our Shot*. n.d. https://thisisourshot.info/about-us (Accessed April 14, 2024).

19. #Vacunateya. 2024. https://vacunateya.com (Accessed April 14, 2024).

20. Two cases of meningococcemia confirmed. *University of Oregon*. 2015. https://around.uoregon.edu/content/two-cases-meningococcemia-confirmed (Accessed April 14, 2024).

21. Herriman R. University of Oregon outbreak: 3rd meningitis case reported. *Outbreak News Today*. 2015. https://outbreaknewstoday.com/university-of-oregon-outbreak-3rd-meningitis-case-reported-25954 (Accessed April 14, 2024).

22. Sherwood C. Meningococcemia outbreak sickens three at the University of Oregon. *Reuters*. 2015. www.reuters.com/article/idUSKBN0LF027 (Accessed April 14, 2024).

23. CD Summary: MENINGOCOCCUS SEROGROUP B: STILL THERE, STILL DANGEROUS. Oregon Health Authority. *Oregon Public Health Division*.

2015. www.oregon.gov/oha/PH/
DISEASESCONDITIONS/
COMMUNICABLEDISEASE/
CDSUMMARYNEWSLETTER/
Documents/2015/ohd6404.pdf (Accessed
April 14, 2024).

24   Oregon tumbler Lauren Jones suddenly
passes away. *Statesman Journal.* 2015.
www.statesmanjournal.com/story/
sports/college/univ-oregon/2015/02/17/
oregon-tumbler-lauren-jones-suddenly-
passes-away/23597259/ (Accessed April
1, 2024).

25   Seeger M, Sellnow T, Ulmer R.
*Communication and Organizational
Crisis.* London, Bloomsbury Academic,
2003.

26   Capitano B, Dillon K, LeDuc A, Atkinson
B, Burman C. Experience Implementing a
University-Based Mass Immunization
Program in Response to a Meningococcal
B Outbreak. *Hum Vaccin Immun*
2019;**15**(3):717–24.

27   Sixth U of O meningococcal disease case
confirmed. *Lincoln County Register.* 2015.
www.thenewsguard.com/regional/sixth-
u-of-o-meningococcal-disease-case-
confirmed/article_55727d54-ce48-11e4-
a1c0-c738365a7ee1.html#:~:text=Oregon
%20Health%20Authority%20officials%
20say,before%20or%20during%20spring
%20break (Accessed April 1, 2024).

28   Aleccia J. After deadly outbreak, Oregon
school to do mass vaccinations. *The
Seattle Times.* 2015. www.seattletimes
.com/seattle-news/health/university-of-
oregon-to-do-mass-vaccinations-in-
deadly-outbreak/ (Accessed April 1,
2024).

29   Vanderford ML, Nastoff T, Telfer JL,
Bonzo SE. Emergency Communication
Challenges in Response to Hurricane
Katrina: Lessons from the Centers for
Disease Control and Prevention. *J Appl
Commun Res* 2007;**35**(1):9–25.

30   Vuocolo S, Balmer P, Gruber WC, Jansen
KU, Anderson AS, Perez JL, York LJ.
Vaccination Strategies for the Prevention
of Meningococcal Disease. *Hum Vaccin
Immun* 2018;**14**(5):1203–15.

31   Candrilli S, Kurosky S. The Response to
and Cost of Meningococcal Disease
Outbreaks in University Campus Settings:
A Case Study in Oregon, United States.
RTI Press. 2019. www.ncbi.nlm.nih.gov/
books/NBK565440 (Accessed April 14,
2024).

32   Liedle C. The organism has basically
diffused throughout the university
campus. *KVAL News Channel 13.* 2015.
https://kval.com/news/local/the-
organism-has-basically-diffused-
throughout-the-university-campus
(Accessed April 1, 2024).

33   Hanrahan M. 6th student in Oregon
infected with meningitis bacteria. *USA
Today.* 2015. www.usatoday.com/story/
news/nation/2015/03/19/meningitis-
outbreak-oregon/25049737/ (Accessed
April 1, 2024).

34   Mass vaccinations at University of
Oregon start slowly. *The Columbian.*
2015. www.columbian.com/news/2015/
mar/03/mass-vaccinations-at-university-
of-oregon-start-sl/ (Accessed April 1,
2024).

35   Misinformation and disinformation.
American Psychological Association. 2023.
www.apa.org/topics/journalism-facts/
misinformation-disinformation
(Accessed April 21, 2024).

36   National Academies of Sciences,
Engineering, and Medicine. *Navigating
Infodemics and Building Trust during
Public Health Emergencies: Proceedings of
a Workshop in Brief.* Washington, DC,
The National Academies Press, 2023.

37   Borges do Nascimento IJ, Pizarro AB,
Almeida JM, Azzopardi-Muscat N,
Gonçalves MA, Björklund M, Novillo-
Ortiz D. Infodemics and Health
Misinformation: A Systematic Review of
Reviews. *Bull World Health Organ*
2022;**100**(9):544–61.

38   Managing the COVID-19 infodemic:
Promoting healthy behaviours and
mitigating the harm from
misinformation and disinformation.
World Health Organization. 2020. www
.who.int/news/item/23-09-2020-

managing-the-covid-19-infodemic-promoting-healthy-behaviours-and-mitigating-the-harm-from-misinformation-and-disinformation (Accessed April 10, 2024).

39. The COVID-19 Infodemic (Editorial). *The Lancet* 2020;20(8):375.

40. First WHO Infodemic Manager Training. *World Health Organization*. 2020. www.who.int/teams/epi-win/infodemic-management/1st-who-training-in-infodemic-management (Accessed April 21, 2024).

41. Diagrams of Rumor and Rumor Control, World War II rumor project collection 1943. *Library of Congress*. 1942. www.loc.gov/item/afc1945001_ms01006 (Accessesd April 21, 2024).

42. Nagar A, Grégoire V, Sundelson A, O'Donnell-Pazderka E, Jamison, AM, Sell TK. *Practical playbook for addressing health misinformation*. Baltimore, MD, Johns Hopkins Center for Health Security, 2024.

43. SteelFisher GK, Findling MG, Caporello HL, Lubell KM, Vidoloff Melville KG, Lane L, et al. Trust in US Federal, State, and Local Public Health Agencies during COVID-19: Responses and Policy Implications. *Health Aff* 2023;**42**(3):328–37.

44. Public Health Connects Speaker Series: A conversation with Dr. Kate Starbird. *YouTube*. 2023. www.youtube.com/watch?v=s2t5S1Ziv0Y (Accessed April 14, 2024).

45. CDC. *Crisis and Emergency Risk Communication October 2014*. Atlanta, GA, CDC, 2014.

46. Prue C, Lackey C, Swenarski L, Gantt J. Communication Monitoring: Shaping CDC's Emergency Risk Communication Efforts. *J Health Commun* 2003;**8**(Suppl. 1):35–49.

47. Lariscy RW, Avery EJ, Sweetser KD, Howes P. Monitoring Public Opinion in Cyberspace: How Corporate Public Relations Is Facing the Challenge. *Public Relations J* 2009;3(4):1–17.

48. Ghidottim N. Why Brands Need Social Media Listening. 2020. www.prsa.org/article/why-brands-need-social-media-listening (Accessed April 21, 2024).

49. Hadi TA, Fleshler K. Integrating Social Media Monitoring into Public Health Emergency Response Operations. *Disaster Med Public Health Prep* 2016;**10**(5):775–80.

50. Pomeranz JL, Schwid AR. Governmental Actions to Address COVID-19 Misinformation. *J Public Health Policy* 2021;**42**(2):201–10.

51. Hancock J. Missouri AG aligns with St. Louis conspiracy theorist in social media lawsuit. *The Missouri Independent*. 2022. https://missouriindependent.com/2022/11/21/missouri-ag-aligns-with-st-louis-conspiracy-theorist-in-social-media-lawsuit/ (Accessed May 10, 2024).

52. United States Course of Appeals for Fifth Circuit: Missouri v Murthy (Opinion). 2023. www.supremecourt.gov/opinions/23pdf/23-411_3dq3.pdf (Accessed October 24, 2024).

53. Murthy v. Missouri: *SCOTUSblog*. n.d. www.scotusblog.com/case-files/cases/murthy-v-missouri-3 (Accessed April 21, 2024).

54. Quinn M. Supreme Court to hear free speech case over government pressure on social media sites to remove content. *CBS News*. 2024. www.cbsnews.com/news/supreme-court-social-media-sites-government-content-misinformation-censorship/ (Accessed April 10, 2024).

55. Mello MM. Vaccine Misinformation and the First Amendment – The Price of Free Speech. *JAMA Health Forum* 2022;3(3):e220732.

56. Syllabus Murthy, Surgeon General, et al., v. Missouri et al. 2023. www.supremecourt.gov/opinions/23pdf/23-411_3dq3.pdf (Accessed April 10, 2024).

57. Intro.9.2 Murthy v Missouri: The First Ammendment and Government Influence on Social Media Companies' Content Moderation. *Constitution Annotated*. n.d. https://constitution

.congress.gov/browse/essay/intro.9-2-3/ ALDE_00000075 (Accessed October 24, 2024).

58 *Study Guide for the Examination for Accreditation in Public Relations*. Wilmington, DE, Universal Accreditation Board/Public Relations Society of America, 2021.

59 Testing and testing priorities for suspected cases. *American Hospital Association*. 2020. www.aha.org/news/headline/2020-03-26-cdc-updates-covid-19-testing-and-preparedness-guidelines (Accessed April 21, 2024).

60 Spiro ES, Starbird K. Rumors Have Rules. *Issues Sci Technol* 2023;39(3):47–49.

61 Centers for Disease Control and Prevention. Epidemiologic and Clinical Characteristics of Monkeypox Cases – United States. 2022. www.cdc.gov/mmwr/volumes/71/wr/mm7132e3.htm (Accessed July 1, 2023).

62 Monkeypox Update: FDA Authorizes Emergency Use of JYNNEOS Vaccine to Increase Vaccine Supply. *Food and Drug Administration*. 2022. www.fda.gov/news-events/press-announcements/monkeypox-update-fda-authorizes-emergency-use-jynneos-vaccine-increase-vaccine-supply. (Accessed July 1, 2023).

63 Owens LE, Currie DW, Kramarow EA, Siddique S, Swanson M, Carter RJ, et al. JYNNEOS Vaccination Coverage among Persons at Risk for Mpox – United States, May 22, 2022–January 31, 2023. 2023. www.cdc.gov/mmwr/volumes/72/wr/mm7213a4.htm (Accessed November 24, 2024).

64 Centers for Disease Control and Prevention. U.S. Map & Case Count. 2022. www.cdc.gov/poxvirus/mpox/response/2022/us-map.html (Accessed July 1, 2023).

65 Essajee NM, Oddo-Moise H, Hagensee ME, Lillis RA, Maffei J, Butler I, et al. Characteristics of Mpox Infections in Louisiana in the 2022 Outbreak. *AIDS Res Hum Retroviruses* 2023;39(11):587–92.

66 CDC. *Crisis and Emergency Risk Communication October 2018*. Atlanta, GA, CDC, 2018.

67 Louisiana Department of Health. LDH identifies first monkeypox case in a Louisiana Resident. 2022. https://ldh.la.gov/news/monkeypox (Accessed November 24, 2024).

68 Louisiana Department of Health. Technical briefing: First monkeypox case identified in Louisiana resident. 2022. www.youtube.com/watch?v=BI7OdCtd-zE (Accessed November 24, 2024).

69 Louisiana Department of Health. 2021 STI Data and Rankings, Louisiana. 2021. https://ldh.la.gov/assets/oph/HIVSTD/Tables-Profiles/2021-STI-Rankings-Release.pdf (Accessed November 24, 2024).

70 Centers for Disease Control and Prevention. CDC activates emergency operations center for monkeypox response. 2022. www.cdc.gov/media/releases/2022/s0628-monkeypox-eoc.html (Accessed November 24, 2024).

71 Louisiana Department of Health [@ladepthealth]. Visiting #SouthernDecadence and need resources? *Instagram*. 2022. www.instagram.com/p/CiDOnyzO3zi/?img_index=1 (Accessed November 24, 2024).

72 Louisiana Department of Health. New Orleans Health Department, CDC host Southern Decadence Health Hub. MPox Information. 2022. https://ldh.la.gov/news/decadence-health-hub (Accessed July 1, 2023).

73 Maccash D. Vaxxtravaganza, a free monkeypox vaccination event, set for bourbon street Wednesday. *NOLA.com*. 2022. www.nola.com/entertainment_life/festivals/vaxxtravaganza-a-free-monkeypox-vaccination-event-set-for-bourbon-street-wednesday/article_32818f70-232b-11ed-86f7-17830c7e688f.html (Accessed July 1, 2023).

74 Louisiana Department of Health [@ladepthealth]. Monkeypox Q&A: Is it a sexually transmitted infection? *Instagram*. 2022. www.instagram.com/p/Cgjo4V9uYo7/?hl=en (Accessed July 1, 2023).

75 Louisiana Department of Health. Mpox information. n.d. https://ldh.la.gov/page/mpox (Accessed November 24, 2024).

76 Woodruff E. Hundreds line up for New Orleans' first mass monkeypox vaccination event. *NOLA.com*. 2022. www.nola.com/news/healthcare_hospitals/hundreds-line-up-for-new-orleans-first-mass-monkeypox-vaccination-event/article_6200b682-1821-11ed-8ef1-db4023677361.html (Accessed July 1, 2023).

Part II Communicating during a Health Emergency

Chapter 8

Communicating during Long Public Health Emergencies
Creating Health Communication Campaigns

Chapter Objectives
- Describe the importance of including health communication campaigns in long-term health emergencies.
- List five steps for developing a health communication campaign.
- Recall the differences between emergency risk communication and health communication campaigns.
- Recall at least two theories to guide campaign development.
- Describe the health belief model.
- Be able to identify a communication objective, audience segments, key messages, channels, and communication products for a health communication campaign.

Including Health Communication Campaigns in Long-Term Health Emergencies

This chapter does not seek to summarize or reproduce knowledge from the field of health communication campaigns. Instead, this chapter aims to highlight the basics of health communication campaigns and how these campaigns can be utilized during the maintenance phase of a health emergency for long-term health emergency responses. Additionally, incorporating health communication campaigns into emergency risk communication is essential for communication health interventions, especially pharmaceutical interventions.

Health communication campaigns are used in many areas of public health such as tobacco use cessation and breast cancer awareness, but often they are not discussed within the realm of emergency risk communication. This is because emergency risk communication focuses on immediate harms and threats and reducing the public's risk of encountering those harms; most of the time, public health emergencies are not multiyear outbreaks but rather emergencies that are mitigated within weeks or months. However, COVID-19 demonstrated that long-term outbreaks (i.e., outbreaks lasting years) require the incorporation of health communication campaigns as a messaging tactic within the emergency response.

For emergency risk communicators engaging in multiyear emergencies, there are three key reasons to include health communication campaigns in long-term health emergency responses. First, health communication campaigns support the Crisis and Emergency Risk Communication (CERC) principle of Promote Action. During the initial part of the maintenance phase, the public is engaging in information-seeking to learn more about the health threat, who is affected, and what they can do to protect their own health. As health emergencies continue for months or years – as we saw with COVID-19 – health communication campaigns are needed to help guide the public to take action. Second, health communication campaigns enhance communication and encourage intended audience behaviors related to the public health intervention. Fundamentally, health communication campaigns are designed to engage behavior change at the community level. During a long-term health emergency, in which the public may need to engage in multiple health interventions, health communication campaigns can support emergency communication activities and help move the public toward taking an action to protect their health. Third, health communication campaigns can help emergency risk communicators understand how values, beliefs, and cultural norms can impact on when people will take a health action, if at all.[1] Vaccine hesitancy emerged during COVID-19 among the US population and impacted vaccine uptake. As a result, the US Ad Council and the COVID Collaborative helped address vaccine hesitancy through a health communication campaign called "It's Up to You."[2] In early 2021, survey research showed that "40% of Americans have not made a decision about getting vaccinated against COVID-19. This hesitant 'movable middle' will be the focus of our initiative."[2] By November 2021, as a result of the "It's Up to You" health communication campaign, the Ad Council reported: "When we first started the project, only 30% of US adults were planning to get vaccinated right away against COVID-19. As of today, over 80% have received at least one dose."[2]

Overview of Health Communication Campaigns

Let's look at the main principles and characteristics of a health communication campaign. Health communication campaigns are "purposive attempts to inform or influence behaviors in large audiences within a specified time period using an organized set of communication activities and featuring an array of mediated messages in multiple channels generally to produce noncommercial benefits to individuals and society."[1] To design and create a health communication campaign, there are five steps to follow[1,3,4]:

1. Conduct a community analysis.
2. Design and initiate the campaign.
3. Implement the campaign and stage a kickoff event.
4. Engage in program maintenance, effectiveness analysis, and consolidation.
5. Disseminate the results.

Conduct a Community Analysis

When designing a health communication campaign, it is important to understand the community and why the community needs in-depth and robust communication to enact behavior change. This type of community analysis and review is a type of formative research, ensuring that the program is feasible, appropriate, and acceptable and allowing us to learn about the intended audience.[5] Reviewing community health assessments or national surveillance data can provide health status information and key demographics about the community.[3] Additionally, research the values, beliefs, and cultural norms of the community to understand how the community lives, works, and exists in its social and physical environments.[1,4] To develop deep insights into the potential pathways of behavior change, however, additional research is often needed to assess the audiences' current knowledge, attitudes, and beliefs, their readiness for change, their communication preferences and habits, as well as relevant social, political, and policy environments that may facilitate or hinder behavior change. Learnings from these research efforts are synthesized to inform campaign objectives, which may aim directly at behavior change or any of its antecedents in the campaign's conceptual framework.[3]

Community-based participatory research directly engages community members, creating a horizontal and inclusive approach to gathering information. Instead of establishing a dichotomy of *outsider* and *insider* or *problem-solvers* and *problems*, engaging with the community establishes a space for co-creation and co-ownership of the health communication campaign. It also increases the likelihood of creating materials that will resonate with the audience by using the audience's own words, phrases, and images relating to its physical environment and community members, even down to colors and font styles.

Design and Initiate the Campaign

Identify relevant theories to guide the design of the communication campaign. Later in this chapter, theories will be highlighted that provide the foundation for health communication campaigns, but there are many communication, social science, and behavioral theories that can be used to help design a health communication campaign. Using a theory to guide the campaign design is beneficial because it can outline areas to consider when creating the measurable objectives and strategies of the campaign. There are two such types of strategy: content strategies and executional strategies.[3] *Content strategies* focus on the content – mainly the words – of the message that will be used during the campaign. Content strategies often identify specific beliefs that are associated with the intended health action. The campaign content may promote or contain the community's beliefs depending on their impacts on the intended health action.[3] In contrast, *executional strategies* focus on the framing of the content. For example, different theories or frameworks such as messaging framing or visual communication will be used to help determine how to display or package the content.[3] Both strategies aim to ensure that the message content will resonate with the intended audience.

In addition to creating the objectives and strategies of the campaign, be sure to identify and delineate audiences, communication channels, communication activities, communication products, timelines, and budgets (see Chapters 3, 4, and 5 for more information on audiences, channels, and products).

Once an approach is outlined for the campaign, ensure that evaluation methods and metrics have been thoroughly considered (see Chapter 10 for more on specific evaluation activities). This ensures that the campaign can be measured throughout its implementation and at its end to determine whether it has met its intended goals. Providing metrics is a key activity for demonstrating the effectiveness of a campaign's activities. When developing communication materials, be sure to enlist members from the community in message testing, including focus groups, to ensure that the language, images, and colors resonate with the intended audiences. Once a program has been designed and created, the next phase is program launch and implementation.

Implement the Campaign and Stage a Kickoff Event

Campaign implementation is often marked by a program launch/kickoff event with a media push.[4] The kickoff event is often a celebratory event designed to gain global attention and to leverage news media coverage to increase the reach and exposure of the communication campaign. For example, for former First Lady Michele Obama's "Let's Move" campaign was designed to reduce child obesity. Its kickoff event took place on the South Lawn of the White House and involved schoolchildren learning physical skills like running, soccer, and tennis from Washington-area sport teams including the Capitals and the Redskins.[6,7]

Engage in Program Maintenance, Effectiveness Analysis, and Consolidation

Once the campaign has been implemented, it is important to engage in process evaluation to ensure that the program is performing as it was intended. Process evaluation often includes monitoring campaign reach, message comprehension, audience engagement, and audience surveys.[3] Use data from the process evaluation to ensure that the campaign is operating as designed by the campaign plan and make adjustments accordingly. For example, if there appears to be a lack of engagement in planned activities, review the impediments to participation and remove any barriers to engagement. If there appears to be a lack of engagement on social media or message confusion, review the social media comments and posts and determine whether messages need to be updated or changed. As the campaign continues, there may be opportunities to consolidate activities or integrate more community volunteers to support campaign operations. Again, use process evaluation data to guide decision-making throughout the program implementation phase to ensure efficient use of resources and effective campaign operations are achieved.

Disseminate the Results

Upon the conclusion of the campaign, enact the formal evaluation plan that was designed in the early stages of campaign planning. Analyze any data, interpret the results, and create a final report that can be shared with leadership and key stakeholders. Including both qualitative and quantitative methods can help triangulate data results, producing more robust analyses and evidence-based results.[3] The case study included at the end of this chapter looks at a published article that analyzed the effectiveness of the COVID-19 health communication campaign "We Can Do This."

Ensure that you communicate the key findings and impacts of the health communication campaign. By sharing the impacts of the health communication campaign, the health agency and campaign designers can demonstrate the value and importance of these types of activities, which builds a foundation for future campaign work. Consider holding a wrap event, in which the campaign results are shared with campaign planners, workers, volunteers, and participants and the end of the campaign is celebrated with those who helped to create and implement it.

Differences between Health Communication Campaigns and Emergency Risk Communication

Health communication campaigns fundamentally differ from emergency risk communication activities. One of the biggest differences relates to time. During a health emergency, communicators need to work quickly to understand the evolving situation,

Table 8.1 Differences between emergency risk communication and health communication campaigns

Emergency risk communication	Health communication campaigns
Short time frame for action	Time for formative research careful consideration of evaluation metrics and processes
Immediate media attention	Need to gain the media's attention
Instructive	Behavior change
Immediate health threat	Prevention and/or detection efforts for known health threats (e.g., heart disease, breast cancer screenings)

address the uncertainty of the situation, and address heightened media attention.[8,9,10] Health communication campaigns are not designed to address emergency situations but rather known health issues such as heart disease or cancer. One of the core design principles of health communication campaigns is to conduct formative research and engage in message testing. Health emergencies don't often allow for in-depth message testing before emergency messages are shared with the public.

In addition, during health emergencies, there is heightened media attention regarding what the health emergency is, who is impacted, and information about the health threat. In contrast, health communication campaigns often need to gain the media's attention. Since the focus of a health communication campaign is not new or novel, communication needs to focus on gaining the attention of the media and the target audience.

Furthermore, emergency risk communication is often instructive, whereas health communication campaigns focus on sustained behavior change over time. During the initial stages of a health emergency, key messages focus on addressing uncertainty and promoting action for people to protect their health. In this context, emergency risk communication messages are instructive: Do *this* to prevent *that* – for example, do not eat red Roma tomatoes because they might cause salmonella.[11] During health communication campaigns, the focus is on sustained behavior change such as tobacco use cessation, eating more vegetables, engaging in more physical activity, or increasing cancer screenings for a particular age group. Stopping a current negative behavior or beginning a new positive behavior is no small feat.[12]

Finally, the focus of emergency risk communication is on an immediate and evolving health threat. In contrast, health communication campaigns address prevention or detection efforts for known health threats, such as lung cancer from smoking, heart disease, or breast or colon cancer.

It is important for emergency risk communicators to understand the differences between emergency risk communication and health communication campaigns (see Table 8.1). By understanding these differences, emergency risk communicators can harness the power of health communication campaign principles and use them during long-term health emergencies.

Theories to Guide Health Communication Campaigns

When designing health communication campaigns, there are many communication and behavior-based theories that campaign designers can draw upon, such as diffusion of innovation, self-efficacy, the extended parallel process model (EPPM), the theory of reasoned action, the health belief model (HBM), and ecological models. Depending on the campaign's objectives, different theories can be used to help design and plan the health communication campaign. This section highlights three theories and how they can be used to help plan a health communication campaign during a long-term health emergency.

Diffusion of Innovation

The theory of diffusion of innovation was developed by Everett Rogers to understand the processes involved in the communication of a new idea or practice – the innovation – through a social system.[13] Due to the novelty of innovation – whether it is a new idea or practice – diffusion is affected by the uncertainty or lack of predictability about what will happen. Additionally, the innovation is designed to change previous thinking or processes via long-term and systematic changes. Diffusion of information can occur in both centralized and decentralized systems. In a centralized system, leaders often determine what, when, and how the diffusion will occur within the system. In contrast, in a decentralized system, horizontal networks self-determine the speed and degree of diffusion adoption.[13] In both centralized and decentralized systems, interpersonal networks play a major role in the adoption or rejection of an innovation.

Rogers offers the following public health example about a failed boil water campaign in Los Molinos, Peru. A local public health worker was tasked with persuading village housewives to boil water to prevent waterborne illnesses over a 2-year period. The public health worker met with the housewives of 200 families from a village several times over the course of a year, and at the end of the program only 11 housewives had been convinced to regularly boil their water.[13] Ultimately, the boil water program failed, and diffusion of innovation theory offers insights as to why it failed. Diffusion of innovation is heavily dependent on social and interpersonal networks, so determining which people adopted this behavior and why can provide insights into why the entire village did not begin to adopt the boil water behavior.

First, the public health worker targeted two individuals: a sick housewife and a housewife who was new to the community. By working primarily with these two women, the public health worker overlooked the social fabric of the community and the community's opinion leaders. The sick housewife and the woman who was new to the community had little social influence within the community and "were not respected as social models of water-boiling behavior of other women."[13]

Second, the housewife who was new to the community adopted the boil water behavior not because of a belief that the boiled water would prevent illness, but to gain social acceptance from the public health worker, whom the housewife believed had a higher social status than herself. It is important to understand that adopting a new health behavior may have nothing to do with preventing illness but rather with social inclusion. This insight can help health communicators understand that providing accurate and informative health information may not be enough for individuals to take action.

Third, the public health worker was perceived as a social stranger by lower-status housewives. In contrast, the health worker being of a middle status allowed them to engage more easily with middle-status housewives. The key takeaway here is that communication was more effective between the public health worker and housewives who had a similar social status and cultural background.

Overall, the boil water program did not take into account the cultural beliefs of the villagers: "An important factor affecting the adoption rate of any innovation is its compatibility with the values, beliefs, and past experiences of the social system."[13]

Self-Efficacy and the Extended Parallel Process Model

Self-efficacy directly impacts behavior change as it impacts the likelihood with which one feels that one can be successful in changing one's behavior to produce outcomes, indicating that "cognitive processes play a prominent role in the acquisition and retention of new behavior patterns."[14] These cognitive processes include seeing actions modeled by others, observing the actions and feedback responses of others engaging in the new behavior, the realization over time that actions have consequences, individual motivation to change behavior based on external reinforcement of the behavior change, and self-motivation to change based on personal and internal standards.[14]

The EPPM builds upon the work of Bandura to further understand how threat perception and self-efficacy impact decision-making.[15] In Bandura's work, the focus was on how much self-efficacy must be present in order for an individual to take action. The EPPM offers insights into how fear appeals could help frame messages to avoid or stop engaging in behaviors that threaten one's health status such as smoking, not wearing a seat belt or bike helmet, or unsafe sex practices. Fear appeals frame messages in terms of perceived susceptibility and vulnerability, awareness of hazards (including gains and losses), and perceived threat to the individual. The downside of fear appeals is that two different cognitive processes can be engaged by such messages – one positive and one negative. The positive reaction is that the individual hears the message and feels the desire to control or avoid the health threat. The negative reaction is that the individual hears the message and emotionally reacts to the message by denying or avoiding the health threat. The key for message designers is to find a balance between an individual's susceptibility to the health threat with their self-efficacy to take action.

Education Entertainment

Another approach to health communication campaigns is to educate the community through education entertainment by inserting credible health information and public service announcements into popular television and streaming shows.[16] Education entertainment approaches call upon social modeling, parasocial interaction, and expectancy value.[1,17,18] Social modeling and parasocial interaction explain how watching characters on a screen can impact one's personal life. For example, if an audience member has a particular affinity for a character and the character engages in particular behaviors, then that character is engaging in social modeling. An audience member may then adopt the character's behaviors. Additionally, parasocial interaction explains how audience members come to feel a close and interpersonal relationship with characters or television personalities. Even though the interaction is often one-way, the audience member comes to feel a close personal connection to the character or television personality, as if they were a friend.

Expectancy value theory was developed by Jacquelynne Eccles and her colleagues.[19,20] The theory hypothesizes that achievement-related choices are motivated by a combination of people's *expectations of success* and *subjective task value*.[19,20] Eccles' work focused on defining expectations of success in particular, such as how one thinks one will do on an upcoming project or task. One's expectation of success is based upon one's subjective view of one's desire to do the task, or subjective task value. Subjective task values are defined as attainment value, intrinsic value, utility value, and cost. Attainment value is defined as how important it is to the individual to do well. Intrinsic value is defined as how much personal enjoyment is obtained from engaging in the task. Utility value is defined as how useful the task is to support future goals. Cost is defined as the amount of time taken away from other tasks.[21,22]

During the COVID-19 pandemic, the popular medical television show *Grey's Anatomy* portrayed how the fictionalized characters within the show had to deal with the very real COVID-19 pandemic. The show mirrored many of the same real-world issues hospitals were facing, such as shortages of personal protective equipment (PPE), burnout, increased volumes of deaths, strict isolation and quarantine procedures, and a lack of ventilators. The show's main character, Meredith Grey, contracted COVID-19 and eventually had to be placed on a ventilator, which were of course in very short supply. Hard decisions had to be made and personal ethics were tested as hospital workers at Grey Sloan Memorial Hospital responded to the pandemic. Popular culture critics and fans reported mixed reviews of this season of *Grey's Anatomy*, which brought real life onto the screen. The reviews ranged from criticism of the show retraumatizing those who had undergone experiences of COVID-19 to appreciating the willingness of the show to capture reality on screen and provide exemplars of courageous hospital workers.[23–26]

Unintended Consequences of Health Communication Campaigns

When designing health communication campaigns, designers are looking to ensure the intended audiences engage in a specific behavior.[27] However, there can be spillover effects among audiences beyond those targeted by these campaigns, as well as effects that the designers did not intend to happen. These unintended effects can impact different variables, including those relating to level (the individual or society at large), time (short or long), audience (intended or unintended), content (specific or diffuse), and valence (desirable or undesirable). Cho and Salmon outlined 11 types of unintended effects from health communication campaigns (see Table 8.2).[27]

It is important for emergency risk communicators to understand how unintended consequences can occur and how these consequences might impact the overall media environment. For example, backlash to a health communication campaign could impact other programs within the health department. Although not all unintended consequences are negative, emergency risk communicators must remember the power that communication holds and how external communication activities can impact the agency, the community it serves, and even society at large.

Table 8.2 Untended consequences of health communication campaigns

Unintended effect	Definition
Obfuscation	Confusion and misunderstanding of health risk and risk prevention methods
Dissonance	Psychological discomfort and distress provoked by the incongruence between the recommended health states and the audiences' actual states
Boomerang	The reaction by an audience that is opposite to the intended response of persuasion messages
Epidemic of apprehension	Unnecessarily high consciousness and concern over health produced by the pervasiveness of risk messages over the long term
Desensitization	Repeated exposure to messages about a health risk may over the long term render the public apathetic
Culpability	The phenomenon of locating the causes of public health problems in the individual rather than in social conditions
Opportunity cost	The choice of communication campaigns as the solution for a public health problem and the selection of certain health issues over others may diminish the probability of improving public health through other choices
Social reproduction	The phenomenon in which campaigns reinforce existing social distributions of knowledge, attitudes, and behaviors
Social norming	Social cohesion and control and accompanying marginalization of unhealthy minorities brought about by campaigns
Enabling	Campaigns inadvertently improve the power of individuals and institutions and promote the images and finances of industries
System activation	Campaigns influence various unintended sectors of society, and their actions mediate or moderate the effects of campaigns on the intended audience

Author's note: The following article is included in this chapter to highlight how health communication campaigns are a critical component of emergency risk communication. The CERC framework that has been used throughout this book lacks the inclusion of health communication campaigns as a critical component in emergency risk communication responses – especially those responses that last for multiple years. This chapter seeks to underscore the importance of including health communication campaigns in emergency risk communication responses. Although the following article deviates from the format used in other chapters of including a student-written case study, including this publication provides readers with an example of a health communication campaign implemented during an emergency risk communication response.

The Initial Relationship between the United Sates Department of Health and Human Services' Digital COVID-19 Public Education Campaign and Vaccine Uptake: Campaign Effectiveness Evaluation

Christopher J. Williams, PhD, Elissa C. Kranzler, PhD, Elissa C. Kranzler, PhD, Joseph N. Luchman, PhD, Benjamin Denison, PhD, Sean Fischer, PhD, Thomas Wonder, PhD, Ronne Ostby, MA, Monica Vines, MS, Jessica Weinberg, MPP, Elizabeth L. Petrun Sayers, PhD, Allison N. Kurti, PhD, Sarah Trigger, MPH, Leah Hoffman, MPH and Joshua F. A. Peck, BA

Introduction

The COVID-19 pandemic has led to more than 104 million COVID-19 cases and over 1 million COVID-19 deaths in the United States as of April 3, 2023.[28] COVID-19 vaccines are safe and effective[29] and are estimated to have prevented more than 66 million COVID-19 cases and 17 million COVID-19-related hospitalizations, saving more than 2 million lives and almost US $900 billion in health care costs in the United States from mid-December 2020 through the end of March 2022.[30] Vaccination research predating the COVID-19 pandemic has demonstrated that it is necessary not only to make vaccines available and accessible but also to address vaccine hesitancy, which is the "delay in acceptance or refusal of vaccination despite the availability of vaccination services."[31]

Vaccine hesitancy is a critical barrier to vaccine uptake,[32] suggesting that interventions that aim to decrease vaccine hesitancy may result in increased vaccine uptake. In the context of COVID-19, research has shown that vaccine hesitancy predicts vaccine uptake[33] such that groups of individuals who were initially less vaccine-hesitant were more likely to report subsequent vaccination. Other research suggests that widespread COVID-19 vaccine uptake requires the application of multicomponent interventions that raise knowledge and awareness to address vaccine hesitancy and influence behavior change.[34,35] Between April 2021 and April 2022, nearly 148.6 million people received a first-dose COVID-19 vaccination in the United States.[32]

Public education campaigns, which reach and engage large population segments through a mix of media channels, have demonstrated a measurable impact on a range of health behaviors[36,37] and have successfully influenced vaccine hesitancy and vaccine uptake in other contexts.[34] In response to the COVID-19 pandemic, the US Department of Health and Human Services (HHS) launched the "We Can Do This" public education campaign ("the campaign")[38] in April 2021 to increase COVID-19 vaccine confidence (the likelihood of vaccination) and, ultimately, vaccine uptake. (In December 2020, the HHS launched the "Slow the Spread" campaign, which encouraged mask wearing and social distancing.)

The "We Can Do This" campaign aims to influence COVID-19 vaccine confidence and uptake through the dissemination of advertisements (e.g., 30-second videos and static images with text) that address key attitudinal and behavioral constructs relevant to these outcomes across a mix of traditional and new media channels. These channels include television, radio, and print media; site direct (digital advertising directly purchased on websites), programmatic (digital advertising purchased through automated marketplace platforms to reach audiences across a range of websites, apps, and platforms), and paid social media (advertising bought directly on social media platforms) advertisements; earned media; partnerships; and influencer engagement. To reach diverse audiences, the campaign has engaged simultaneously with the general population and with specific racial and ethnic audiences through tailored communications in more than 14 languages, including English and Spanish.

Between April 5 and September 26, 2021, according to Nielsen Digital and Total Ad Ratings (see *Journal of Medical Internet Research* online article for Multimedia Appendix 1), the campaign is estimated to have reached more than 90% of US adults an average of 20.9 times across measured television and digital channels (Nielsen Digital Ad Ratings, unpublished data, 2021). In addition to the campaign's national reach, it also delivered extra ads to markets, zip codes, and population segments with higher proportions of vaccine-hesitant adults and higher COVID-19 prevalence. As the vaccination uptake rate varied across designated market areas (DMAs), the campaign also took vaccination rates into account when deciding where to deliver these extra ads to help encourage first-dose vaccination.

To date, there have been no published evaluations of the impact of this campaign on COVID-19 vaccine uptake. This study is the first to assess the association between digital campaign media dose – an understudied avenue for public education campaign dissemination – and an individual's likelihood of receiving their first COVID-19 vaccination dose.

Methods

Overview

To evaluate the potential association between the campaign and vaccine uptake, we used individual-level survey data and market-level campaign media dose data. Digital campaign media dose refers to the aggregation of all digital ads that were placed in a DMA at a given time. The individual-level data were derived from the COVID-19 Attitudes and Beliefs Survey (CABS), a nationally representative, probability-based longitudinal survey of US adults (aged 18+ years) administered every 4 months to the same individuals through the AmeriSpeak probability-based research panel of the National Opinion Research Center (NORC).[39] The 35-minute web-based survey measures adherence to COVID-19-preventive behaviors, including COVID-19 vaccination, and respondents' sociodemographic characteristics. Analysis was conducted with data from the 3,642 respondents who completed survey waves 1–3, as wave 3 was the first wave in which respondents provided the date of their first COVID-19 vaccination. (Details about survey administration and a table of unweighted descriptive statistics are included in *Journal of Medical Internet Research* online article for Multimedia Appendix 1.) Paid campaign media dose data were collected for digital platforms (i.e., site direct, social media, and programmatic advertisements; described in *Journal of Medical Internet Research* online article for Multimedia Appendix 1) from campaign launch on April 1 to November 7, 2021, the last date of CABS wave 3 completion. This represents all the paid digital media doses administered during this period as part of the campaign.

Ethics Approval

We sought institutional review board (IRB) approval for this study from the Biomedical Research Alliance of New York, an external IRB service accredited by the Association for the Accreditation of Human Research Protection Programs. The study protocol and materials were reviewed and approved by Biomedical Research Alliance of New York's social and behavioral IRB (Federalwide Assurance FWA00000337, protocol 20-077-821).

Informed Consent, Respondent, Confidentiality, and Compensation

Although all respondents provided consent as part of their registration into their associated panel, we ensured that all qualifying respondents provided informed consent to participate in the study. The consent language was available on the web, programmed into the final part of the screener. After screening respondents, we directed those eligible (i.e., respondents who did not screen out) to read the consent language. If they decided to participate, eligible respondents electronically provided consent and were directed to the web-based survey. Although this study presented minimal risk of harm to subjects, all respondents were informed at the beginning of the survey that any questions that make them feel uncomfortable may be skipped or ignored. We included links to mental health resources for respondents to access if they experienced any distress from participating in the study.

To ensure respondent confidentiality, (1) data transfer was conducted via a secure, password-protected site; (2) all screening-related information was not tied to any personal identifiable information, but identified and matched by the assigned unique ID; (3) datasets and reports did not contain any personal identifiable information; and (4) respondents were not tied to individual responses, and any data used in reporting were not to be attributed to specific respondents. Data were tightly controlled behind firewalls with password-protected access by senior researchers. All final data were stored in a secure environment that does not have access to the internet and requires a separate access code by researchers. Researchers were trained to never export data from this secure server.

Respondents who decided to participate were offered US $10 in the first wave of the CABS and US $18 for each subsequent wave of the survey.

Measures

Dependent Variable

The dependent variable was dichotomous, indicating whether a respondent reported receiving the first dose of a COVID-19 vaccination in each broadcast week. The unit of analysis was the respondent-broadcast week; we used broadcast weeks, which run from Monday to Sunday, because that is how advertising is purchased. Within the dataset, there was an observation for each CABS respondent in each broadcast week starting the week of November 30, 2020, as this date marks the beginning of the first broadcast week in which a vaccine was publicly available. If a respondent did not report having been vaccinated in a broadcast week, then they were included as an observation in the subsequent broadcast week. If a respondent reported having been vaccinated in a broadcast week, then they were not included as an observation in the subsequent broadcast week. Some respondents (n = 241) reported vaccination dates that occurred before the date of the US Food and Drug Administration (FDA) emergency use authorization (EUA). Under the assumption that these individuals misstated the year of vaccination, it was changed from 2020 to 2021 in these instances. As a robustness test, we conducted analyses in which individuals who reported a vaccination date before the FDA EUA were dropped. As the results were similar, we retained them in the analysis.

Independent Variable

The independent variable was paid campaign digital media dose, representing the change in the total number of site direct, programmatic, and social media advertisement impressions (impressions are the digital publishers' estimates of the number of times an advertisement is seen or heard) in a DMA (a DMA region is a group of counties and zip codes that form an exclusive geographic area in which the home market television stations are the predominant stations in terms of total hours viewed; DMA is a proprietary construct of the Nielsen Company) per 100,000 people between $week_{t-2}$ and $week_{t-1}$. This operationalization allowed us to assess the short-term relationship between increasing digital media dose in a DMA and the individual-level likelihood of first-dose vaccination. We used the change in impressions between $week_{t-2}$ and $week_{t-1}$ because we expected a lag between one's decision to get vaccinated and vaccine receipt due to logistics (e.g., navigating appointment availability and scheduling), such that adding or decreasing campaign dose would not immediately influence vaccinations. The change in dose in each DMA reflects that the campaign varied the distribution of advertising over both week and markets; therefore, markets had a lower, same, or higher dose of advertising from week to week. Respondents were assigned a digital dose by broadcast week based on their DMA of residence.

Covariates

To account for the potential influence of factors exogenous to the campaign that could still be correlated with changes in media dose, analyses controlled for the change in weekly COVID-19 cases and deaths and the change in weekly cable news COVID-19 coverage by DMA between $week_{t-2}$ and $week_{t-1}$. Cable news is used as a measure of COVID-19 salience, and although this is only one form of media, it can serve as a proxy for all media discussion of the topic due to the intermedia agenda-setting effect.[40] To account for the potential influence of sociodemographic characteristics on first-dose vaccination, we controlled for respondent age, sex, race/ethnicity, education, household income, political ideology, rurality, essential worker status, and preexisting health conditions as reported in CABS wave 3. A model accounting for whether an individual is insured is included in Multimedia Appendix 1 (see *Journal of Medical Internet Research* online article for Multimedia Appendix 1). The results for the main independent variable are nearly identical; however, we chose not to include this variable in the main model as it is correlated with other demographic variables.

We expected that individuals may have predispositions that may influence the effectiveness of the campaign and their likelihood to get a vaccination, so we controlled for respondent vaccine confidence (i.e., a respondent's reported vaccine uptake or likelihood that they will get vaccinated against COVID-19) as reported in CABS wave 1. Details about COVID-19 cases and deaths data, COVID-19 cable news coverage data, sociodemographic variables, and vaccine confidence, including a discussion of the coding of these variables, are provided in Multimedia Appendix 1 (see *Journal of Medical Internet Research* online article for Multimedia Appendix 1).

Statistical Analysis
Before conducting analyses, we examined the independent and dependent variable distributions to inform our analytic approach. The earliest a respondent reported receiving the first dose of a COVID-19 vaccine was December 2, 2020 (see *Journal of Medical Internet Research* online article for Multimedia Appendix 1 for a discussion of robustness tests relevant to vaccination date). Figure 1 presents a histogram of the dates that respondents reported first-dose vaccination (see *Journal of Medical Internet Research* online article for Figure 1). The largest percentage of first-dose vaccinations occurred in March 2021, with the first-dose vaccination rate dropping steadily through April to July 2021. First-dose vaccination increased slightly in August 2021 before dropping off substantially in October 2021. If an individual was not vaccinated by the date on which they completed CABS wave 3, then their last observation in the dataset was the broadcast week of their wave 3 survey completion date.

The change in digital media dose by DMA, the main independent variable, ranged from −155,716.4 to 117,041.3, with a mean of 520.6 (SD [standard error] 14, 281.69). Table S1 (see *Journal of Medical Internet Research* online article for Multimedia Appendix 1) presents descriptive statistics for all variables in the analysis.

To assess the relationship between digital media dose and first-dose COVID-19 vaccination, we estimated a series of multilevel logistic regression models, with varying intercepts by DMA to account for the nesting of respondents within DMAs. The SEs [standard errors] of these models are clustered by DMA. The intraclass correlation coefficient for the main model was 0.03, indicating that about 3% of the variance in the outcome variable varies across DMAs.

We estimated four regression models in a stepwise manner. Model 1 (baseline model) estimates the relationship between change in digital media dose between $week_{t-2}$ and $week_{t-1}$ and the likelihood of first-dose COVID-19 vaccination. In model 2, we estimated the baseline model, including controls for exogenous COVID-19-relevant factors. In model 3, we also controlled for the sociodemographic characteristics of survey respondents. In model 4, we included an additional control for respondents' vaccine confidence as reported in wave 1. As there may have been certain time periods in which a DMA was more likely to see changes in digital impressions and individuals were more likely to receive a vaccination, we included week dummy variables in all models. All models were weighted and design adjusted (see Survey Weighting in *Journal of Medical Internet Research* online article Multimedia Appendix 1). Analyses were conducted using *Stata* (version 17; StataCorp).[41] Multimedia Appendix 1 (see *Journal of Medical Internet Research* online article) includes a discussion of the regression model specification for the primary model below (model 4).

Results

Relationship between Digital Advertising Media Dose and the Likelihood of Vaccination
Table 1 (see *Journal of Medical Internet Research* online article for Table 1) presents results from all regression models. As the models used in this study are multilevel logit models, the coefficients cannot be directly interpreted in terms of substantive effect. Rather, we calculate marginal effects (see below) to understand the substantive effects of each variable. Results for model 1 show a positive and statistically significant relationship between the weekly change in digital impressions and the likelihood of first-dose vaccination ($\beta = 0.000014$; $Z = 3.22$; $P = 0.001$), indicating that an increase in digital impressions within a DMA was associated with a higher likelihood of a respondent in that DMA reporting having received a first-dose COVID-19 vaccination in the subsequent week.

There were no substantive differences between models 1 and 2 in the effects of change in digital media dose on the likelihood of first-dose COVID-19 vaccination; the effect on the likelihood of first-dose vaccination continued to be positive ($\beta = 0.000014$; $Z = 3.16$; $P = 0.002$) after controlling for factors exogenous to the campaign. The change in new COVID-19 cases was negative and significant ($\beta_{cases} = -0.0006$; $Z = -1.99$; $P = 0.047$), whereas the change in deaths was negative and insignificant ($\beta_{deaths} = -0.01$; $Z = -1.18$; $P = 0.24$). The total change in COVID-19 cable news coverage was positive and insignificant ($\beta = 0.172$; $Z = 0.24$; $P = 0.81$). (The week dummy variable format makes it difficult to fully assess the effect of COVID-19 cable news coverage.)

The relationship between change in digital media dose and the likelihood of first-dose vaccination was positive and statistically significant for both models 3 and 4 ($\beta_{model3} = 0.000013$; $Z = 3.12$; $P = 0.002$ and $\beta_{model4} = 0.000014$; $Z = 3.13$; $P = 0.002$, respectively) after controlling for respondents' sociodemographic characteristics and vaccine confidence. In fact, there was a minimum difference seen in the effect of the change in digital media dose when controlling for sociodemographics. This indicates that individual sociodemographics do not change the overall effect of the campaign, which is as expected given that any one individual's age, income, ideology, etc., is in all likelihood not correlated with the campaign's decision to increase or decrease digital dose in the DMA in which that individual lives.

Taken together, models 1–4 consistently indicated that an increase in the number of digital impressions in a DMA between $week_{t-2}$ and $week_{t-1}$ was associated with an increased likelihood that an individual in that DMA received their first dose of a COVID-19 vaccine in the subsequent week.

Substantive Effects of Digital Dose on the Likelihood of Vaccination
To examine the substantive relationship between the change in digital campaign impressions and the likelihood of first-dose COVID-19 vaccination, we estimated the expected probability of first-dose vaccination across levels of weekly change in digital impressions while holding all other variables at their means. More than 95% of all observations fell between −30,000 and 30,000 impressions, although this variable ranged from about −155,000 to a high of about 117,000 in some markets (see *Journal of Medical Internet Research* online article for Figure 2).

Figure 3 (see *Journal of Medical Internet Research* online article for Figure 3) illustrates the expected probability of first-dose vaccination as a function of the change in digital media dose when this variable falls between −30,000 and 30,000 impressions. The solid pink line is the expected probability of an individual receiving a first-dose vaccine, given the change in digital impressions in their DMA in the previous week, while holding all other variables at their means. The dashed lines represent the 95% CI.

When digital impressions in a DMA decreased by 30,000 between $week_{t-1}$ and $week_{t-2}$, the chance of a respondent in that DMA receiving a first-dose COVID-19 vaccine in $week_{t-0}$ was about 1.2%. When digital impressions did not change between $week_{t-1}$ and $week_{t-2}$, the chance of a respondent receiving the first dose of a COVID-19 vaccine was one-third greater (1.7%). When digital impressions increased by 30,000 between $week_{t-1}$ and $week_{t-2}$, the chance of a respondent receiving a first-dose COVID-19 vaccine was 2.6%. In other words, increasing digital impressions from 0 to 30,000 in a given week increased the likelihood of being vaccinated by 53%. Increasing digital impressions from −30,000 to 30,000 in a given week more than doubled (125% increase) the likelihood of being vaccinated. The average marginal effect on the likelihood of receiving a first-dose COVID-19 vaccination in a broadcast week given a change of 1 additional impression is 0.0000433%.

Discussion

Principal Findings

This study assessed the relationship between paid campaign digital media and the likelihood of COVID-19 vaccination in a representative sample of US adults. Results demonstrate a positive and significant relationship between the weekly change in digital impressions and the likelihood of first-dose vaccination, providing initial evidence that the digital campaign has been effective in increasing COVID-19 vaccination among US adults. This association remained statistically significant after controlling for a series of covariates, including COVID-19 cases and deaths as well as respondents' sociodemographic characteristics and baseline vaccine confidence, indicating that results are robust to the inclusion of other factors. It is possible that the association is a factor of both getting people who would otherwise not be vaccinated to do so and shortening the time to vaccination, both of which are of substantial importance during a pandemic. Future research could use event-history modeling to explore these possibilities.

Results indicate that when change in digital impression exposure is held at 0, older respondents compared to younger respondents, those with higher incomes compared to those with lower incomes, and those with higher education compared to those with lower levels of education were significantly more likely to receive first-dose COVID-19 vaccination. These findings, which are independent of the campaign's effects, align with recent research demonstrating that willingness to vaccinate is higher among individuals aged 65 years and older compared to younger groups[42]; that lower-income individuals are less willing to get vaccinated compared to those with higher incomes[43]; and, relative to individuals with less education, those with a college degree or higher reported greater vaccine acceptance.[44] Results also demonstrate that, independent of digital campaign exposure, politically conservative respondents were significantly less likely to be vaccinated compared to more liberal respondents, echoing findings from other research that show political conservatism is negatively associated with intentions to get vaccinated and vaccine uptake.[45,46]

Importantly, much of the extant literature examines longer-term effects (e.g., recalled campaign exposure or campaign impressions aggregated over longer periods of time) on behavior change,[47,48,49] whereas this study examines the relationship between weekly change in digital impressions and vaccination uptake. Focusing on the short-term effects of digital dose may represent a more conservative approach, likely underestimating the total effect of the digital campaign on COVID-19 vaccination. Further, this study is somewhat limited in scope, as it focuses only on the relationship between the digital campaign and vaccine uptake and does not account for additional media channels through which the campaign was disseminated (e.g., television and out-of-home advertising), all of which may impact the relationship between the campaign and vaccine uptake. Although this is a first assessment of the impact of digital impressions on COVID-19 vaccine uptake, a fruitful avenue for future research may involve the incorporation of other media channels through which the campaign was disseminated, to test the association between campaign impressions and vaccinations more comprehensively.

Limitations
This study's results reflect a discrete period and single media channel and may not reflect the influence of the campaign on the likelihood of vaccination during other time periods or channels through which the campaign has been disseminated (e.g., print and radio). The recalled date of first-dose vaccination was subject to recall bias and may not reflect respondents' actual date of vaccination. All impressions data were aggregated by DMA; however, the dependent variable was provided at the respondent level. Weekly changes in media dose by DMA functioned as a measure of probable dose, exogenous to our survey data, but does not represent confirmed campaign exposure among respondents. It is possible that weighting methodologies could influence findings; however, sensitivity checks found little change in the association (see *Journal of Medical Internet Research* online article for Multimedia Appendix 1). Previous evaluations[47,48,49] have examined effects of campaign exposure aggregated over longer periods, whereas this study examined short-term effects (i.e., week-over-week change) of the campaign on vaccine uptake. This is likely a conservative approach, which could lead to an underestimation of campaign effects.

Although our models included potential influencing factors for vaccine uptake, the variable list was not exhaustive, and analyses may have been subject to the influence of unmeasured confounders. For more than 2 years, US adults have been exposed to information and conversations about COVID-19 vaccination from government sources (e.g., federal agencies and state and municipal health departments), health care representatives (e.g., health care professionals and pharmaceutical companies), community-based organizations, and friends and family. Concurrently, many government, travel, and employer vaccination mandates and policies were implemented during the study period. It is possible that first-dose vaccination in our study sample was influenced by one or several other factors not included in our models. Further, the change in the campaign's digital dose may have differential effects based on geography, with the campaign being more successful in certain regions of the country. This may be an interesting area for future research.

Conclusions
The COVID-19 pandemic represents one of the largest public health crises of our era.[50] Public education campaigns can help promote COVID-19 vaccine uptake.[51] Results from this study offer the first evidence of a large-scale digital COVID-19 public education campaign's initial impact on vaccine uptake. The size and length of the HHS COVID-19 "We Can Do This" public education campaign make it uniquely situated to examine the

impact of a digital campaign on COVID-19 vaccination, which may help inform future vaccine communication efforts and broader public education efforts. These findings suggest that campaign digital dose has attenuated the burden of COVID-19 in the United States; future research may be useful in assessing campaign impact on reduced COVID-19-attributed morbidity and mortality and other benefits.

Public Health Implications
This study's findings show that the HHS COVID-19 public education campaign was associated with a greater likelihood of individual vaccination in any given week during the period from April 1 to November 7, 2021. People who reported living in areas with more digital campaign impressions were more likely to be vaccinated, as increasing digital impressions from −30,000 to 30,000 in a given week more than doubled (125% increase) the likelihood of being vaccinated. These findings indicate that, similar to public education campaign influence on other health behaviors,[36,37] the HHS COVID-19 public education campaign has played a key role in influencing COVID-19 vaccine uptake in the United States. Public education campaigns have promise to influence other COVID-19 vaccination behaviors, such as encouraging parents to get their eligible children vaccinated and encouraging eligible adults to get a COVID-19 booster.

Acknowledgments
This work was supported by the US Department of Health and Human Services (HHS) using National Institutes of Health (NIH) contract #75N98019D00007 under orders 75N98022F00001, 75N98021F00001, and 75N98020F00001. The authors gratefully acknowledge our colleagues at the HHS Office of the Assistant Secretary for Public Affairs (ASPA); the HHS Office of the Assistant Secretary for Planning and Evaluation (ASPE), especially Trinidad Beleche, Nicholas Holtkamp, and Lok Wong Samson; the Centers for Disease Control and Prevention (CDC), especially Lynn Sokler; and the Fors Marsh-led team of agencies contributing to the implementation and evaluation of this campaign. We thank the thousands of research respondents who made this study possible.

This publication represents the views of the authors and does not represent US HHS position or policy.

Source: This is an open-access article distributed under the terms of the Creative Commons Attribution License (https://creativecommons.org/licenses/by/4.0/), which permits unrestricted use, distribution, and reproduction in any medium, provided the original work, first published in the *Journal of Medical Internet Research*, is properly cited. The complete bibliographic information, a link to the original publication on www.jmir.org/2023/1/e43873 as well as this copyright and license information must be included. Originally published in the *Journal of Medical Internet Research* (www.jmir.org), March 5, 2023.

Quick Response Communications Planning

When health communication campaigns are used during the maintenance phase of long-term health emergency responses it is imperative to leverage campaign design principles (see earlier in this chapter) to ensure the development of communication objectives and the identification of key audiences, key messages, channels, and communication materials and products. The following subsections include descriptions of each of these topics and examples that are related to the HHS "We Can Do This" health communication campaign that was used during the COVID-19 health emergency.

Communication Objectives

A communication objective is a measurable, time-bound, and audience-focused action.[52] Often communication strategies and objectives are designed to create awareness, educate, or persuade audiences.[52] The following is an example of a communication objective from the "We Can Do This" campaign.

"We Can Do This" was a national initiative to increase public confidence in and uptake of COVID-19 vaccines while reinforcing basic prevention measures. Through a nationwide network of trusted messengers and consistent, fact-based public health messaging, the campaign helped the public make informed decisions about their health and COVID-19, including steps to protect themselves and their communities. The effort was driven by communication science and provided tailored information for at-risk groups.[53]

Although this communication objective lacked a reference to time, it does include references to measuring audience behavior.

Audiences

As outlined in Chapters 3 and 4, identify your audiences and audience segments and their information needs. Understanding *which* audience needs *what* type of information will help you to organize and strategize on your key messaging.

Audience segments for the "We Can Do This" health communication campaign included:

- General market
- Asian-American-Pacific Islander
- Parents
- Health care professionals
- Older adults
- Young adults and students
- Rural communities
- Latino-Hispanic
- Teachers/school administrators
- Black-African Americans
- LGTBQ+
- People with disabilities
- American-Indian-Alaska Natives

Key Messages

Communication objectives will provide you with a broad strategy about who you want to communicate with and the information you would like to provide. Key messages are the specific messages that the agency wants to communicate that are aligned with the communication objectives. For example, if the communication objective is create awareness about an infectious diseases, there are specific key messages that need to be created. During the initial phase of an emergency, the key messages will need to address uncertainty, make a commitment to those affected by the health emergency, provide messages of self-efficacy, and express empathy.

Key message topics for the "We Can Do This" health communication campaign included:
- Building vaccine confidence
- Boosters
- COVID-19 vaccination information
- Updates on COVID-19 vaccines
- Long COVID
- COVID-19 treatment
- Vaccine benefits
- Preventive measures
- Vaccine safety
- Pregnancy, breastfeeding, and fertility
- Vaccine misinformation
- Building campaign confidence

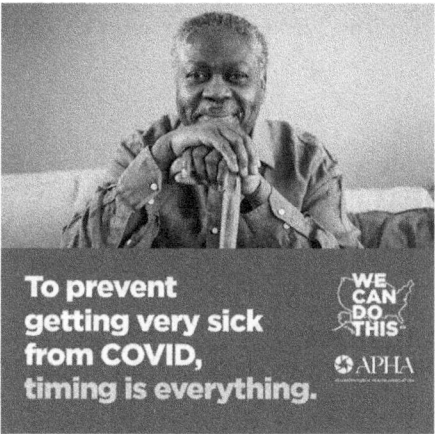

Figure 8.1 Social media graphic "Timing Is Everything" designed for sharing in the "We Can Do This" national health communication campaign
Source: www.apha.org/Topics-and-Issues/Communicable-Disease/Coronavirus/We-Can-Do-This

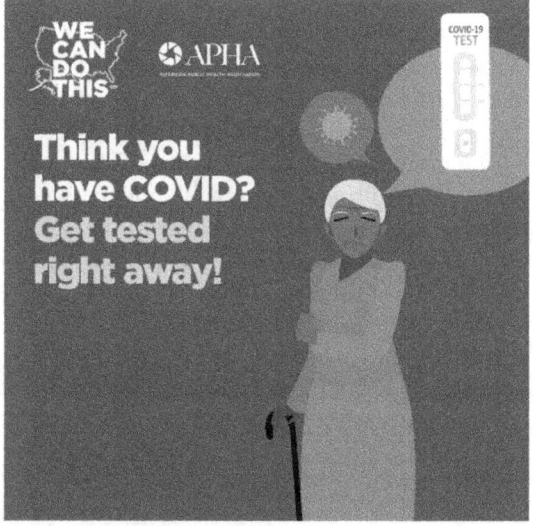

Figure 8.2 Social media graphic "Get Tested" designed for sharing in the "We Can Do This" national health communication campaign
Source: www.apha.org/Topics-and-Issues/Communicable-Disease/Coronavirus/We-Can-Do-This

Channels

As outlined in Chapter 5, think through what channels are available to you for sharing information and which audiences use what channels.

Communication channels for the "We Can Do This" health communication campaign included:
- COVID.gov website
- Weekly emails
- Webinars
- Social media

Communication Products

As outlined in Chapter 5, think through what communication materials need to be developed, such as talking points, web page copy, and visuals such as charts and graphs.

Communication products for the "We Can Do This" health communication campaign included:
- Informational content
- Posters and flyers
- Toolkits for specific audiences and in multiple languages (employers, older adults, parents)
- Social media graphics (see Figures 8.1 and 8.2)
- Videos

Key Tips for Spokespeople, Partner Agencies, and Call Centers

During every phase of a health emergency, spokespeople, partner agencies, and call centers need to receive consistent and coordinated information from the health agency. Here are key some key tips for those who are spokespeople or who work at partner agencies or call centers during the maintenance phase of a health emergency.

Spokespeople: When health communication campaigns are used during a long-term health emergency, the campaigns will use specific key messages to communicate about the health communication program. These key messages may differ from emergency risk communication information about the response operations of the health emergency. It is important for spokespeople to be up to date on all public messaging related to the emergency response operations and health communication campaign activities. This ensures that spokespeople can stay on message during all external communication activities.

Partner agencies: Partner agencies can help amplify health communication campaign messages by participating in media events, attending kickoff events, and sharing communication materials with their audiences. Coordinate with the campaign organizers to ensure partner activities support the objectives of the campaign.

Call centers: When communication campaigns begin, it is important for call centers to be aware of the new messages that will be shared. Ensure that call centers have access to key messages and know where to direct individuals if the call centers receive inquiries from the public about the health communication campaign. Coordinate with campaign organizers to determine whether the call centers ought to provide metrics about the number and type of inquiries received during the health communication campaign.

Theory Callout: Health Behavior Model

The Health Belief Model (HBM) was created in the 1950s by Irwin M. Rosenstock, Godfrey M. Hochbaum, S. Stephen Kegeles, and Howard Leventhal, who were social psychologists working at the US Public Health Service, where their work focused mainly on prevention.[54,55] Rosenstock and colleagues were curious about why few people were getting screened for tuberculosis even though mobile X-rays were readily available. They developed a model that would take into account the behavior of individuals who were not yet suffering from a severe disease.[55]

The main constructs of the theory relate to a person's perceptions, modifying factors, and likelihood of action. The person's individual perceptions plus external modifying factors impact whether they will actually take an action to protect their health. Within the HBM, individual perceptions are made up of how concerned and interested someone is regarding their own health, their beliefs about how vulnerable they are to the health threat, and their beliefs about the consequences of the health threat. Modifying factors include demographic variables such as gender, sex, socioeconomic status, geographic location, age, perceived threat, and cues to action. Likelihood to take action is defined as the perceived benefits compared against the perceived barriers to taking the health action. If someone perceives that there is a threat to their health and there is an external cue (e.g., modifying factor) for them to take action, plus the person believes that the perceived benefits outweigh the perceived barriers, they are likely to take the recommended health action.[32]

A recent study revealed that the HBM "has a good predictive ability of COVID-19 related behavior" and found that perceived benefit was a significate predicator of behavioral action.[56] For emergency risk communicators, the HBM is a good tool to use when planning and designing health communication campaigns during a long-term health emergency.

End-of-Chapter Reflection Questions

1 Think about a time when you created a health communication campaign for a public health program. Identify how the program was developed and implemented and evaluate the campaign.

2 Reflect upon the vaccine health campaigns during COVID-19. How were the health campaigns developed, implemented, and evaluated? What worked well for your agency? What needs improvement?

3 Reflect on your agency's policies regarding appropriate paperwork for engaging with vendors. Is everything in place to ensure that you can rapidly engage with an outside agency to develop a health communication campaign?

4 How would you engage your community-based organizations in a health education campaign to support behavior change? List three community-based organizations you can count on to support your agency. List three different community-based organizations you'd like to develop relationships with.

References

1. Rice R, Atkins C. *Public Communication Campaigns*, 4th edition. Thousand Oaks, CA, Sage Publications, Inc., 2012.
2. The History of Our COVID-19 Vaccine Education Initiative. *Ad Council*. 2024. www.adcouncil.org/our-impact/covid-vaccine/our-covid-19-vaccine-retrospective (Accessed March 7, 2024).
3. Zhao X. Health Communication Campaigns: A Brief Introduction and Call for Dialogue. *Int J Nurs Sci* 2020;7:S11–15.
4. *Making Health Communication Programs Work*. Washinton, DC, Health and Human Services, n.d.
5. CDC. *Types of Evaluation*. National Center for HIV/AIDS, Viral Hepatitis, STD, and TB Prevention, editor. Atlanta, GA, CDC, n.d.
6. White House. Let's Move South Lawn Series Kickoff. *YouTube*. 2010. www.youtube.com/watch?v=8MDfrB0i0Zk (Accessed March 23, 2024).
7. Let's Move! Partnership for a Healthier America. www.ahealthieramerica.org/articles/let-s-move-84 (Accessed March 23, 2024).
8. *Crisis and Emergency Risk Communication Manual*. Atlanta, GA, Centers for Disease Control and Prevention, 2014.
9. CDC. *Crisis and Emergency Risk Communication October 2018*. Atlanta, GA, CDC, 2018.
10. Seeger M, Sellnow T, Ulmer R. *Communication and Organizational Crisis*. London, Bloomsbury Academic, 2003.
11. Vidoloff K, Petrun E. Communication Successes and Constraints: Analysis of the 2008 Salmonella Saintpaul Foodborne Illness Outbreak. *Journal of the Northwest Communication Association* 2010;39(1):65–90.
12. Marcus BH, Forsyth LH. The Challenge of Behavior Change. *Med Health R I* 1997;80(9):300–302.
13. Rogers E. *Diffusion of Innovations*. New York, London, Free Press, 1983.
14. Bandura A. Self-Efficacy: Toward a Unifying Theory of Behavioral Change. *Psychol Rev* 1977;84:191–215.
15. Stephenson MT, Witte KD. Creating Fear in a Risky World: Generating Effective Health Risk Messages. In: Rice R, Atkins C, editors. *Public Communication Campaigns*, 3rd edition. Thousand Oaks, CA, Sage Publications, 2001; 88–102.
16. Orozco-Olvera V, Shen F, Cluver L. The Effectiveness of Using Entertainment Education Narratives to Promote Safer Sexual Behaviors of Youth: A Meta-Analysis, 1985–2017. *PLoS ONE* 2019;14(2):e0209969.
17. Bandura A. Social Cognitive Theory of Mass Communication. In: Bryant J, Zillmann D, editors. *Media Effects: Advances in Theory and Research*, 2nd edition. Mahwah, NJ, Lawrence Erlbaum Associates, 2002; 121–53.
18. Horton D, Wohl R. Mass Communication and Para-Social Interaction: Observations on Intimacy at a Distance. *Psychiatry* 1956;19(3):215–29.
19. Eccles JS, Wigfield A. Motivational Beliefs, Values, and Goals. *Ann Rev Psychol* 2002;53(1):109–32.
20. Eccles JS, Adler TF, Futterman R, Goff SB, Kaczala CM, Meece JL, Midgley C. Expectancies, Values, and Academic Behaviors. In: Spence J, editor. *Achievement and Achievement*

Motivation. San Francisco, CA, W. H. Freeman, 1983; 75–146.

21 Wigfield A, Tonks S, Lutz KS. Expectancy-Value Theory. In: Wentzel K, Wigfield A, editors. *Handbook of Motivation at School*. New York, Routledge, 2009; 55–75.

22 Leaper C. More Similarities than Differences in Contemporary Theories of Social Development? A Plea for Theory Bridging. *Adv Child Dev Behav* 2011;40:337–78.

23 Piester L. Why I Probably Won't Ever Rewatch *Grey's Anatomy*'s Pandemic-Filled Season 17. *E-News*. 2021. www.eonline.com/news/1276345/why-i-probably-wont-ever-rewatch-greys-anatomys-pandemic-filled-season-17 (Accessed March 7, 2024).

24 Power E. *Grey's Anatomy* catches Covid-19 – but it's nothing serious. *The Irish Times*. 2021, March 31.

25 Shukla S. "*Grey's Anatomy*" Season 17 review: It displays courage and goodwill of the medical community during the COVID pandemic. *WION*. 2021. www.wionews.com/entertainment/hollywood/news-greys-anatomy-season-17-review-it-displays-courage-and-goodwill-of-the-medical-community-during-the-covid-pandemic-343146 (Accessed March 7, 2024).

26 St. James E. 17 seasons in, *Grey's Anatomy* reimagined itself for the pandemic. But only a little bit. *Vox*. 2021, www.vox.com/culture/22465064/greys-anatomy-finale-season-17-recap-review-covid-19-beach (Accessed March 7, 2024).

27 Cho H, Salmon CT. Unintended Effects of Health Communication Campaigns. *J Communication* 2007;57(2):293–317.

28 COVID Data Tracker. *Centers for Disease Control and Prevention*. 2022. https://covid.cdc.gov/covid-data-tracker (Accessed March 7, 2024).

29 COVID-19 Vaccination. *Centers for Disease Control and Prevention*. 2021. www.cdc.gov/coronavirus/2019-ncov/vaccines/effectiveness/work.html (Accessed April 4, 2024).

30 Schneider EC, Shah A, Sah P, Vilches T, Pandey A, Moghadas S, Galvani AP. Impact of U.S COVID-19 vaccination efforts: an update on averted deaths, hospitalizations, and health care costs through March 2022. *The Commonwealth Fund*. 2022. www.commonwealthfund.org/blog/2022/impact-us-covid-19-vaccination-efforts-march-update (Accessed March 23, 2024).

31 MacDonald NE, SAGE Working Group on Vaccine Hesitancy. Vaccine Hesitancy: Definition, Scope and Determinants. *Vaccine* 2015;33(34):4161–64.

32 Aw J, Seng JJB, Seah SSY, Low LL. COVID-19 Vaccine Hesitancy – A Scoping Review of Literature in High-Income Countries. *Vaccines (Basel)* 2021;9(8):900.

33 Wagner AL, Porth JM, Wu Z, Boulton ML, Finlay JM, Kobayashi LC. Vaccine Hesitancy during the COVID-19 Pandemic: A Latent Class Analysis of Middle-Aged and Older US Adults. *J Community Health* 2022;47(3):408–15.

34 Jarrett C, Wilson R, O'Leary M, Eckersberger E, Larson HJ, SAGE Working Group on Vaccine Hesitancy. Strategies for Addressing Vaccine Hesitancy – A Systematic Review. *Vaccine* 2015;33(34):4180–90.

35 Finney Rutten LJ, Zhu X, Leppin AL, Ridgeway JL, Swift MD, Griffin JM, et al. Evidence-Based Strategies for Clinical Organizations to Address COVID-19 Vaccine Hesitancy. *Mayo Clin Proc* 2021;96(3):699–707.

36 Wakefield MA, Loken B, Hornik RC. Use of Mass Media Campaigns to Change Health Behaviour. *Lancet* 2010;376(9748):1261–71.

37 Anker AE, Feeley TH, McCracken B, Lagoe CA. Measuring the Effectiveness of Mass-Mediated Health Campaigns through Meta-Analysis. *J Health Commun* 2016;21(4):439–56.

38 Weber MA, Backer TE, Brubach A. Creating the HHS COVID-19 Public Education Media Campaign: Applying Systems Change Learnings. *J Health Commun* 2022;27(3):201–07.

39. Technical overview of the AmeriSpeak® panel NORC's probability-based household panel. *NORC*. 2022. https://tinyurl.com/2p97y2v6 (Accessed May 10, 2024).

40. Vu HT, Guo L, McCombs ME. Exploring "the World Outside and the Pictures in Our Heads". *Journal Mass Commun Q* 2014;91(4):669–86.

41. StataCorp. Stata Statistical Software: Release 17. www.stata.com (Accessed March 23, 2024).

42. Kelly BJ, Southwell BG, McCormack LA, Bann CM, MacDonald PDM, Frasier AM, et al. Predictors of Willingness to Get a COVID-19 Vaccine in the U.S. *BMC Infect Dis* 2021;21(1):338.

43. El-Mohandes A, White TM, Wyka K, Rauh L, Rabin K, Kimball SH, et al. COVID-19 Vaccine Acceptance among Adults in Four Major US Metropolitan Areas and Nationwide. *Sci Rep* 2021;11(1):21844.

44. Yasmin F, Najeeb H, Moeed A, Naeem U, Asghar M, Chughtai N, et al. COVID-19 Vaccine Hesitancy in the United States: A Systematic Review. *Front Public Health* 2021;23(9):770985.

45. Latkin C, Dayton L, Miller J, Yi G, Balaban A, Boodram B, et al. A Longitudinal Study of Vaccine Hesitancy Attitudes and Social Influence as Predictors of COVID-19 Vaccine Uptake in the US. *Hum Vaccin Immunother*. 2022;18(5):2043102.

46. Berg MB, Lin L. Predictors of COVID-19 Vaccine Intentions in the United States: The Role of Psychosocial Health Constructs and Demographic Factors. *Transl Behav Med* 2021;11(9):1782–88.

47. McAfee T, Davis KC, Alexander RL, Pechacek TF, Bunnell R. Effect of the First Federally Funded US Antismoking National Media Campaign. *Lancet* 2013;382(9909):2003–11.

48. Farrelly MC, Duke JC, Nonnemaker J, MacMonegle AJ, Alexander TN, Zhao X, et al. Association between the Real Cost Media Campaign and Smoking Initiation among Youths – United States, 2014–2016. *MMWR Morb Mortal Wkly Rep* 2017;66(2):47–50.

49. Farrelly MC, Nonnemaker J, Davis KC, Hussin A. The Influence of the National Truth Campaign on Smoking Initiation. *Am J Prev Med* 2009;36(5):379–84.

50. WHO coronavirus (COVID-19) dashboard. *World Health Organization*. 2022. https://covid19.who.int (Accessed May 10, 2024).

51. COVID-19 vaccine effectiveness research. *Centers for Disease Control and Prevention*. 2022. www.cdc.gov/vaccines/covid-19/effectiveness-research/protocols.html (Accessed April 7, 2024).

52. *Study Guide for the Examination for Accreditation in Public Relations*. New York, Universal Accreditation Board/Public Relations Society of America, 2021.

53. APHA. COVID-19. 2024. www.apha.org/Topics-and-Issues/Communicable-Disease/Coronavirus/We-Can-Do-This (Accessed March 7, 2024).

54. Jones CL, Jensen JD, Scherr CL, Brown NR, Christy K, Weaver J. The Health Belief Model as an Explanatory Framework in Communication Research: Exploring Parallel, Serial, and Moderated Mediation. *Health Communication* 2015;30(6):566–76.

55. Rosenstock I. Historical Origins of the Health Belief Model. *Health Education & Behavior*. 1974;2(4):328–35.

56. Zewdie A, Mose A, Sahle T, Bedewi J, Gashu M, Kebede N, Yimer A. The Health Belief Model's Ability to Predict COVID-19 Preventive Behavior: A Systematic Review. *SAGE Open Med* 2022;10:20503121221113668.

Part III — Communicating and Planning after a Health Emergency

Chapter 9

Pivoting from Crisis Management to Recovery
Communicating the End of a Health Emergency

Chapter Objectives
- Describe the four components of a recovery message.
- Describe the importance of educating the public after a health emergency.
- List how to communicate with policymakers after a health emergency.
- Identify recovery messages by analyzing a real-world example.
- Recall the importance of memorials after health emergencies.
- Identify three ways to care for organizational staff after a health emergency.
- Be able to write communication objectives, identify audiences, develop key messages, identify channels, and identify communication products that are needed for recovery messaging.
- Recall the mindfulness framework.

Chapters 6, 7, and 8 focused on initial and maintenance messages and health communication campaigns that occur from the beginning of an emergency through the weeks, months, and even years of a health emergency response. Theoretically, the transition from the maintenance phase to the recovery phase occurs when the public health threat has been mitigated. From a public health perspective, this phase is not about responding to or managing a health threat but focusing on what has happened and how the community moves forward. The Federal Emergency Management Agency (FEMA) defines the recovery phase as aiming to "provide assistance to individuals and communities overwhelmed by all hazards, including acts of terrorism, natural disasters or other emergencies."[1] The National Disaster Recovery Framework outlines the principles, roles and responsibilities, structures, and processes needed to ensure a community affected by a disaster can restore, redevelop, and revitalize its health, social, economic, and environmental domains to create a more resilient community.[2]

For the purposes of this chapter, the term "recovery" will be used to describe messages that occur during the Crisis and Emergency Risk Communication (CERC) resolution phase. A key tenet of recovery messaging is signaling that the health emergency or crisis is over – that there is no additional threat to health or public safety. Recovery messaging has distinct characteristics: signal the new normal, identify that the health threat has been mitigated, express empathy, continue with commitment statements, educate the public, and engage with policymakers. During recovery, a sense of collective and community healing is needed, and memorials and anniversary observances should occur. Recovery messaging can help boost community resilience, providing the ability to come back stronger after a major disaster or emergency.

Health departments often have to pull away from a health emergency to investigate another outbreak or natural disaster that has occurred, or perhaps priorities will shift away from the current health emergency. When this happens, recovery messaging often does not occur; however, considering the commitment messages that were given during the initial and maintenance phases of an emergency, it behooves the health agency – especially when considering credibility, trust, transparency, and respect – to engage in recovery messaging with the public and those affected by the emergency.

Recovery emergency risk communication during COVID-19 was inconsistent and varied. Part of this is due to the expiration of official government emergency declarations allowing emergency funding to be released to support the coronavirus response. When those emergency declarations expired, there was often a misperception by the public that the health threat was over; however, this merely meant that emergency funding and emergency authorizations were ending, but the threat to health from COVID-19 was still present.[3]

Recovery Messages: What They Are and How to Write Them

There are four message components of a recovery message that will support the CERC principles of being right, being credible, expressing empathy, promoting action, and showing respect.

Recovery message components include:
- Signal the move toward a "new normal."
- Indicate the health threat has been mitigated.
- Express empathy.
- Continue to state the agency's commitment to the community.

Signal the Move toward a "New Normal"

During the recovery phase, there is a sense that things may not return to how they were before the health emergency.[4] Messaging during this phase needs to focus on what the health agency has learned while managing this health threat. Something will have changed at the individual level, whether that is a behavior change to not eat a certain type of food or new habits such as coughing into a sleeve, wearing a mask, or physically distancing when certain outbreaks occur. At a community level, when looking at natural disasters with health impacts such as flooding, tornadoes, earthquakes, and wildfires, the physical environment might have changed. Such changes to people's physical environment and way of life have impacts on how they interact with each other and how they view the world. Further, these changes to the physical environment often mean that it takes a long time to rebuild and develop a new normal.

For health emergencies, recovery messages that signal the new normal draw attention to the current status of community health risk. For example, during June 2022, in the midst of the COVID-19, the US Centers for Disease Control and Prevention (CDC) messaging reframed community risk levels by using a metaphor of a weather map.[5,6,7] Just as an individual would check the weather forecast for the day, CDC's new messaging included a graphic to help people understand community risk levels based on a color-coded map. The color coding for a particular geographic region would let an individual know whether the risk of contracting COVID-19 was high or low in that area and so determine what kind of self-protective action was needed.

The following is an excerpt from a speech given by the World Health Organization (WHO) Director General in May 2023 regarding the end of the declared COVID-19 pandemic. This is an example of how an organization signals that a "new normal" is occurring as a health emergency comes to an end.

> **Example Message: WHO Signal toward the "New Normal"**
> But COVID-19 has been so much more than a health crisis. It has caused severe economic upheaval, erasing trillions from GDP, disrupting travel and trade, shuttering businesses, and plunging millions into poverty. It has caused severe social upheaval, with borders closed, movement restricted, schools shut, and millions of people experiencing loneliness, isolation, anxiety, and depression.
>
> COVID-19 has exposed and exacerbated political fault lines, within and between nations. It has eroded trust between people, governments, and institutions, fueled by a torrent of mis- and disinformation. And it has laid bare the searing inequalities of our world, with the poorest and most vulnerable communities the hardest hit, and the last to receive access to vaccines and other tools.
>
> For more than a year, the pandemic has been on a downward trend, with population immunity increasing from vaccination and infection, mortality decreasing, and the pressure on health systems easing. This trend has allowed most countries to return to life as we knew it before COVID-19.
>
> For the past year, the Emergency Committee – and WHO – have been analyzing the data carefully and considering when the time would be right to lower the level of alarm.
>
> Yesterday, the Emergency Committee met for the 15th time and recommended to me that I declare an end to the public health emergency of international concern. I have accepted that advice.
>
> It is therefore with great hope that I declare COVID-19 over as a global health emergency. However, that does not mean COVID-19 is over as a global health threat.
>
> Last week, COVID-19 claimed a life every 3 minutes – and that's just the deaths we know about. As we speak, thousands of people around the world are fighting for their lives in intensive care units. And millions more continue to live with the debilitating effects of post-COVID-19 condition.
>
> This virus is here to stay. It is still killing, and it's still changing. The risk remains of new variants emerging that cause new surges in cases and deaths.
>
> The worst thing any country could do now is to use this news as a reason to let down its guard, to dismantle the systems it has built, or to send the message to its people that COVID-19 is nothing to worry about. What this news means is that it is time for countries to transition from emergency mode to managing COVID-19 alongside other infectious diseases.
>
> I emphasize that this is not a snap decision. It is a decision that has been considered carefully for some time, planned for, and made on the basis of a careful analysis of the data.
>
> If need be, I will not hesitate to convene another Emergency Committee should COVID-19 once again put our world in peril. While this Emergency Committee will now

cease its work, it has sent a clear message that countries must not cease theirs. On the Committee's advice, I have decided to use a provision in the International Health Regulations that has never been used before, to establish a Review Committee to develop long-term, standing recommendations for countries on how to manage COVID-19 on an ongoing basis.

In addition, WHO this week published the fourth edition of the Global Strategic Preparedness and Response Plan for COVID-19, which outlines critical actions for countries in five core areas: collaborative surveillance, community protection, safe and scalable care, access to countermeasures, and emergency coordination.[8]

Indicate the Health Threat Has Been Mitigated

This key message focuses on telling the community that the health threat has been mitigated – that it is less severe than it was during the maintenance phase of the emergency. Typically, this means there is no longer a threat to the general public's health.

Express Empathy

As outlined in previous chapters, emotionally mature individuals are likely to be more empathetic, meaning they are more in touch with their own deep feelings and can imagine, or mentalize, the feelings of others.[9] Empathy can be used in messaging throughout all of the phases of a health emergency.

For leaders and spokespeople engaging in emergency risk communication, being able to understand or at least imagine the feelings of others is critical during an emergency response. Further, empathetic individuals can deliver more authentic messages that resonate deeply with an audience. Psychologist Paul Ekman talked about empathy with the Dalai Lama and differentiated between various types of empathy and compassion. Through their conversations, empathy isn't just about knowing what the other feels, but also relates to the ability to feel with them.[10] Psychologist Daniel Goleman elucidates this further, offering that empathy can take on three different forms: cognitive, emotional, and compassionate.[9]

- *Cognitive:* Simply knowing how the other person feels and what they might be thinking.
- *Emotional:* When you feel physically along with the other person, as though their emotions were contagious.
- *Compassionate:* We not only understand a person's predicament and feel with them, but are spontaneously moved to help, if needed.

Continue to State the Agency's Commitment to the Community

As outlined in previous chapters, commitment statements have two parts: explaining what the agency is doing to find new information about the health emergency and letting the community know that the health agency will be there until the end of the health emergency. As the health agency moves into the resolution phase of the health emergency, recovery messaging ought to continue to express the commitment that the health agency has made to the community and provide updates on the progress that has been made during the health emergency. By demonstrating that the health agency followed through on its commitment, the agency can maintain its credibility and trust with the community affected by the health emergency.

Example Messaging: Health Threat Has Been Mitigated, Express Empathy, and Continue Commitment to Community after an Ebola Outbreak in Uganda

The CDC joins the Government of Uganda and the global public health community in marking the end of the Ebola outbreak in Uganda. Forty-two days, or two incubation periods, have passed since the last case of Ebola was reported, marking the end of the outbreak. In addition, entry screening and public health monitoring of travelers to the United States who have been in Uganda in the prior 21 days will lift effective today, Wednesday, January 11.

"I commend the Government of Uganda, local health workers, and global public health partners who worked to end the country's Ebola outbreak," said CDC Director Rochelle P. Walensky, M.D., M.P.H. "I also want to thank the CDC staff on the front lines in Uganda and around the world who worked countless hours to accelerate an end to the outbreak."

"Our heartfelt sympathies are with the people who lost loved ones to this disease. CDC remains committed to partnering with the Ugandan Ministry of Health in support of survivor programs and in helping strengthen global preparedness and response capacities that can prevent or extinguish future Ebola outbreaks."

CDC will continue to support the Ugandan Ministry of Health in continuing surveillance, infection prevention and control, and response activities to help ensure rapid detection and response to any future cases and outbreaks.[11]

Public Education Campaigns and Engaging Policymakers

Similar to the maintenance phase, during which long-term health emergencies require health communication campaigns to encourage people to take action through health interventions, the recovery phase represents another space to use two specific communication strategies: Educate the public via a public education campaign and engage with policymakers regarding the importance of public health work. Additionally, any lessons learned or after-action reviews can be shared with the public and policymakers during the recovery phase to support organizational learning (see Chapter 10).

Educate the Public

As outlined in Chapter 8, health communication campaigns are vital ways to encourage the community to take action to protect their health. The ending of a health emergency represents another opportunity to use a health communication campaign to continue to educate the public about similar health threats, reinforce the identity of the health department as a trusted source during health emergencies, and highlight the capabilities of the health department to respond to health emergencies.

Engaging in a health communication campaign after a health emergency is important because the health department has the attention of the public, meaning there is a primed audience. The term "priming" comes from research into media effects and specifically agenda-setting by the mass media.[12] For emergency risk communicators, the application of priming to recovery messages means that while the health emergency has people's attention, the health department has an opportunity to continue to communicate about the agency's work to build trust with the public regarding its capabilities and responsiveness.

When building a public education campaign after a health emergency there are several important questions to consider:
- Where are our strengths?
- Where can we build with our community around the positive aspects of our response, and where are the weaknesses or things that are seen negatively by our community?
- How do we build back and move forward as we're building toward this new normal?
- What lessons did the agency learn that we want to share with the public?

It is important to consider the current sentiment within the community. If the agency stumbled or experienced multiple failures from which it did not recover, the tone and messaging of the campaign will be different than that of a campaign that highlights all of the successes of the agency.

Example Messaging: Public Education

In Uganda's capital city, Kampala, a public education campaign coordinated by the Ministry of Health and WHO was implemented after the end of the Ebola outbreak to continue to educate people about Ebola. The campaign worked with community organizers and *boda boda* – or taxi drivers – to help raise awareness, address rumors, and help people report any suspect cases of Ebola.

The campaign involved leaflets, posters, and walking the streets. The key messages included telling people that Ebola is fatal, its signs and symptoms, how to avoid Ebola, and what to do if they find someone in their community who is ill.[13]

Engaging with Policymakers

Engaging with policymakers falls within the role of health policy within a health agency. Often the health director and a policy team monitor and evaluate the performance of health programs and report these metrics to elected officials, including the governor and legislature, state health departments, and health advisory boards. For example, in Oregon, within the Oregon Health Authority (OHA), the Office of Health Policy "conducts impartial policy analysis, research, and evaluation, and provides technical assistance to support health reform planning and implementation in Oregon."[14] Two specific areas of policy work include[14]:

- Developing and analyzing policy as legislatively directed on priority topics such as the key elements of health system transformation, rural health care initiatives, health care financing, and others.
- Analyzing emerging health policy issues and regulations and working with national and other state experts to bring best practices and new ideas to Oregon.

Similarly, the Washington State Health Department and the Executive Office of Policy, Planning, and Evaluation work areas include:

- Offering policy advice, strategies, and standards for internal and external partners.
- Leading and supporting agency-wide initiatives with community impact and design, such as reaccreditation, foundational public health services, and operationalizing the agency's Transformational Plan.
- Supporting the creation of regulations and policies that help the public and the agency implement new laws and programs.

- Measuring impact through policy design and evaluation.
- Creating an overarching policy agenda that aligns actions with strategic priorities.[15]

After a major emergency, changes to public policy often occur.[16] Such events are called "focusing events." A focusing event is "sudden; relatively uncommon; can be reasonably defined as harmful or revealing the possibility of future greater harms; has harms that are concentrated in a particular area or community of interest; and that is known to policy-makers and the public simultaneously."[16] Such focusing events can cause changes to the exposure and attention given to social and political changes and result in groups mobilizing to highlight or constrict these issues.[16] Instead of the focusing event of COVID-19 mobilizing support to provide more funding to public health and to invest in public health preparedness to establish a resilient and capable system that is able to respond to future outbreaks, in the United States the reaction has been to reduce and minimize the public health system.

During COVID-19 in the United States, state governments enacted emergency orders to shut down economic operations such as restaurants, close schools, require the wearing of masks, and vaccine mandates; these orders varied state by state, often influenced by the dominant political party at the governor level.[17] Since 2022, there has been an effort to limit the authority of public health agencies, governors, and state or local health officials in the United States.[18] In 2023, through federal budget negotiations, approximately $27 billion of appropriated COVID-19 dollars were pulled back through a rescission. These dollars, which were unspent but had been appropriated to be used for COVID-19 activities in multiple federal agencies, were redistributed to other parts of the federal budget.[19] Underfunding public health has been a long-standing issue, and in recent years Public Health Emergency Preparedness funding has undergone major cuts.[20] The lack of sufficient funding for public health was exacerbated during COVID-19, revealing the health system's inability to respond to emerging threats, the lack of technology and data systems for disease surveillance, and the inadequate support to maintain a robust workforce.[21]

For emergency risk communicators, it is important to coordinate with public health leadership and the health policy team to understand the responsibilities of the health agency set forth within the established statues. After an emergency, engaging with elected officials is important in order to share metrics and program evaluations regarding the successes and challenges of the health emergency response. When engaging with elected officials, it is important to keep in mind the messaging needs of this particular audience and to frame the messages so that they will resonate with them. Communicating about investments in public health with policymakers is supported by the "10 Essential Public Health Services" framework developed by CDC.[21]

The following messaging recommendations for engaging with elected officials are provided by the Berkley Media Studies Group[22,23]:

1. Frame public health as indispensable and use metaphors when possible.
2. Lead with strengths and achievements, not deficits and weaknesses.
3. Boost the public's confidence in public health by using precise, active language and compelling images that demonstrate the field's competence.
4. Use plain but descriptive language so anyone can understand what's at stake.
5. Emphasize how these bills block public health's job of keeping the community healthy and safe.

Further, when writing key messages, there are three message components to use to develop values-based messages related to health policy:
- A short description of the problem
- A specific solution along with who is responsible for implementing the solution
- A values statement that reminds the audience why this matters

Example
- *Description of problem:* The public health system our country needs cannot be built on the boom-and-bust cycle of emergency funding.[24]
- *Solution:* The system needs long-term, flexible funding. Short-term and inflexible funding lines for public health make investing in essential infrastructure, workforce, and cross-cutting approaches to prevention, including addressing the social determinants of health, impossible.[24]
- *Values:* We must invest in the public health programs and workforce needed to prevent illness and injury. Doing so would reduce the amount of money that we currently spend on treating preventable disease.[24]

Informing elected officials about the work of the health agency is different from lobbying elected officials. There is a distinction that must be drawn regarding how public health leaders and employees gain support from policymakers. Public health officials cannot engage in direct lobbying of elected officials, but public health officials can talk about the importance of public health and provide metrics and statistics about the effectiveness of current health policies.[23,25,26,27] It is good for any government employee to review their state's government ethics laws on lobbying to ensure any actions taken do not violate state laws. It is possible for health agencies to provide stakeholders and advocates with the latest data and metrics so that when they lobby elected officials they can advocate for why more funds ought to be shifted to the health agency for future public health preparedness.

Mini-Case Study: Oregon Health Authority's COVID-19 Resilience RISE Plan

Signal the Move toward a "New Normal"

OHA developed the COVID-19 RISE (Resilience in Support of Equity) plan detailed five main goals for supporting people in Oregon through the ongoing coronavirus monitoring, but the agency also highlighted that the health threat was no longer a crisis-level pandemic. Here, OHA signaled it was ready to go back to normal public health operations. This signal of moving back to normal public health operations is our signpost or signal of moving into the recovery phase.

> **Messaging Example**
> After more than two years of taking effective, science-based public health actions to slow the spread of COVID-19, Oregon has reached a new phase in the pandemic. The Omicron surge has passed. The spread of the SARS-CoV-2 virus has dramatically tapered. Now:
> - More than 8 in 10 people in Oregon have at least short-term protection against severe COVID-19 disease through vaccination, a prior infection or both.
> - COVID-19 infections have dropped 94% since the peak of the Omicron surge.
> - COVID-19 hospitalizations have dropped to pre-Omicron levels.[23]

Indicate the Health Threat Has Been Mitigated

In the Oregon RISE plan, the agency cited actions they had taken to respond to COVID-19, the number of lives saved, the number of cases, the number of deaths that Oregon experienced, and its ranking in terms of vaccinations (i.e., the percentage of eligible residents who had received a booster). OHA also provided hospital and mask data. This information provided evidence of how OHA managed the health emergency and began to pivot the messaging to focus on recovery through community resilience.

> **Messaging Example**
> Given our population's current level of immunity, Oregon now can lift nearly all the public health requirements that helped prevent the worst forecasts of Omicron-fueled hospitalizations and deaths from becoming a reality. As hospitalizations decline, people in Oregon no longer need to rely on statewide policy interventions to reduce their risk. It is now possible for us to manage COVID-19 at personal and community levels.
> But the pandemic is not yet over. Like a wildfire that has been contained but not fully extinguished, the COVID-19 pandemic still poses risks to many of us. Like a wildfire, the pandemic has left a stark and smoldering aftermath for communities trying to recover.[28]

Educate the Public

The Oregon RISE program also provided information on developing community resilience. It was an outreach program to build a bridge from the health emergency into a new normal. The message's focus was to educate the public about how OHA had managed the health emergency and how it would now pivot into recovery, focusing on community resilience and a new normal.

> **Messaging Example**
> This plan – Oregon RISE: Resilience in Support of Equity – outlines the near-term priorities Oregon will pursue to monitor COVID-19, shield people at highest risk, reinvigorate our communities and repair our social fabric. Oregon's top priority will be to support the capacity and follow the lead of the communities that have been hardest hit by COVID-19: communities of color and tribal communities. Before the pandemic, systemic racism and oppression fueled trauma, higher rates of chronic disease and other conditions potentially leading to loss of life and livelihood. The COVID-19 pandemic intensified and worsened these unjust and systemic health inequities and at the same time amplified the power of resilience, culture and social cohesion within these communities. It's also our priority to protect people who remain more vulnerable to severe disease from COVID-19, including older adults and people with underlying health conditions. In the coming months after public health interventions lift, our goal will be to save lives by strengthening the resilience of people, schools and communities so they can protect themselves from COVID-19. Our five-point plan includes:
> - Protect communities who have been hardest hit by COVID-19.
> - Protect people who are most vulnerable to COVID-19.
> - Expand access to vital health care and support a thriving workforce.
> - Keep schools open for students, staff and families, and help students recover instructional time.
> - Restore social cohesion by listening to local communities and helping people protect themselves and others.[28]

Community Renewal and Social Resilience: Living Memorials and Public Ceremonies

When faced with uncertain or unbelievable circumstances, people engage in a process of sensemaking – a way to comprehend what seems incomprehensible.[29] As people engage in sensemaking to process the impacts of a health emergency on a community, emergency risk communicators can engage in recovery messaging that focuses on the new normal. For example, postcrisis renewal communications should contain future-oriented, positive messages that focus on rebuilding despite the crisis.[4] The foundation for renewal depends upon social resilience – a combination of the physical environment of the community and the social capacity of community members to withstand and recover from a health emergency.[30] The CERC principles of expressing empathy and showing respect need to be woven throughout recovery messages that focus on loss, coping, and resilience.

A key component of recovering from any disruption to daily living is to make sense of what occurred and to engage in ritualized actions to recognize and commemorate the loss.[31] Ritualized actions can include wearing ribbons, posting signs, temporary art installations, permanent memorials, and ceremonies. Ceremonies can be private and individual, such burying remains or holding wakes, funerals, memorials, or celebrations of life that resonate with the cultural and spiritual practices of the deceased.[32] For the purposes of emergency risk communication and health emergencies, physical memorials and public ceremonies will be discussed in the following paragraphs.

Memorials offer a physical site that symbolizes a community's collective loss and painful experience.[33] Memorials can also serve as catalysts for individuals to acknowledge, remember, and deal with a loss they have trouble expressing or would prefer to avoid.[33] Memorials can symbolize the memory and become a physical manifestation of remembering what happened.[34] Examples of memorials that represent national and international events include the Holocaust Memorial, Berlin; the Judenplatz Holocaust Memorial, Vienna; the Peace Memorial Park, Hiroshima; the Vietnam War Memorial, Washington, DC, United States; the Berlin Wall Memorial, Berlin; the 9/11 Memorial and Museum, United States; the Flight 93 National Memorial, Pennsylvania, United States; and the National 9/11 Pentagon Memorial, Virginia, United States. Research has shown memorials can offer healing effects for those personally affected by the trauma of the event.[33] During COVID-19, normal ritualized ceremonies of burying remains and holding wakes, funerals, and memorials were halted due to health concerns; the negative impacts of this disruption were solidly felt in nursing facilities.[35] The increased number of deaths within a short period of time coupled with public shaming caused fear and anxiety among health care workers, and the residents – isolated because of health care guidelines designed to keep them healthy and safe – suffered community losses resulting in intense and challenging grief.[35] To support their healing and mourn their losses, a nursing facility in Washington state created a memorial garden to honor those who had passed due to COVID-19. The intention of the garden was to offer an opportunity for residents, families of the deceased, and health care workers to work through their grief, whether it was prolonged, traumatic, complicated, or disenfranchised, and reestablish a sense of community through a physical memorial to remember those who had passed.[35] Other permanent COVID-19 memorials are now underway: In Long Beach, California, the city government and a community-based advisory group selected a memorial design called "Twin Arches" to honor and commemorate the lives lost to COVID-19. The design will include two arches that will memorialize those who died during COVID-19, creating an interactive and self-reflective space for those visiting the memorial.[36]

In London, community groups and families of the deceased collaborated to develop the National COVID-19 Memorial Wall.[37] The wall is located near the River Thames and across from the Houses of Parliament. The wall consists of more than 220,000 hand-painted red hearts symbolizing those who died by COVID-19. In the United States, Senators Markey and Warren continue to introduce legislation to create a "COVID-19 Victims Memorial Day" for the first Monday in March. Creating a national memorial day would recognize the nation's mourning, honor those who had passed, and provide a reminder to Congress "to renew its commitment to protecting communities from this ongoing public health crisis."[38]

In addition to permanent memorials, there are spontaneous memorials. These are often seen in the immediate aftermath of a tragedy: "spontaneous memorials can have a communicative value due to their materiality and immediacy to help transition grief to mourning."[34] The death of Princess Diana of Wales brought attention to the phenomenon of spontaneous memorials, and such temporary memorials are common after events such as mass shootings, terrorist attacks, natural disasters, and similar events that include many fatalities in a public setting.[39] Research has revealed the psychological benefits of spontaneous memorials, including individual processing of grief, strengthening of a sense of community, and taking back or confronting the site of the incident.[39]

During COVID-19, other types of temporary commemorations and ceremonies included the *New York Times* front page being full of names to honor the 100,000 Americans who had died from COVID-19 in 2020.[40] In February 2021, US President Biden and Vice President Harris held an outdoor candle-lit ceremony at the White House to honor the 500,000 Americans who had died from COVID-19.[41] In the fall of 2021, a temporary art installation of 600,000 white flags was installed on the National Mall in Washington, DC, to honor those who had died from COVID-19.[42]

While temporary and physical memorials symbolize the loss associated with a tragedy, communication provides the bridge between the memorial and the individual or the community. When memorials are unveiled or anniversary observances occur, communication through words and actions connects the listeners to the meaning of the memorial or anniversary event. CERC principles advise emergency risk communicators to engage in empathetic and respectful communication during health emergencies.

The following paragraphs offer suggestions for providing empathetic and respectful communication while speaking at memorials and anniversary observances. These techniques come from the public speaking principles for giving a speech of dedication, which is a particular type of speech designed for unveiling a memorial.[43,44]

- Open with a message of empathy and comfort. People gathered for this event have experienced a loss, and coming together again will likely trigger feelings of sadness. Consider sharing a poem, a quote, or a short story that would resonate with the audience.
- Explain how you are involved and why you were asked to be part of the event.
- Explain what is being dedicated or honored during the event.
- Explain who and what agencies were involved to make this memorial or special event happen.

- Finally, explain why the dedication is important to the community. Weave in messages of empathy and honoring those whose lives were lost. Close with a poem, quote, or short story that would resonate with the audience.

Caring for Your Staff

Another important aspect of the recovery phase is internal communications with health department staff. In Chapter 10, we'll discuss specifics of how staff engage in organizational learning after a health emergency, but this section is focused on caring for and maintaining a resilient workforce. After a fire at Texas A&M University that killed 12 students, the university administration directed professors to continue with business as usual. A&M professor Katherine Miller expressed, "Emotion is an integral part of the workplace," and professionals often lack socialization for dealing with emotions at work.[31]

COVID-19 was challenging for everyone, but it was especially challenging for public health workers who had been training and preparing for decades to respond to such a health emergency. Due to a lack of leadership, the early missteps at CDC regarding testing, the silencing of health officials who wanted to warn the public, the sheer size, gravity, and reality of responding to a novel virus and global pandemic, the length of the outbreak, the implementation of strict isolation and quarantine measures, the mandating of vaccines, protests at health directors' homes, and the politicization of public health, it is no wonder public health officials and health care workers began quitting and retiring early.

While sifting through what she knew theoretically from emotional labor academic papers and research, Miller realized that her direct experience did not necessarily match up with what she theoretically knew about stress, burnout, and emotional labor during a traumatic event.[31] While her research on emotional labor looked at people working in service organizations who engaged in detached concern in order to keep working, Miller realized she was not able to continue with business as usual are the fire at her university. Instead, she learned three key lessons about dealing with people after a traumatic event:

1 Emotion is real and needs to be recognized.
2 Shared experiences help people to process grief.
3 Identification with an organization can lead to community identification.

For public health leaders, these lessons are relevant during and after a health emergency in order to understand how the workforce is processing the situation.

As a leader, caring for a health department's staff after a major health emergency is a necessity. While caring for staff would fall under the human resources department, as a leader it is imperative to set the vision and intention of how you lead and manage your organization, but especially how humans are treated within that system. In addition to setting that vision and intention, a leader must set an example and embody how they want others to act and behave. For example, during COVID-19, not only were health department staff responsible for responding to the coronavirus outbreak, but they were also experiencing the outbreak themselves. Just like those whose health and safety they were trying to protect, health department staff lives were also disrupted: moving work online; managing children who were attending school online or setting up homeschooling; and navigating relationships with everyone at home or navigating relationships through a screen.

COVID-19 revealed not only cracks in the health care system, but also cracks in how we manage our stress, emotions, and caring for others. In her book *Showing Up*, Jen Marr explains that tragedies compel people who want to give comfort to those affected by the tragedy, but they often do so in unhelpful ways.[45] She cites that after the Sandy Hook Elementary shooting, the town of 27,000 people received 56,000 stuffed animals and 9 tractor trailers full of paper snowflakes and letters. While well-intentioned behavior, Marr suggests that during such tragedies comfort and empathy are what are needed most.

While after-action reviews and hotwashes (see Chapter 10) highlight strengths and areas of improvement for processes and procedures, often the human experience is not given space in relation to staff processing or making sense of what has happened. Through communication, leaders can provide an opportunity for staff to be heard and seen after major health emergencies. The following are tips and strategies from Marr on how leaders can "show up" for their staff using the Circle of Comfort strategy when engaging one-to-one with people:

- *Becoming present and awareness-building*: Remove other distractions in the office space – Turn of computer monitors, silence email notification beeps or close laptops, put phones down, and turn off notifications. Allow yourself to be fully present with the other person.
- *Situational analysis*: Similar to active listening, begin to evaluate and process what the other is sharing. Consider their situation and whether any action is needed. Sometimes organizational resources such as employee assistance programs may be appropriate resources. At other times, staff may simply want to know that their boss/manager/supervisor has heard them.
- *Personalized action and connection*: If action is needed, consider – in addition to organizational resources – what might be a simple action of "just for you" care that is appropriate to the situation. For leaders, this may involve checking in on your direct reports and asking how they are doing or sending a personal message or email to employees. Keep in mind that, for true connection, a heart-centered message written by a leader instead of by the communication staff is more authentic and more likely to resonate with employees.
- *Reflection*: Reflect on what has unfolded or transpired. Allow this connection and comfort to be seen.

Engaging in comfort and empathy at the workplace builds trust and allows relationships to grow.[45]

Quick Response Communications Planning

During the recovery phase, it is important to review communication objectives, key audiences, key messages, channels, and communication materials and products and update the communications strategy from what was established in the initial health emergency phase. The following subsections include descriptions of each of these topics and examples that are related to the recovery phase of a health emergency.

Communication Objective

A communication objective is a measurable, time-bound, and audience-focused action.[46] Often communication strategies and objectives are designed to create awareness, educate, or persuade the audience.[46]

The following communication objective examples have been updated to reflect objectives that could be used during the recovery phase. These objectives have been updated from previous chapters that focused on objectives for the initial and maintenance phases of the health emergency.

Example 1

    Measles: The county health department will announce the end of the outbreak and continue to promote vaccine education.

Example 2

    Foodborne illness: The county health department will end outbreak investigation activities and will work with fair organizers and food vendors on food safety education.

Example 3

    Unknown novel infection: The county health department will continue to monitor cases and hospital infections and will continue to promote boosters for avian influenza during the fall vaccination education campaign.

Audiences

As outlined in Chapters 3 and 4, identify your audiences and audience segments and their information needs. Understanding *which* of audience needs *what* type of information will help you to organize and strategize on key messaging. Using the audience segment variables outlined in Chapter 3, the following examples develop audience segments that will receive emergency risk communication messages during the recovery phase of the emergency.

Example 1 Measles

    Audiences continue to include schoolchildren and their parents, adults who have not received the measles, mumps, and rubella (MMR) immunization, school district officials, health care providers, community-based advocacy groups, and elected officials. There were no changes to the audience groups during the recovery phase. See Table 9.1 for audience segments for this example.

Table 9.1 Audience segments by risk variable for a measles outbreak

Variable	Definition	Audience segment
Risk level	Who is most at risk based on current health threat?	Schoolchildren (plus parents as children are minors) Adults who have not received the MMR immunization
Location or proximity	Who is closest to the risk or health threat?	Schoolchildren by vaccination status (plus parents as children are minors)
Employment	Is there a particular industry that is affected by the health crisis?	School district officials and health care providers
Values	What does the audience segment value, believe in, and support?	Informed Consent Action Network (group does not support vaccination) Vaccinate Your Family (group does support vaccination)
Organizational affiliations	What organizations do individuals in this segment belong to or associate with?	Local elected officials

Example 2 Foodborne illness

Audiences continue to include but are not limited to fair attendees, fair organizers, food cart vendors, health care providers, fair attendees from other counties in the state, and food suppliers who gave products to food vendors. There were no changes to the audience groups during the recovery phase. See Table 9.2 for audience segments for this example.

Table 9.2 Audience segments by risk variable for a foodborne illness outbreak

Variable	Definition	Audience segment
Risk level	Who is most at risk based on current health threat?	Fair attendees who ate at food carts
Employment	Is there a particular industry that is affected by the health crisis?	Fair organizers Food cart vendors Health care providers
Location or proximity	Who is closest to the risk or health threat?	Fair attendees from other counties in the state
Employment	Is there a particular industry that is affected by the health crisis?	Food suppliers who gave products to food vendors

Example 3 Unknown novel infection

Audiences still include but are not limited to individuals who live in a particular county, individuals who have underlying health conditions, incident management teams from other government agencies, the media, elected officials, and advocacy groups. There were no changes to the audience groups during the recovery phase. See Table 9.3 for audience segments for this example.

Table 9.3 Audience segments by risk variable for an unknown novel infection

Variable	Definition	Audience segment
Risk level	Who is most at risk based on current health threat?	Individuals who live in a particular county
Location or proximity	Who is closest to the risk or health threat?	Individuals who live in a particular county
Health condition	Who has current health conditions that may be at a heightened risk (e.g., age, underlying medical conditions, pregnant)?	Individuals who live in a particular county and who have specific underlying medical conditions
Employment	Is there a particular industry that is affected by the health crisis?	Health care providers
Organizational affiliations	What organizations do individuals in this segment belong to or associate with?	Incident management teams from other government agencies The media Elected officials
Values	What does the audience segment value, believe in, and support?	Anti-Mask League (group does not support wearing masks)

Identify Key Messages

Communication objectives will provide you with a broad strategy about who you want to communicate with and the information you'd like to provide. Key messages are the specific messages that the agency wants to communicate that are aligned with the communication objectives. For example, if the communication objective is to create awareness about an infectious disease, there are specific key messages that need to be created. During the recovery phase of the emergency, the key messages include signaling toward a new normal and that the health threat has been mitigated.

Example 1 Measles

Key Message 1: Signal toward a new normal.

- We want to thank the community and our school district officials for the time, attention, and steadfastness that have been demonstrated throughout this outbreak.
- We have learned there are distinct differences in our community regarding vaccinations. Each side has their own deeply held convictions about what is right and what is the right action for their children.
- As we move forward, we must embrace the likelihood of more outbreaks like this. The county health department will continue to do its work to protect the health and safety of our community while respecting the rights of our individual citizens.
- We ask all of our community members to remain respectful of each other's choices whether we agree with them or not.

Key Message 2: Health threat has been mitigated.

- The good news is that, based on the case monitoring we have been conducting and the incubation period for measles, this outbreak is officially over.
- The county health department will continue to provide information to community education groups over the next 3 weeks.
- We've also made a plan with the school district to engage in a community education campaign about school vaccinations. We will provide more information on that as it becomes available.

Example 2 Foodborne illness

Key Message 1: Signal toward a new normal.

- For anyone who became ill during this outbreak, you know firsthand the health challenges associated with a foodborne illness. And many of you will likely educate your friends and colleagues about food safety tips, especially when eating outside your home.
- The county health department and the county fair will be teaming up over the next several months to provide public education on food safety and in-depth food safety training for food handlers.
- We look forward to sharing more information about these efforts with you when it becomes available.

Key Message 2: Health threat has been mitigated.

- This outbreak has required a long investigation to find its source. We are satisfied with CDC's determination that the source of the outbreak was not from our community but tied to an international supplier.
- We are happy to announce the outbreak is officially over.

Example 3 Unknown novel infection

Key Message 1: Signal toward a new normal.

- Our community has spent several months living with avian influenza and its impacts on our daily lives. We've had to relive some parts of the COVID-19 response. But we also did better than we did with our COVID-19 response.
- Through community collaborations and partnerships, our efforts to build and support community resilience paid off.
- Instead of the intense learning losses our K–12 students experienced during COVID-19, we were able to provide educational support throughout this outbreak, ensuring successful learning retention for our children.
- We also spent more time focusing on ensuring social cohesion during this outbreak, with many of our senior-focused nonprofit organizations reporting a tripling in the amount of volunteering during this outbreak.
- We've done so much to make sure we remained a community during this outbreak.
- And although we will begin to decrease some of our public health actions, we need to remain steadfast with our booster vaccinations to ensure we keep this illness at bay.

Key Message 2: Health threat has been mitigated.

- As with COVID-19, the health threat of avian influenza may never be completely gone.
- Like seasonal influenza, this illness will continue to circulate in our communities each year.
- The county health department will continue to work to monitor cases and hospitalizations with our local partners. This information will continue to be posted on our website.

Identify Channels

As outlined in Chapter 5, think through what channels are available to share information and what audiences use which channels.

Example 1 Measles

The following audiences and communication channels would remain the same during the recovery phase to alert people to the end of the health emergency. Specific channel selection would be needed when developing the community education program. See Table 9.4 for channel identification for this example.

Table 9.4 Communication channels for each audience segment during a measles outbreak

Audience segment	Communication channel
Schoolchildren (plus parents as children are minors) Adults who have not received the MMR immunization	Email to parents Email to school workers School website Health department website Health department social media channels Media relations
Schoolchildren by vaccination status (plus parents as children are minors)	Email to parents
School district officials and health care providers	Conference calls or virtual meetings with school officials Health Alert Network message for clinicians

Example 2 Foodborne illness

The following audiences and communication channels would remain the same during the recovery phase to alert people to the end of the health emergency. Specific channel selection would be needed when developing the food safety education program and food handler education program. See Table 9.5 for channel identification for this example.

Table 9.5 Communication channels for each audience segment for a foodborne illness outbreak

Audience segment	Communication channel
Fair attendees who ate at food carts	Media relations Fair social media channels
Fair organizers Food cart vendors Health care providers	Face-to-face meetings Emails Health Alert Network message for clinicians

Example 3 Unknown novel infection

The following audiences and communication channels would remain the same during the recovery phase to alert people to the end of the health emergency. In this example, media relations, the agency's website, social media channels, and the Health Alert Network system would be the best channels to use in this type of health emergency. See Table 9.6 for channel identification for this example.

Table 9.6 Communication channels for each audience segment for an unknown novel infection

Audience segment	Communication channel
Individuals who live in a particular county	Media relations Health department website Health department social media channels
Individuals who live in a particular county and who have specific underlying medical conditions	Media relations Health department website Health department social media channels
Health care providers	Health Alert Network message

Communication Products

As outlined in Chapter 5, think through what communication materials need to be developed, such as talking points, web page copy, and visuals such as charts and graphs.

Example 1 Measles

The following communication channels and products would remain the same during the recovery phase to alert people to the end of the health emergency. Specific channel selection and communication products would be needed when implementing the community education program. See Table 9.7 for a list of communication products for this example.

Table 9.7 Communication products that can be sent on communication channels for a measles outbreak

Communication channel	Communication product
Email to parents Email to school workers School website Health department website Health department social media channels Media relations	Letter and email copy about outbreak Web page copy Social media messages (include visuals, hashtags, and web URLs for more information) Talking points
Email to parents Conference calls or virtual meetings with school officials Health Alert Network message for clinicians	Letter and email copy about outbreak Talking points Health Alert Network message copy

Example 2 Foodborne illness

The following communication channels and products would remain the same during the recovery phase to alert people to the end of the health emergency. Specific communication channel and product selection would be needed when developing the food safety education program and food handler education program. See Table 9.8 for a list of communication products for this example.

Table 9.8 Communication products that can be sent on communication channels for a foodborne illness outbreak

Communication channel	Communication product
Media relations Fair social media channels	Talking points Social media messages (include visuals, hashtags, and web URLs for more information)
Face-to-face meetings Emails Health Alert Network message for clinicians	Talking points Email copy Health Alert Network message copy

Example 3 Unknown novel infection

The following communication channels and products would remain the same during the recovery phase to alert people to the end of the health emergency. Specific channel selection would be needed when developing the community education campaign. See Table 9.9 for a list of communication products for this example.

Table 9.9 Communication products that can be sent on communication channels for an unknown novel infection

Communication channel	Communication product
Media relations Health department website Health department social media channels	Talking points Web page copy Social media messages (include visuals, hashtags, and web URLs for more information)
Media relations Health department website Health department social media channels	Talking points Web page copy Social media messages (include visuals, hashtags, and web URLs for more information)
Media relations Health department website Health department social media channels	Talking points Web page copy Social media messages (include visuals, hashtags, and web URLs for more information)
Health Alert Network message	Health Alert Network message copy

Key Tips for Spokespeople, Partner Agencies, and Call Centers

During every phase of a health emergency, spokespeople, partner agencies, and call centers need to receive consistent and coordinated information from the health agency. Here are some key tips for those who are the spokespeople or who work at partner agencies or call centers during the recovery phase of a health emergency.

Spokespeople: During the recovery phase of a health emergency, it is important to engage in empathetic and mindful communication with stakeholders, partner agencies, and employees. Whether the health emergency response was a success or failure, as the spokesperson and the face of an agency there is a unique role to play to humanize the organization, maintain or rebuild trust, and continue to demonstrate the commitment of the health agency to protecting the public's health and preventing further health harms. Consider establishing town halls to gather feedback from external and internal audiences and to give people an opportunity to be heard on what's working and what needs improvement. Monitor community feedback and take note if any organizations are planning memorials or public ceremonies to commemorate the health emergency. Review organizational policies and programs that support mindfulness and stress reduction for employees and revisit organizational values to support workforce development for career advancement and overall well-being.

Partner agencies: During the recovery phase of a health emergency, operations will begin scaling down, and there will be a return to a steady state of operations. Inquire about hotwashes and after-action reviews and when they will take place. Prepare feedback and notes to share with the lead agency on what worked and what did not. Monitor community feedback and take note if any organizations are planning memorials or public ceremonies to commemorate the health emergency.

Call centers: During the recovery phase of a health emergency, operations will begin scaling down and there will be a return to a steady state of operations. Inquire about when the call center will stand down and what the transition period will be when the call center stops taking calls about the health emergency. Ensure there is a plan to direct public inquiries back to the health department or other agency.

Theory Callout: Mindfulness

Mindfulness is defined as the awareness that emerges through paying attention on purpose, in the present moment, and nonjudgmentally to the unfolding of experience moment by moment.[47] Mindfulness comes from the teachings of the Buddha and provides the foundation for understanding how the nature of the mind, emotionality, and suffering can impact mindfulness, or one's attention to the true nature of how things are.[47] The Mindfulness-Based Stress Reduction (MBSR) program developed by Dr. Jon Kabat-Zinn helps reduce stress through the development of formal mindfulness meditation techniques.[47] Research studies have provided evidence for stress reduction through MBSR in individuals with chronic depression, generalized anxiety disorders, panic disorders, diabetes, hypertension, and HIV.[48] Mindfulness provides important insights for emergency risk communicators. First, mindfulness – paying attention on purpose, moment to moment, and without judgment – is useful not only for public health leadership but also for all public health employees to consider during the recovery phase of a health emergency. For external communications, mindfulness can play a role in stakeholder engagement and the evaluation of the agency's interactions with stakeholders. Stakeholders will provide feedback – both positive and negative – to the agency; how can that feedback be received and integrated in a mindful way to better serve the community in the future? Second, for internal communications, leadership needs to take account of the status of the health department workforce. Some 46% of all employees in state and local health agencies left their jobs between 2017 and 2021.[29] Challenges stemming from the COVID-19 pandemic, including criticism, harassment, and personal thefts, likely exacerbated job retention issues.[29] Mindfulness can help guide leadership to analyze organizational issues that lead to job loss and to develop solutions to retain, train, and sustain the job force. Third, providing access to the MBSR program as workforce development training represents an evidence-based intervention that is known to reduce stress and support personal well-being. Providing this resource to public health staff demonstrates the value of mindfulness within the agency and supports building a resilient workforce.

An Analysis of the Georgia Department of Public Health's Response to COVID-19
Jessica Worthington, MPH

In December 2019, a virus now known to be SARS-CoV-2 – or COVID-19 – was first identified in Wuhan, China, through a small cluster of cases. The emergence of this novel coronavirus disrupted the global landscape, challenging all nations across the globe to confront unprecedented health, economic, and social obstacles. As the virus rapidly spread across continents, countries scrambled to implement various strategies to curb its transmission and mitigate its consequences. Among the affected regions in the United States, the southeast faced significant challenges in managing the outbreak. This case study presents a detailed analysis of the COVID-19 pandemic through the lens of public health and the corresponding communication-based response provided by the Georgia Department of Public Health (DPH). By utilizing the principles and phases of CERC, this case study seeks to provide an in-depth understanding of the situation in Georgia.

An Overview of the Crisis
From the beginning of the pandemic, Georgia reported a substantial number of COVID-19 cases, with over 2.3 million confirmed cases in the state resulting in 35,493 deaths. The first two cases in Georgia were identified on March 1, 2020, in the Metro Atlanta area of Fulton County, and they were announced to the public on the morning of March 2 by the governor and DPH.[49] As the pandemic spread across the entire landscape of the state, 20% of all Georgia residents would eventually become infected.

According to an article in *The Atlanta Journal-Constitution* on the Georgia COVID-19 timeline, the exponential increase in cases during the first wave overwhelmed the health care systems, leading to shortages of medical supplies and hospital beds.[50] One of the underlying factors contributing to the rapid spread of COVID-19 in Georgia was the initial delay in implementing containment measures. The government's response to the outbreak was criticized for being slow and insufficient, with widespread concerns about inadequate testing and contact tracing.[50] Moreover, conflicting messages and mixed compliance with social distancing guidelines added to the challenges in controlling the spread of the virus.[49] However, over the next several months, between March and June 2020, the situation improved as the government enforced stricter measures and implemented a phase-based reopening plan.[50] Businesses were gradually allowed to resume operations, with precautionary measures such as mandatory face mask usage and capacity limits.[50] These measures, combined with increased testing capacity, helped to flatten the curve and prevent a complete collapse of the health care system.

Response and Government Measures
The response to the COVID-19 pandemic in Georgia involved a mix of federal, state, and local government actions. CDC, based in Atlanta, played a crucial role in providing guidelines and support at the federal level. Under Governor Brian Kemp's leadership, the state government declared a state of emergency and issued a series of executive orders to tackle the crisis. These orders included measures that implemented social distancing guidelines, restrictions on public gatherings, and statewide shelter-in-place orders.[50] According to an article by Ariel Hart in *The Atlanta Journal-Constitution*, one of the notable challenges faced in Georgia was the lack of a coordinated statewide approach.[49] Instead, the response was largely decentralized, with individual counties and local authorities implementing their own measures. This decentralized approach resulted in inconsistencies across the state, making it difficult to mitigate the spread effectively. This highlights the importance of a unified response to a public health crisis.

Health Care System Capacity and Resources
The COVID-19 pandemic tested the capacity and resilience of Georgia's health care system. During the initial wave, the surge in cases strained hospitals and health care facilities, leading to concerns about resource shortages.[49] The shortages of personal protective equipment (PPE), ventilators, and hospital beds became significant concerns for health care workers and policymakers.[49] The state government took measures to increase capacity in order to alleviate the strain on the health care system.[50] As outlined in an article in *The Atlanta Journal-Constitution* about the Georgia COVID-19 timeline, temporary field hospitals were set up and additional health care workers were recruited to meet the growing demand.[49] Moreover, the government collaborated with private-sector entities to ramp up the production of PPE and essential medical supplies.

Timeline of Key Disaster or Crisis Events
The following timeline provides an overview of COVID-19 in Georgia, beginning with its first announcement and covering the milestone moments until the end of the public health emergency.[50,51]

The First Announcement of COVID-19 and Initial Measures (March 2020)
On March 2, 2020, the Georgia DPH confirmed the state's first two cases of COVID-19. Following the announcement, Governor Brian Kemp declared a state of emergency on March 14, activating various emergency response measures. These measures included social distancing recommendations, restricting the size of public gatherings, and implementing hygiene protocols emphasizing frequent handwashing and sanitization.

Surge in Cases and the Implementation of Stay-at-Home Orders (April–June 2020)
Despite initial measures, Georgia witnessed a surge in COVID-19 cases in April. As a response, Governor Kemp issued a statewide stay-at-home order, effective from April 3 to April 30, aimed at mitigating the spread of the virus. The order encouraged residents to stay at home unless they were performing essential tasks such as seeking medical care or buying groceries.

Reopening Georgia and Controversial Decision (May 2020)
In a controversial move, Governor Kemp allowed businesses to gradually reopen on April 24, 2020, starting with gyms, hair salons, and bowling alleys. This decision garnered both praise and criticism, with concerns raised regarding the potential for increased transmission rates. However, Governor Kemp defended the decision, highlighting the importance of reviving the economy while ensuring public safety.

Surge in Cases and Mandatory Mask Policy (July–September 2020)
As COVID-19 cases surged again in Georgia during July, Governor Kemp signed an executive order on July 15 mandating the use of face masks in public places. This measure aimed to limit the transmission of the virus and protect vulnerable populations. Additionally, local governments were granted the authority to adopt stricter measures if necessary.

Vaccine Rollout and Eased Restrictions (December 2020–February 2021)
Amid ongoing challenges, Georgia began its vaccination campaign. On December 14, 2020, the first doses of the Pfizer–BioNTech vaccine were administered in the state. The vaccination efforts prioritized health care workers, elderly individuals, and those with underlying medical conditions. Subsequently, restrictions on businesses and public gatherings gradually eased, aligned with the state's prioritized vaccination phases.

Declining Cases and Phased Return to Normalcy (March–May 2021)
As vaccination rates increased, Georgia witnessed a decline in COVID-19 cases throughout the spring of 2021. This decline led to the relaxation of many restrictions, allowing businesses to operate at higher capacities and the resumption of public events with appropriate safety measures in place. However, following the advice of health officials, Governor Kemp emphasized the ongoing need for vigilance and adherence to best practices.

End of the Public Health Emergency in Georgia (June 2021)
On June 22, 2021, Governor Kemp signed an executive order and announced the end of the public health emergency related to COVID-19 in Georgia. This decision came into effect on July 1, 2021. It is important to note that although the public health emergency had been concluded on a state level, relevant health agencies, such as DPH, continued to monitor the situation and provide guidance to the public. The state continued to emphasize the importance of remaining cautious and responsive to any emerging risks or surges.[52]

CERC Principles and Phase-Based Messaging
Overall, the principles and phases of CERC, developed by CDC, provide a comprehensive framework for effective communication during crises and emergencies.[53] The six core principles of CERC are Be First, Be Right, Be Credible, Express Empathy, Promote Action, and Show Respect. These principles aim to foster trust, address public concerns, and facilitate the dissemination of essential information during emergencies or crises. By adhering to these principles and following the designated phases, communication professionals can effectively guide public responses, ultimately ensuring the safety and well-being of those affected. The principles and phases of CERC provide a valuable foundation to promote informed decision-making.

The principle of Be First emphasizes the importance of providing information to the public as quickly as possible during a crisis or emergency.[53] This helps to establish trust and allows the public to take immediate action to protect themselves. Be Right means ensuring that the information communicated is accurate and based on reliable sources. This principle recognizes the importance of avoiding speculation or guesswork, which can lead to confusion and erode trust in communication efforts.[53] Be Credible involves establishing trust with the public by providing transparent and honest information.[53] This principle emphasizes the importance of communicating in a way that is perceived as trustworthy, which can be achieved through open and consistent communication. Express Empathy acknowledges the emotional impact of a crisis or emergency on the public.[53] This principle recognizes the need to show understanding and support for individuals who may be experiencing fear, anxiety, or grief due to the situation. Promote Action encourages the public to take necessary steps to protect themselves and their communities.[53] This principle recognizes that communication efforts should provide information and motivate the public to engage in behaviors that will mitigate the impact of the crisis or emergency. Show Respect recognizes the diversity within the affected population and the importance of tailoring communication efforts to meet their specific needs.[6] This principle emphasizes the need to understand cultural, linguistic, and other factors that may affect the public's understanding and response to the crisis or emergency.

CERC Phases
The CERC framework incorporates four distinct phases that align with different emergency stages: preparation, initial, maintenance, and resolution.[53] Each phase necessitates specific communication strategies to effectively respond to the changing needs of the public and

address their concerns. In the preparation phase, communication professionals engage in preparedness activities to ensure the readiness of communication plans and strategies. This includes developing response plans, identifying key stakeholders, and conducting risk assessments to anticipate and mitigate potential communication challenges.

During the initial phase, communication efforts focus on promptly providing accurate information to the public, addressing immediate concerns, and guiding them on protective actions.[53] Communication in this phase is critical for establishing trust and ensuring the public has the information necessary to make informed decisions. The maintenance phase involves continuous communication to address evolving public concerns, provide updates on the situation, and ensure that the public remains informed and engaged.[53] This phase also requires monitoring public sentiment, addressing rumors and misinformation, and adapting communication strategies as needed. The resolution phase marks the end of the crisis or emergency and shifts communication efforts towards closure, evaluation, and facilitating the recovery process.[53] Communication professionals play a crucial role in rebuilding trust, addressing any lingering concerns, and conveying lessons learned from the crisis or emergency to prevent future occurrences. Overall, the principles and phases of CERC provide a comprehensive framework for effective communication during crises and emergencies. By adhering to the principles and following the phases, communication professionals can establish trust, provide timely and accurate information, and facilitate appropriate public responses to ensure the safety and well-being of the affected population.

DPH's Response to COVID-19 during the Initial Phase

Georgia DPH's response to COVID-19 during the initial phase was marked by an urgent and proactive approach, emphasizing the need for timely information dissemination, risk communication, and community engagement. The department recognized the importance of gaining public trust, maintaining transparency, and addressing the uncertainties surrounding the novel coronavirus. These actions align with the CERC principles that advocate for providing accurate, consistent, and timely information.

Be First

DPH successfully adhered to the CERC principle of Be First. It effectively communicated on the emerging situation, promptly sharing information about the virus, how it was preparing to address a potential outbreak, symptoms to look out for, and prevention measures. This is best demonstrated in a social media post DPH made on February 28, 2020. In this post, DPH announced the formation of a "Coronavirus task force" and reassured the public that the agency and state were preparing for future outbreaks while the case count in Georgia remained at zero. This proactive approach aimed to ensure that the public had access to essential knowledge, fostering a shared understanding of the pandemic's severity and the necessity of public health measures.

Be Right and Be Credible

While DPH demonstrated the CERC principles of Be Right and Be Credible through individual social media posts throughout all phases of the pandemic, these two CERC principles undertaken in the initial phase were the areas that I believe proved to be the greatest challenge that DPH faced. DPH best illustrates the principle of Be Right in a social media post from February 26, 2020. In this Facebook post DPH let the public know it was working closely with CDC to prepare for a possible pandemic in Georgia. This alignment with CDC aimed to showcase DPH's dedication to furnishing scientifically validated information and seeking counsel from subject matter experts in anticipation of uncertain circumstances. At this point in time, DPH's commitment to evidence-based communication was helping to build its credibility and counter misinformation or fear during a time when no cases had yet been identified in the state.

In April 2020, during the initial phase of the pandemic, DPH launched its COVID-19 dashboard. This dashboard was intended to serve as an online platform for citizens to access real-time data and statistics related to the virus in the state. However, after the platform's initial launch, the public frequently noticed changes and irregularities in the graphs and data posted on DPH's website and dashboard.[54,55]

Numerous news outlets reported on the dashboard's shortcomings, making it clear that the launch was deeply flawed, with *The Atlanta Journal-Constitution* highlighting significant discrepancies between the number of COVID-19 cases reported by the state and those shown on the dashboard.[54] In one particular graph posted on DPH's website, there was a dramatic change in impact numbers posted on April 22, with unexplained updates and corrections made to the same graph as recorded on April 28. According to *Atlanta Magazine*, these dramatic examples of inconsistent data created confusion and eroded public trust in the department's ability to manage the crisis effectively.[55] The dashboard, which was supposed to be a reliable source of information, became a subject of criticism and raised concerns about the state's capacity to handle the pandemic. Among the contributing factors to this communication failure was the lack of testing and verification procedures before the dashboard's launch. According to numerous open record emails and pieces of documentation, DPH admitted to failing to conduct comprehensive testing on the dashboard's functionality, resulting in inaccurate, incomplete, and misleading data being presented to the public.[55]

Before launching the dashboard, DPH's failure to engage with potential users, such as health care professionals, epidemiologists, and the public, left crucial insights unaddressed, leading to them producing a less user-friendly and effective platform than they might have done otherwise.[55] Furthermore, the lack of transparency in the decision-making processes surrounding the development and launch of the dashboard also played a significant role in its failure.[55] The public should have been made aware of the methodologies used to collect and analyze COVID-19 data, and this lack of transparency cast doubt on the accuracy and reliability of the information provided. As *Atlanta Magazine* pointed out, this undermined the public's perception of the state's commitment to transparency and its ability to handle the health crisis.[55] These examples of the COVID-19 dashboard and an incorrectly published graph called the organization's credibility into question. They undercut the foundation laid by DPH, eroding public trust and hindering the state's credibility in terms of the CERC principles of Be Right and Be Credible in communicating crucial information to the public effectively.[53]

Maintenance and Recovery Phases

During the maintenance phase, the department shifted its focus toward encouraging public health actions, combating misinformation, and communicating with a diverse audience. In its messaging, DPH continued to provide regular updates, adapt guidelines based on evolving evidence, and implement targeted interventions in high-risk settings. The department also actively engaged with community organizations and stakeholders to facilitate effective collaboration.

Promote Action
DPH heavily relied on social media to effectively promote action during both the maintenance and recovery phases. At the onset of the maintenance phase, the focus on action primarily entailed DPH advocating proper hygiene practices, the use of face masks, and

social distancing through social media campaigns. As the vaccination campaign gained momentum, online messaging adopted a new approach to address vaccine hesitancy by actively encouraging and coupling the vaccination process with sound public health practices. It was crucial to emphasize to the public that while vaccines played a significant role in the recovery process, they were not the sole decisive factor on this trajectory.

Show Respect
Throughout the maintenance and recovery phases, the principles Express Empathy and Show Respect were consistently observed in social media messaging, exemplifying the remaining two CERC principles. DPH's commendable efforts in this regard were demonstrated through various social media posts. These posts acknowledged and showed appreciation for the contributions of nurses and first responders, made note of the need to prioritize mental health, and emphasized a need for unity during the challenging period of the pandemic. DPH's consistent and ongoing demonstration of empathy through active engagement on social media was particularly noteworthy.

Regarding the CERC principle of Show Respect, DPH demonstrated its ability to embody this beyond online platforms and posts. While DPH incorporated multilingual content into its social media platforms, one of its most inclusive actions was in organizing a live webinar for the general public to discuss the impacts of COVID-19 on the Hispanic and Latino communities. This approach displayed astuteness, uniqueness, and inclusiveness, effectively reaching a demographic typically underserved or overlooked throughout the state. Moreover, it utilized a creative strategy and approach to enhancing engagement and inclusivity.

Discussion of Implications
During the maintenance and recovery phases, DPH utilized various communication channels to disseminate information, such as press conferences, social media, and public service announcements. However, for communication to be effective, it is crucial to establish a two-way exchange that encourages dialogue between authorities and the impacted population.[56] Unfortunately, DPH primarily emphasized one-way communication, with a focus on information dissemination, providing few adequate provisions for feedback and engagement. Notably, many of DPH's Facebook posts featured a caption at the bottom indicating that the public's ability to comment on the posts had been turned off or "limited," narrowing the audience from whom DPH was able to receive direct engagement. This same message was displayed on numerous social media posts, including a post featuring a video with the Attorney General. Social media has immense potential as a tool and resource. For instance, online forums and live chats can facilitate real-time interaction with the public, fostering transparency and trust, thereby meeting the crucial need for immediate two-way communication.[57] However, by restricting public comments, the message being conveyed is that the opinions and feedback of the public are of less value than the opinions and feedback of those in positions of authority. In the future, DPH should consider removing limitations on social media comments and instead focus on creating an active and engaged social media experience whereby the public can ask questions and receive real-time responses from genuine experts.

Credibility Matters
One of the primary insights gleaned from evaluating DPH's communication strategy is that credibility is a highly cherished asset that, once compromised, is exceedingly challenging to restore. Following the episode surrounding the COVID-19 dashboard and incorrect graph postings, DPH encountered significant difficulties in regaining its credibility and trust with

the public.[54,55] Regrettably, instead of acknowledging its errors and moving forward, DPH opted for the more arduous path of denial and shifting blame.[54,55] A notable example of this is when DPH Commissioner Kathleen Toomley abruptly terminated the conversation during an interview with a WABE radio station reporter when she was asked a question about the COVID-19 dashboard and subsequent data inconsistencies.[54,55]

Consequently, every time there was a subsequent delay in reporting or failure to meet data release deadlines during the remainder of the pandemic, memories of the ill-fated dashboard launch resurfaced. Just as the pandemic persisted for multiple years, so did this narrative. In future endeavors, DPH should exercise greater caution when integrating new technologies. While technology can play a constructive role and provide supportive online resources during a crisis, research, testing, and a soft unveiling of technological resources should be prioritized and conducted prior to any official launch. It is imperative to recognize that the importance of being first should not come at the cost of prioritizing accuracy and credibility.

Failure to Meet
Lastly, from a communications perspective, it is important to address Georgia DPH's board of directors' failure to meet during the COVID-19 pandemic. An exposé featured in an *Atlanta Journal-Constitution* publication dated May 2021 unveiled that, spanning a continuous 15-month interval preceding the article's publication, DPH's board had refrained from convening through virtual or in-person sessions. The last meeting of this board can be traced back to February 2020.[58]

The pandemic demanded swift action and coordination from health authorities to provide essential services and guidance to the population. However, the DPH board's failure to convene hindered its ability to respond effectively.[58] Because the board did not meet, DPH lacked a unified front and a holistic decision-making process, resulting in delayed and fragmented responses to the crisis.[58]

Comparing this to the CERC principles, the DPH board's failure to meet undermines the principles of Be First, Be Right, and Be Credible. The timely dissemination of accurate and credible information is pivotal during a crisis.[53] Unfortunately, Georgia residents were left without the necessary guidance and information on testing locations, safety precautions, and vaccination plans due to DPH's lack of communication. Consequently, confusion and misinformation arose among the population, leading to increased risks and unnecessary anxiety.

The CERC principle of Be Credible emphasizes transparency and the importance of building trust with stakeholders.[53] The DPH board's failure to meet undermined this principle, eroding trust among various entities managing the crisis. This lack of collaboration negatively affected the response to the pandemic and hindered the proper allocation of resources and the implementation of evidence-based strategies.[58] In the same way that all Americans had to adjust to a new way of doing business during the pandemic, so should have DPH. With the prevalence and availability of online meeting tools and platforms, board members and DPH staff had the resources to ensure the continuity of operations regarding state government needs and requirements. In the future, DPH should develop, with its board's support, an update to its operational bylaws addressing how board meetings will be handled in the future during times of crisis. This will serve to outline expectations for future agency staff and board members.

Conclusion
By assessing DPH's response using the CERC principles, this analysis provides valuable insights for improvements in future crisis communication efforts during public health emergencies. The effective application of these principles can better engage the public,

promote adherence to preventive measures, and ultimately contribute to better public health outcomes.[53] As the landscape of COVID-19 continues to evolve, continuous evaluation and enhancement of crisis communication strategies will be crucial for navigating future challenges effectively.

By implementing these recommendations, DPH could improve communication throughout all phases of emergency and crisis communication, thereby mitigating the negative impacts discussed in this case study. Effective crisis communication is crucial when managing unforeseen disasters and events. It is essential for public health agencies to prioritize clear, timely, and accurate communication to protect and promote the health of the population effectively.[53]

End-of-Chapter Reflection Questions

1 Write your own recovery messages for an infectious disease outbreak. Identify recovery message components with in your message.
2 Consider how your agency moves from one crisis to another. How do you communicate about the end of a health emergency?
3 Reflect on memorials you've seen to commemorate a disaster or emergency. What stands out to you about these memorials? If your community were to create a memorial, how would you or your agency be involved?
4 How does your agency work with staff after a large public health emergency? What kinds of support are provided to employees?

References

1 FEMA. Recovery. 2023. www.fema.gov/about/offices/recovery (Accessed April 10, 2024).
2 FEMA. National Disaster Recovery Framework. n.d. www.fema.gov/emergency-managers/national-preparedness/frameworks/recovery (Accessed April 10, 2024).
3 CDC. End of the Federal COVID-19 Public Health Emergency (PHE) Declaration. 2023. https://archive.cdc.gov/#/details?url=https://www.cdc.gov/coronavirus/2019-ncov/your-health/end-of-phe.html (Accessed April 10, 2024).
4 Ulmer R, Sellnow T, Seeger M. *Effective Crisis Communication: Moving from Crisis to Opportunity*. Thousand Oaks, CA, Sage Publications, 2010.
5 An Update on the Ongoing Federal Response to COVID-19: Current Status and Future Planning. Hearing before the Senate Health, Education, Labor, and Pensions Committee. 2022. www.help.senate.gov/newsroom/photos/an-update-on-the-ongoing-federal-response-to-covid-19-current-status-and-future-planning (Accessed April 10, 2024).
6 People's CDC. COVID-19 Weather Report. 2022. https://peoplescdc.org/2022/06/14/peoples-cdc-weather-report (Accessed April 10, 2024).
7 CDC. COVID Data Tracker. 2024. https://covid.cdc.gov/covid-data-tracker/#county-view?list_select_state=all_states&list_select_county=all_counties&data-type=Vaccinations (Accessed April 10, 2024).
8 WHO Director-General's opening remarks at the media briefing: 5 May 2023. *World Health Organization*. 2023. www.who.int/director-general/speeches/detail/who-director-general-s-opening-remarks-at-the-media-briefing—5-may-2023 (Accessed May 24, 2024).

9. Goleman D. *Emotional Intelligence*. New York, Bantam Book, 1995.

10. Dalai Lama TG, Ekman P. *Emotional Awareness: Overcoming the Obstacles to Psychological Balance and Compassion: A Conversation between the Dalai Lama and Paul Ekman*. New York, St. Martin's Essentials, 2008.

11. Ebola Outbreak Over in Uganda: Media Statement. *Centers for Disease Control and Prevention*. 2023. www.cdc.gov/media/releases/2023/s0111-ebola-outbreak.html (Accessed April 10, 2024).

12. Scheufele DA, Tewksbury D. Framing, Agenda Setting, and Priming: The Evolution of Three Media Effects Models. *J Commun* 2006;57(1):9–20.

13. OHA. Office of Health Policy Portland, Oregon. n.d. www.oregon.gov/oha/HPA/HP/Pages/index.aspx (Accessed April 10, 2024).

14. Executive Office of Policy, Planning and Evaluation. *Washington State Department of Health*. n.d. https://doh.wa.gov/about-us/executive-offices/policy-planning-and-evaluation (Accessed April 10, 2024).

15. Birkland TA. Focusing Events, Mobilization, and Agenda Setting. *J Public Policy* 1998;18(1):53–74.

16. Zhang X, Warner ME, Meredith G. Factors Limiting US Public Health Emergency Authority during COVID-19. *Int J Health Plan Manage* 2023;38(5):1569–82.

17. Levin D. Efforts to Rollback Public Health Authority: Tracking the Legislation and Assessing the Impact. *The Network for Public Health Law*. 2024. www.networkforphl.org/resources/efforts-to-rollback-public-health-authority-tracking-the-legislation-and-assessing-the-impact (Accessed April 10, 2024).

18. Bustillo X, Keith T. Debt limit deal claws back unspent COVID relief money. *NPR*. 2023. www.npr.org/2023/05/31/1178996725/debt-ceiling-deal-unspent-covid-relief-money-democrats-republicans (Accessed April 10, 2024).

19. The Impact of Chronic Underfunding on America's Public Health System: Trends, Risks, and Recommendations, 2023. *Trust for America's Health*. 2023. www.tfah.org/report-details/funding-2023/ (Accessed April 10, 2024).

20. Johns M, Rosenthal J. Fact Sheet: How Investing in Public Health Will Strengthen America's Health. The Center for American Progress. 2022. www.americanprogress.org/article/how-investing-in-public-health-will-strengthen-americas-health/ (Accessed April 10, 2024).

21. Castrucci BC. The "10 Essential Public Health Services" Is the Common Framework Needed to Communicate About Public Health. *Am J Public Health* 2021;111(4):598–99.

22. Krasnow ID, Cuestra SM. Using values and framing to create messages that motivate. *Berkeley Media Studies Group*. 2019. www.bmsg.org/using-values-and-framing-to-create-messages-that-motivate (Accessed April 10, 2024).

23. Championing public health amid legal and legislative threats: Framing and language recommendations. *Berkeley Media Studies Group*. 2022. www.bmsg.org/resources/publications/championing-public-health-amid-legal-and-legislative-threats-framing-and-language-recommendations (Accessed April 10, 2024).

24. Public Health Leaders Discuss the Importance of Sustained Public Health Funding in the Post COVID-19 Landscape [press release]. *Trust for America's Health*. n.d. www.tfah.org/article/public-health-leaders-discuss-the-importance-of-sustained-public-health-funding-in-the-post-covid-19-landscape/ (Accessed April 11, 2024).

25. CDC. The State Health Department's Role in the Policy Process. n.d. https://stacks.cdc.gov/view/cdc/41704 (Accessed April 11, 2024).

26. Pollack Porter KM, Rutkow L, McGinty EE. The Importance of Policy Change for Addressing Public Health Problems. *Public Health Rep* 2018;133:9S–14S.

27. Public health policy analyst. *Careers in Public Health.net*. 2024. www

.careersinpublichealth.net/careers/public-health-policy-analyst (Accessed April 10, 2024).

28 *Oregon's COVID-19 Plan: Resilience in Support of Equity (RISE)*. Portland, OR, Oregon Health Authority, 2022.

29 U.S. governmental public health workforce shrank by half in five years, study finds. Harvard University. 2023. www.hsph.harvard.edu/news/hsph-in-the-news/u-s-governmental-public-health-workforce-shrank-by-half-in-five-years-study-finds (Accessed April 10, 2024).

30 Morton M, Nurie N. Editorial: Community Resilience and Public Health Practice. *Am J Public Health* 2013;**103**(7):1158–60.

31 Miller K. The Experience of Emotion in the Workplace: Professing in the Midst of Tragedy. *Manag Commun Q* 2002;**15**(4):571–600.

32 Hidalgo I, Brooten D, Youngblut JM, Roche R, Li J, Hinds AM. Practices Following the Death of a Loved One Reported by Adults from 14 Countries or Cultural/Ethnic Groups. *Nursing Open* 2020;**8**(1):453–62.

33 Wagoner B, Brescó I. Memorials as Healing Places: A Matrix for Bridging Material Design and Visitor Experience. *Int J Environ Res Public Health* 2022;**19**(11):6711.

34 McConville L. *How Translating a Memorial through the Interior whilst Encouraging Participation Can Be Most Effective in Communicating Current Tragedies and Complex Histories whilst Providing a Space for Collective Remembrance*. Unpublished dissertation, University of Edinburgh, 2023.

35 Hoffman M. The Use of Garden Memorial Ritual for Survivors, Families, and Healthcare Workers as a Result of the COVID-19 Pandemic in Nursing Facilities. *Omega (Westport)* 2024;**90**(1):433–39.

36 Del Cid A. COVID-19 Memorial Long Beach Public Works. n.d. www.longbeach.gov/pw/projects/covid-19-memorial/#:~:text=The%20selected%20design%20entitled%20%E2%80%9CTwin,artwork%20and%20engage%20in%20reflection (Accessed February 24, 2024).

37 National Covid Memorial Wall. n.d. www.nationalcovidmemorialwall.org (Accessed February 24, 2024).

38 Markey E. Senators Markey and Warren Reintroduce Resolution Memorializing Those Lost to COVID-19. 2023. www.markey.senate.gov/news/press-releases/senators-markey-and-warren-reintroduce-resolution-memorializing-those-lost-to-covid19#:~:text=Markey%20(D%2DMass.),introduced%20in%20August%20of%202021 (Accessed February 24, 2024).

39 Collins H, Allsopp K, Arvanitis K, Chitsabesan P, French P. Psychological Impact of Spontaneous Memorials: A Narrative Review. *Psychol Trauma* 2020;**14**(7):1230–36.

40 Barry D, Buchanan L, Cargill C, Daniel A, Delaquérière A, Gamio L, et al. U.S. Deaths Near 100,000, An Incalculable Loss. *The New York Times*. 2020, May 24.

41 Detrow S. Watch: President Biden Delivers Emotional Remembrance of 500,000 COVID-19 Victims. *NPR*. 2021. www.npr.org/2021/02/22/970155352/white-house-to-honor-victims-of-the-coronavirus-in-evening-ceremony (Accessed May 23, 2024).

42 Franklin J. More than 600,000 White Flags on the National Mall Honor Lives Lost to COVID. *NPR*. 2021. www.npr.org/sections/coronavirus-live-updates/2021/09/17/1037011493/covid-national-mall-white-flags-art-exhibit-memorial-pandemic-dead (Accessed May 23, 2024).

43 Types of Special Occasion Speeches. *Oklahoma State University*. n.d. https://open.library.okstate.edu/speech2713/chapter/18-2-types-of-special-occasion-speeches-2 (Accessed February 24, 2024).

44 York S. *Remembering Well: Rituals for Celebrating Life and Mourning Death*. Hoboken, NJ, Jossey-Bass, 2000.

45. Marr J. *Showing Up: A Comprehensive Guide to Comfort and Connection.* Potomac, MD, New Degree Press, 2022.

46. *Study Guide for the Examination for Accreditation in Public Relations.* New York, Universal Accreditation Board/Public Relations Society of America, 2021.

47. Kabat-Zinn J. *Mindfulness-Based Interventions in Context: Past, Present, and Future.* Washington, DC, American Psychological Association, 2003.

48. Niazi AK, Niazi SK. Mindfulness-Based Stress Reduction: A Non-Pharmacological Approach for Chronic Illnesses. *N Am J Med Sci* 2011;**3**(1):20–23.

49. Georgia COVID-19 timeline: A month by month look at the toll. n.d. *The Atlanta Journal-Constitution.* www.ajc.com/news/coronavirus/anniversary-timeline (Accessed June 16, 2022).

50. Hart A. Georgia's pandemic response ranked among the nation's worst. *The Atlanta Journal-Constitution.* 2022. www.ajc.com/news/coronavirus/georgias-pandemic-response-ranked-among-the-nations-worst/D5SG4WXZORFUXAHSIO4WMYIM7U (Accessed June 16, 2022).

51. State of Georgia. 2020 executive orders. *Governor Brian P. Kemp Office of the Governor.* 2020. https://gov.georgia.gov/executive-action/executive-orders/2020-executive-orders (Accessed June 16, 2022).

52. WTOC Staff. Gov. Kemp says he has signed final executive order extending COVID-19 public health emergency. 2021. www.wtoc.com/2021/06/22/gov-kemp-says-he-has-signed-final-executive-order-extending-covid-19-public-health-emergency (Accessed June 16, 2022).

53. Centers for Disease Control and Prevention. Crisis and Emergency Risk Communication (CERC) Manual. 2008. https://emergency.cdc.gov/cerc/manual/index.asp (Accessed June 16, 2022).

54. Georgia Covid-19 Dashboard Undercounts Total Test Results. *The Atlanta Journal-Constitution.* n.d. www.ajc.com/news/state–regional/georgia-covid-19-dashboard-undercounts-total-test-results/NSlaXia5pS6BvcKZkk5LeP (Accessed June 16, 2022).

55. Landman K, Wells M. Behind Georgia's COVID-19 dashboard disaster. *Atlanta Magazine.* 2021. www.atlantamagazine.com/great-reads/behind-georgias-covid-19-dashboard-disaster (Accessed June 16, 2022).

56. McDavitt B, Bogart LM, Mutchler MG, Wagner GJ, Green HD Jr, Lawrence SJ, et al. Dissemination as Dialogue: Building Trust and Sharing Research Findings Through Community Engagement. *Prev Chronic Dis* 2016;**13**:150473.

57. Veinot TC, Mitchell H, Ancker JS. Good Intentions Are Not Enough: How Informatics Interventions Can Worsen Inequality. *J Am Med Inform Assoc* 2018;**25**(8):1080–88.

58. Trubey JS. As pandemic raged, Georgia Public Health Advisory Board failed to meet. *The Atlanta Journal-Constitution.* 2021. www.ajc.com/news/investigations/as-pandemic-raged-georgia-public-health-advisory-board-failed-to-meet/PEULREDN6ZCR7KLIXESPN6TDMY (Accessed June 16, 2022).

Part III — Communicating and Planning after a Health Emergency

Chapter 10
Evaluating Emergency Risk Communication and Engaging in Public Education for the Next Emergency

Chapter Objectives
- List the four types of program evaluation.
- Recall at least six ways to evaluate communication before and during a health emergency.
- Describe how evaluation can support organizational learning after a health emergency.
- Explain how evaluation can support community resilience and disaster preparedness after a health emergency.
- Compare and contrast academic research approaches to evaluating emergency risk communication.
- Recall the awareness, desire, knowledge, ability, and reinforcement (ADKAR) model and its application to organizational change management.

Program Evaluation

Program evaluation is a core tenet of public health programs. It helps identify if a program is helping those it is intended to, if a program has been implemented correctly or fully, or if there are problems during and after implementation, and it ensures accountability regarding the use of public funds and resources to serve the community. Public funds are often used to develop and implement community programs intended to educate, support, and change behavior for healthier outcomes, so it is necessary for program managers to be able to communicate whether a program was effective or not. Establishing an evaluation framework before a program is implemented is critical because it is difficult to assess or measure the effectiveness of a program, communication message, or health intervention without having preestablished metrics or goals to assess.

In the 2002 Crisis and Emergency Risk Communication (CERC) manual, "evaluation" was listed as a distinct phase that occurs after a health emergency. In the 2014 and 2018 CERC manuals, the Centers for Disease Control and Prevention (CDC) recommended that evaluation ought to occur throughout all phases of a health emergency. Waiting to evaluate communication until after a health emergency represents a missed opportunity for emergency risk communicators to ensure that health messages are resonating with the intended audience segments. Further, emergency risk communicators face other barriers to evaluation after a health emergency, including already working on another emerging issue or a lack of an evaluation plan prior to the start of a health emergency. Additionally, any seasoned emergency risk communicator can attest that evaluating emergency risk communication outcomes is inherently complex due to various factors that can impact emergency risk communication.

This chapter outlines practical ways emergency risk communicators can use evaluation throughout the health emergency to inform and improve emergency risk communication messaging strategies and activities. The chapter starts with a basic orientation to program evaluation and its relevance to emergency risk communication. There are four common types of evaluation found in public health: formative, process, outcome, and impact. The following paragraphs outline these different types of program evaluation.

Formative evaluation is done before a program is implemented to ensure that it is feasible, appropriate, and acceptable.[1] Formative evaluation utilizes focus groups or semistructured interviews to gather information from a group of people associated with the program being evaluated. For example, during COVID-19, researchers engaged in a rapid formative evaluation to gather information from hospital site coordinators where a new personal protective equipment (PPE) program was going to be implemented.[2] Through 20-minute phone or online semistructured interviews, the researchers gathered information about what the site coordinators knew about the intervention, how they perceived the new program would impact their work, and what new tasks would be assigned to them because of the new PPE program. The researchers used the information from this formative evaluation to create recommendations to ensure that the hospital provided comprehensive information about the program, provided feedback to all PPE program participants, and provided appropriate training for all new health care workers.[2]

For emergency risk communicators, formative evaluation can be used to gather information from audience segments to help create key messages about health threats. This type of emergency risk communication involving formative research is often completed during the precrisis phase of the CERC life cycle.

Process evaluation helps the evaluator determine whether the program activities have been implemented as they were intended.[1] Process evaluation can be done throughout the lifetime of the program to ensure the program stays on its intended track or course. For public health programs, process evaluation can be used to monitor and document the frequency of participation in the health program and how well participants are adhering to the program's activities. For example, during the COVID-19 pandemic, process evaluation was used to assess the implementation of the "Time for You" mental health support program for frontline workers.[3] Based on the process evaluation, the researchers learned that the two of the three program offerings needed to be adapted to provide more flexibility in the length and number of sessions to better serve program participants.[3]

In emergency risk communication, process evaluation can be used to assess whether the Joint Information Center (JIC) processes are working as they were intended. For example, if a JIC is created with a small number of people involved, process evaluation could allow researchers to determine that more people are needed to handle media inquiries or additional team members are needed to liaise with stakeholders and partner agencies.

Outcome evaluation, or effectiveness evaluation, measures the effects that the program is having on the population by assessing progress in the outcome objectives that program is meant to achieve. For example, during COVID-19, the National Institutes of Health created the Community Engagement Alliance (CEAL) to address challenges and build trust with burdened communities through participation in clinical trials, provision of feedback on vaccine communication, and adoption of community mitigation practices.[4] The outcome evaluation of the CEAL program used pre- and post-measures from surveys and publicly available COVID-19 data. A formal program evaluation is underway to assess the full effectiveness of the CEAL program.[4]

For emergency risk communication, outcome evaluation often assesses the number of individuals who participated in the health emergency interventions, mass vaccination clinics, or patients who received specific medical treatments to prevent illness.

Impact evaluation is usually completed at the end of a program to assess whether the program achieved its overall goal. For public health programs, this means measuring changes in awareness, knowledge, attitudes, skills, or behaviors.[5] In the Kirkpatrick model, step 3 of the evaluation framework assesses how an employee's behavior changes on the job as a result of attending a training course that was designed to help them develop a new skill.[6]

For emergency risk communication, scholars and practitioners are trying to understand how best to assess the impacts of emergency risk communication. Due to the complexity and mediating factors inherent to emergencies, it is often difficult to attribute impact to emergency risk communication messaging. This chapter later explores current scientific and peer-reviewed research on evaluating the impact of emergency risk communication.

Communication Evaluation

In addition to understanding and participating in program evaluation, emergency risk communicators also need to evaluate communication materials to ensure that they will resonate with the intended audiences (see Table 10.1). The public relations and marketing industry has a variety of tools to evaluate communications, which will be discussed in the following paragraphs.[7]

Focus groups are used by evaluators to gather together a small number of individuals from the community engaged in the program to represent the community at large. As trying to contact every member of a community is not realistic or financially feasible, program teams and evaluators work with a focus group that represents a subset of the community. This enables the program and evaluator to collect information from the community and to test the messages developed for the program and its supportive communications. This process represents a common way to gather information from an audience segment and to test messages.

Table 10.1 Different ways to evaluate communication before and during a health emergency

Focus groups	Intercept interviews
Surveys	Content analysis
Communication audits	In-depth interviews
Complaint reviews	Public inquiries
Observation	Community town halls
Media monitoring and analysis	Literature reviews

For emergency risk communication, focus groups can be used in the precrisis phase to test messages that could be used during an emergency response. Findings from focus groups can be used to create consensus recommendations with partner agencies that will be involved with emergency risk communication activities. Developing consensus recommendations with other responding agencies ensures consistent and coordinated emergency messaging is achieved.[8,9]

Intercept interviews are used to gather information from a member of the public, and they are often used in marketing and public relations fields. For emergency risk communication, intercept interviews could be used at a mass vaccination clinic or point of dispensing site to ask people about their experience, such as how long it took for them to receive their vaccine or medicine and how they heard about the event (i.e., social media, news media, friend, employer, etc.).

Surveys are used to gather information from a large number of the community members and to ask them to respond to key questions about key needs before a program begins or about key details regarding the program of interest. Surveys can be deployed via the internet, phone, and post. The main benefit of surveys is that you can gather large amounts of data that can be generalized to the survey population. The major downside with surveys is that the return rate (or the number of completed surveys) can be low, and then the data acquired potentially are not representative of the community of interest.

For emergency risk communication, surveys can be used to gather data on how the public is perceiving the emergency response, what they know about the health threat, and how likely they are to participate in the health intervention. Surveys can also be deployed soon after an emergency to learn about the public's activities during the event and the public's satisfaction with the agency's response efforts.

Content analysis is a type of analysis that can be completed deductively (i.e., using a framework or theoretical construct to confirm the presence or absence of something) or inductively (i.e., to allow for the emergence of themes or narratives). Content analysis is often used to understand focus group data or in-depth interviews. Content analysis is also often useful when analyzing large volumes of text such as those generated by public inquiries.

For emergency risk communication, content analysis could be used to analyze public inquiries received by the agency's call center. Content analysis of the call center inquiries can reveal information-seeking behavior by the public, such as what questions are they asking about the emergency. If many questions are being asked about vaccines, travel, or symptoms, this is an indication to check the communication strategy and the key messages being shared, potentially indicating that an update to the communication strategy is needed.

Communication audits are done to understand the brand identity or communication policies of an organization and also to assess the amount of information materials that are available for a given program or to revise outdated program materials. To understand brand identity, information is gathered to determine how the identity of the organization is being portrayed through organizational practices such as the use of logos on official documents to how email signatures are formatted. Communication audits also review communication policies such as reviewing and clearing documents for public consumption, identified spokespeople, and media and social media usage for official business.

For emergency risk communication, communication audits are usually conducted before or after an emergency response. When a communication audit is conducted before an emergency, it assesses how much information (e.g., communication materials) is available on a given topic such as influenza, *E. coli*, measles, hepatitis C, and other health threats that could arise in the community. Such audits also assess when the information was created and whether the materials need to be revised and updated. When communication audits happen after an emergency, they are usually part of an after-action review (AAR) to improve organizational processes during an emergency. AARs are discussed in depth in the following section.

In-depth interviews, or key informant interviews, are useful for understanding public perceptions of a program or policy. They are also used to better understand a community's understanding of the issue that a program hopes to address or to better understand the context within which a program will engage with a community and any specific needs that such engagement should address, such as language, culture, social limitations, trauma sensitivity, equity, or connectivity issues.

For emergency risk communication, in-depth interviews are helpful during the precrisis stage to help you understand what a person or audience segment knows about a particular topic and how such knowledge could inform public messaging related to potential health threats.

Complaint reviews provide information regarding complaints filed by external stakeholders or members of the public about an organization. Complaint reviews can also be submitted via social media comments and posts.

For emergency risk communication, complaint reviews can provide insights into where an agency missed an opportunity to respond to the public's needs during an emergency. Complaint reviews can also hold an organization accountable for its emergency response and can lead to internal policy changes to better serve a community in future responses.

Public inquiries through phone calls, letters, emails, or social media posts provide data that can be analyzed for input into communication activities and organizational messaging strategies.

For emergency risk communication, public inquiries can provide many insights into how the public and stakeholders are perceiving a health threat and how an agency is responding to such a situation. When an agency receives public inquiries, those submitting these inquiries are engaging in a behavior called "information-seeking." During emergencies, people will seek out information to make sense of what is happening and to learn what they can do to protect themselves. Public inquiries can provide useful information regarding communication strategy as to whether the current key messages are aligned with an audience segment's information needs. Sometimes, communication strategies may need to be updated if public inquiries are not addressed in the current key messages.

Observation is the process of observing behaviors or the environment and recording the observations as data. For example, when a call center is set up for a health emergency, observations can be helpful for training purposes. A trainer will observe how customer service representatives are engaging with the public. The trainer can provide their findings to the customer service representative and determine whether updates are needed to training materials.

For emergency risk communication, observations are helpful in call centers (as described in the example in the previous paragraph), epidemiological interviews, emergency operation centers, and JICs because managers and training directors can see how procedures are being implemented. If there are inefficiencies in these procedures, changes will need to be made to ensure a better flow of operations is established, which is critical during emergency responses.

Community town halls provide an opportunity to gather information on how an organization is engaging with a community. Community forums can be online platforms such as Facebook groups or Reddit communities where people are engaging on a given topic. Health departments can sponsor virtual or in-person town halls to share and gather information from the public.

For emergency risk communication, town halls can be used to create a two-way dialogue between a health agency and the public. Town halls are often used early during emergency responses to work with affected communities and build organizational credibility, trust, and transparency regarding emergency response efforts.

Media monitoring and analysis are often done to understand how the news media is reporting on an organization and how those media stories impact the public's perception of such an organization. Media monitoring and analysis also include monitoring a health department's social media channels, which is called "social listening": "Social listening, the process of monitoring and analyzing conversations to inform communication activities, is an essential component of infodemic management. It helps inform context-specific communication strategies that are culturally acceptable and appropriate for various subpopulations."[10]

For emergency risk communication, media monitoring and analysis can provide useful insights about audience perceptions based on media framing. For broadcast and digital newspapers, editorial frames – or how the media is reporting on the topic – can influence what the public thinks about a given topic (see Chapter 11 on agenda setting theory). It is imperative for a health department to monitor and analyze what the media is reporting. Further, social listening provides another data source to understand how the public is perceiving a health emergency. Both media reports and social media posts can be used as proxies for audience input and can provide useful information that can be used to update communication strategy.

Literature reviews of peer-reviewed, scientific literature can provide the latest knowledge on evidence-based health interventions or theoretical analyses of communication activities that are relevant to a health issue that is arising. Reviews of gray literature (i.e., reports, working papers, speeches, etc.) can also provide useful information related to such a health emergency.

For emergency risk communication, literature reviews can provide useful theoretical constructs that can inform the messaging strategy or provide more evidence-based information to inform the development of health communication campaigns (see Chapter 8 on health communication campaigns during emergencies). Due to the sheer number of articles that are published, academic scholars might engage in in-depth literature reviews called "scoping reviews." A scoping review uses a systematic approach to identify and synthesize a body of literature.[11]

Turning Evaluation Findings into Learning Opportunities within a Health Agency

At the end of a health emergency, the public health preparedness and response staff will organize an outcome evaluation to assess the effectiveness of the health emergency response. The outcome evaluation will be called an AAR. This type of evaluation is often mandated by government funding and is a common practice outlined by the Federal Emergency Management Agency (FEMA). An AAR leads to the creation of an after-action report that is "a document intended to capture observations of an exercise and make recommendations for post-exercise improvements. The final AAR and Improvement Plan (IP) are printed and distributed jointly as a single AAR/IP following an exercise."[12]

In some cases, a formal AAR does not occur, and instead public health preparedness staff will host a meeting called a "hotwash." A hotwash is a facilitated discussion to capture feedback about any issues, concerns, or proposed improvements participants may have following an exercise, planned event, or real-world incident.[13] Hotwashes tend to be more informal meetings that identify strengths, areas of improvement, and corrective actions regarding the emergency response.[14]

AARs and hotwashes are critical to helping an organizational learn and improve processes and procedures for future emergency responses. The reports that are generated by AARs or hotwashes capture what an organization learned during an emergency response and what needs to be improved, modified, or streamlined for the next emergency response. As organizations consider what procedures and processes need to change in order to improve future emergency response operations, they are engaging in organizational learning.

Organizational learning occurs through identifying problems and ensuring changes are made to address these problems. There are three types of organizational learning after emergencies: retrospective sensemaking, structural reconsideration, and vicarious learning.[15]

Retrospective sensemaking occurs when an organization becomes aware of previously unnoticed or overlooked issues that lead to negative impacts during an emergency response. Wieck, the scholar who developed the theory of sensemaking, calls this type of noticing "biased hindsight."[15] A famous example of this comes from the organizational communication and psychology literature analyzing the ill-fated NASA Challenger launch. Although NASA was aware of potential issues regarding the impact of temperature on the booster rockets, these issues were overlooked until the postaccident investigation, when attention was focused upon what and when NASA became aware of potential threats to the launch.[15,16]

Structural reconsideration occurs when an organization deems it necessary to rearrange internal structures because current structures hinder the flow of information and efficiency of operations. Reorganization of agencies is often difficult without major disruption, so "reorgs" are often seen after major emergencies.[15] CDC is no stranger to structural reconsideration. In April 2022 – amid the COVID-19 response – the CDC Director launched two reviews of the agency: a scientific and programmatic review and a structural review.[17] The former sought to understand how the agency develops and implements science, and the latter gathered feedback on CDC's current processes, systems, and structures. In August 2022, the CDC Director launched "CDC Moving Forward," an initiative to improve how CDC develops science, to create new internal systems and processes, to reorganize the agency's office and department structures, and to identify new programs to better position CDC for future responses.[17]

The third way organizations learn is through *vicarious learning*, which occurs when organizations, agencies, and governments not involved in an emergency observe what is happening to other agencies during the emergency and reflect on how those actions could impact their own organizations.[15,18] This learning occurs through reflection without direct experience of the emergency. During the COVID-19 response, governments across the world watched each other and engaged in vicarious learning. Various countries enacted different levels of quarantine and had different capacities of health care services, which led to different outcomes. Consider how New Zealand's travel restrictions were lauded for stopping the spread of COVID-19 in the country,[19] or how Italy's health care system was crippled[20] during the global coronavirus pandemic.

Training and Exercises

Another important aspect of organizational learning is ensuring staff engage in organizational learning on an individual level through training and through participating in exercises. Organizations will need to distill the learnings from AARs and IP into tangible policies, processes, and procedures. To understand how these new policies, processes, and procedures will be implemented, training and exercises are developed.

Training can take the form of structured learning through live or recorded meetings and lectures. The training material is based upon the recommendations in the AAR and IP and is developed using best practices for adult learning. The outcome of such training is to ensure health department staff are educated and have the appropriate proficiency to conduct any new processes in the next emergency response.

Exercises test and validate plans, policies, procedures, and capabilities. Exercises also identify resource requirements, capability gaps, strengths, areas for improvement, and potential best practices. Exercises are designed to test the entire program or system to ensure that the personnel training adequately conveyed the changes to the program or system.[21] Exercises can take the form of tabletop discussions or full-scale enactments of an emergency. When health department staff participate in exercises, they engage in individual learning that impacts overall organizational learning.

Supporting Community Resilience and Disaster Preparedness after a Health Emergency

In addition to organizational learning, learning occurs at the community level and can lead to community resilience, which is the ability to plan for, absorb, and rapidly recover from disruptive events.[22] In the United States, disaster researchers have studied community resilience after many natural disasters including but not limited to Hurricane Andrew (1992), Northridge Earthquake (1994), Hurricane Katrina (2005), the Joplin, MO, tornado (2011), and Superstorm Sandy (2012).[22] Research on community resilience has evolved to include long-term impacts on communities. While this research has focused primarily on natural disasters, understanding community resilience from a health department perspective is needed – especially as public health officials learn from the 2019 coronavirus pandemic. In emergency risk communication, community resilience often takes the form of engaging with the public through community-based participatory research (CBPR) and public education campaigns after a disaster.

Community-Based Participatory Research

CBPR was developed in the 1940s by social scientist Kurt Lewin, who was looking at how to use research to support planned social change.[23] Key principles of CBPR include:

- Recognize the identity of the community.
- Build upon the resources of the community.
- Promote collaboration and learning among researchers.
- Promote balance and mutual benefits between researchers and the community.
- Focus on community-defined problems, not researcher agenda.
- Engage in cocreating processes to maintain project partnerships.
- Disseminate knowledge from the study to all project partners.
- Require long-term commitment from all involved in the project.

During COVID-19, CDC used this framework to understand the experiences of African American, Native American, and Latinx people.[24] The research revealed several key findings, including: increases in mistrust, anxiety, and fear were observed among these groups; understanding sociocultural context is needed during emergency responses; and adapting communication strategies can help address community concerns.

Disaster Preparedness and Public Education

Organizational and community learnings from health emergencies can be used to educate and prepare for the next emergency. As emergencies unfold through phases – precrisis/steady state, initial, maintenance, and recovery – eventually there comes a stage when the life cycle moves from recovery and postcrisis back to precrisis or steady state. Steady state is described as the time when no emergencies are occurring; this can also be called the precrisis stage. During this time of moving from postcrisis to precrisis, there is an opportunity to educate the public about learnings from the previous emergency and about how they can prepare for future emergencies.

For public health, following COVID-19, there was concerted focus on messaging about the flu, respiratory syncytial virus (RSV), and COVID-19 vaccinations in the fall of 2023. The learnings from the COVID-19 vaccination campaigns, the scientific knowledge of needing additional vaccinations, and the experiential knowledge of flu seasons coupled with the emergence of RSV among children and older adults revealed that educational health campaigns were needed to explain who needed what type of vaccine for fall 2023.[25,26,27]

Other disaster preparedness and public education campaigns include the Department of Homeland Security and FEMA's Emergency Preparedness Month in September,[28] CDC's "Ready Wrigley" campaign focused on family emergency preparedness,[29] and CDC's infamous 2011 "Zombie Preparedness" campaign.[30]

Academic and Theoretical Evaluation of Emergency Risk Communication

In the academic literature, scholars and researchers continue to deal with the following issue regarding evaluating emergency risk communication:

> Evaluation science can improve the knowledge base of ERC [emergency risk communication] by building evidence on which communication strategies, including messages and dissemination platforms, are or are not effective. Despite growing literature in this field, a framework guiding the evaluation of ERC practice and its relationship to population outcomes during emergency situations does not exist.[31]

Scholars have made efforts to provide some frameworks and measures to evaluate emergency risk communication. The following subsections provide an overview of that work.

The CERC Framework

This book has utilized CDC's CERC framework to show how to analyze the presence or absence of these principles in messages in publicly available media artifacts such as press releases, media briefings, news media stories, and social media posts. Each chapter has provided a case analysis of different health emergencies using the CERC framework and phase-based messaging to make sense of how emergency risk communication occurs. Further, there are many published peer-reviewed articles that use CERC to analyze and evaluate emergency risk communication strategies and newspaper frames, and even to support the development of social media messages.[32–41] To further understand the CERC model and the theoretical possibilities of emergency risk communication, academic scholars and communication researchers want to understand how to measure and assess emergency risk communication variables. Such analyses would strengthen the field of study and theoretical understanding of emergency risk communication, thus providing more opportunities to test these theoretical ideas. The following subsections outline current academic research evaluating emergency risk communication within the field of public health.

Risk Communications Evaluation

The risk communications evaluation (RICE) framework looks at outcomes measured in three areas: information environment, population, and the public health system.[31] In this framework, the information environment refers to the aggregate of individuals, organizations, and systems that collect, process, disseminate, or act upon the information received.[31] This includes things such as the actual crisis message or posts on social media, reports by the media, message framing, transparency of messages, and consistency of messaging. Analysis of the information environment can inform public health officials regarding how messages are filtered or elaborated upon by the media or social media, and such information's availability during a crisis may be critical for improving targeted messages.

Individuals interviewed in one study reported several things that contribute to emergency risk communication effectiveness, such as:

> [I]nclusion of risk communication as a technical and integral part of any emergency plan; existing institutional mechanisms for ERC [emergency risk communication], including clear delineations of roles and responsibilities (e.g., spokespersons); existing protocols for quickly vetting and approving the release of the message to the public; and the establishment of an emergency operation center. Interviewees discussed the development of communication plans and the need for such plans to be inherently adaptable to local systems and a variety of scenarios, as each crisis and system possesses unique characteristics.[31]

Next, at the population level, the RICE framework focuses on public surveys, interviews, and focus groups. Using these tools, the variables of information exposure, information-seeking behaviors, information processing, knowledge, attitudes, and beliefs can be assessed. Further, gathering data on when and how the message was delivered, received, and acted upon is very useful to provide feedback to emergency risk communicators regarding message effectiveness. Data can be gathered using large population surveys or small focus groups.

Finally, the third level of evaluation looks at the public health system. At the system level, outcomes are related to changes in policies, mitigation strategies, and social consequences, which can be partially linked to the impact of emergency risk communication. In contrast to the CERC framework, which uses phases or "time" to demark the development of the health emergency, the RICE framework suggests focusing on "measurement of outcomes at the level at which data could be gathered and analyzed, leaving the 'time' component as a function of the type of study design or threat being considered."[31]

Earlier, Faster, Smoother, Smarter Model

Dickman and colleagues propose a risk communication model that evaluates outcomes based upon "identifiable performance parameters related to the dynamics of an outbreak."[42] Specifically, outbreaks that are detected quickly can be controlled quickly, limiting disruption to public health. Within this framework, risk communication is defined as "interactive, holistic, continuous and engaging activity that focuses on dialogue, intelligence gathering, building relationships over time, a knowledge base informed by new and accessible communication technologies (e.g. social media and networks), and supportive environments."[42]

Based on this definition, risk communication activities can be outlined as in Table 10.2.

Based upon these risk communication activities and combining them with the basic tenets of outbreak detection, this risk communication framework evaluates the following performance parameters[42]:

- *Earlier:* Reducing the time lag between the onset of an outbreak and its detection by getting closer to and more engaged with the community and the infectious activities on the ground.

Table 10.2 Components and definitions of the earlier, faster, smoother, smarter model

Risk communication model	Example of risk communication activity
Listening and gathering insights, assessing and sharing	Monitoring social media chats or performing formative research to better understand perceptions, attitudes, knowledge, and behaviors of vulnerable and other populations
Communicating and engaging	Making reliable, up-to-date information available and accessible; selecting appropriate trustworthy communicators, platforms, and channels for distribution of information; integrating key stakeholders into planning and dissemination activities
Coordinating, supporting, and reviewing	Building and supporting ongoing relationships with stakeholders and partners; monitoring and evaluating performance parameters and adjusting practice based on learning

- *Faster:* Reducing the time lag between detection and response activities.
- *Smoother:* Better coordination of national and international response activities.
- *Smarter:* Feeding back to improve decision-making and responses during the current event and leaving a legacy to improve preparedness, control, response, and recovery for future outbreaks.

Emergency Risk Communication Conceptual Model

Seeger and colleagues developed the emergency risk communication conceptual model, which includes three key components: inputs, message development and dissemination, and short-, mid-, and long-term emergency risk communication outcomes.[43] By applying the CERC framework, emergency risk communicators can develop clear, timely, accurate, and actionable health messages that lead to particular outcomes or impacts. The nine potential outcomes or impacts of emergency risk communication messages are:

- Reach of message
- Increased exposure and awareness
- Increased information-seeking and sharing
- Reduced uncertainty
- Increased knowledge and understanding
- Maintained or increased source credibility
- Alignment of risk perception with actual risk
- Increased self-efficacy
- Behavior change[43]

These risk communication outcomes and definitions are outlined in Table 10.3.

Table 10.3 Nine risk communication outcomes and definitions

Risk communication variable	Definition
Reach of the message	How many people received the message
Awareness	How many people became aware of the health threat
Increased information-seeking and sharing	How often people sought out information about the health threat and shared it with others
Reduced uncertainty	A reduction in uncertainty about the health threat
Increased knowledge and understanding	An increase in knowledge about the health threat and reduction in psychological impacts of the health threat
Maintained or increased source credibility	How the organization/agency responding to the emergency was perceived as credible by the audience
Alignment of risk perception with actual risk	People understood the actual risk to their health and not just their perceived risk of the health threat
Increased self-efficacy	Increased numbers of people who believed they could carry out a recommended public health action
Behavior change	Long-term goal of emergency risk communication was to influence behavior among audiences to mitigate the health threat

How to Apply the Emergency Risk Communication Model to Your Agency's Emergency Risk Communication Messages

Seeger and colleagues outlined a model for evaluating emergency risk communication that takes these nine outcomes into consideration. Using CDC's CERC framework, Seeger and colleagues suggested that these nine emergency risk communication outcomes can be impacted through short-term, mid-term, and long-term communication actions.[43] However, these outcomes can also be affected by contextual factors such as crisis conditions, existing knowledge, attitudes and behaviors, demographics and previous experiences of audiences, larger issue context, misinformation, and competing/conflicting messages. This subsection outlines how emergency risk communicators can identify metrics associated with these nine risk communication outcomes to understand the impacts of emergency risk communication on the intended audiences (see Table 10.4 for practical applications of the emergency risk communication model).

Reach of Message

Identifying the reach of messages requires identifying what channels were used to get the message out, then researching the reach of those channels. For example, TV stations have statistics about how many people watch their shows; online newspapers have numbers on how many people are accessing their platforms and can provide estimations of potential reach; and social media platforms (e.g., Facebook, Instagram, X) can provide reach and exposure metrics for business accounts.

Increased Exposure and Awareness

Identifying an increase in exposure and awareness is more challenging regarding emergency risk communication because there is no baseline prior to exposure of emergency health messages. By the time a health agency communicates about a health emergency, the news media or social media will have already been producing content about it. It would be difficult for the health agency to claim that their health emergency messages were truly impactful without knowing the baseline of knowledge of the public prior to them receiving any information about the health emergency. It is possible to gather some type of baseline if the health agency conducts a health communication campaign for a public health intervention. In such a case, the health campaign typically conducts pre- and post-campaign surveys to assess whether the campaign informed, educated, or persuaded people to take an action. Regarding social media, each platform (e.g., Facebook, Instagram, X) typically provides reach and exposure metrics for business accounts.

Increased Information-Seeking and Sharing

Increased information-seeking and sharing relates to how often people sought out information about the health threat and shared it with others. Emergency risk communicators can gather data on the number of calls coming into an emergency hotline or call center. Further, these call centers can also provide reports on the types of calls they received and can categorize the call inquiries (e.g., questions about symptoms of the virus, travel concerns, vaccines). These data provide some insights into the type of information people are looking for.

For information-sharing, emergency risk communicators can track social media shares on Facebook or the number of new email newsletter subscribers after a media

Table 10.4 Overview of emergency risk communication model and practical applications for emergency risk communicators

Construct	Definition	Practical application	Example
Reach of the message + increased exposure and awareness	How many people received the message + how many people became aware of the health threat	Identify reach of channels (TV, radio, web pages, newsletters) that were used to disseminate emergency messages and estimate the potential number of people that could have received the message	Broadcast Channel 6, estimated reach of 1.3 million viewers 88.9 Public Radio, estimated reach of 800,000 listeners GovDelivery email list: 6,740 subscribers Facebook – 1 million impressions on handwashing post From vaccine campaign evaluation, 500 people reported learning about the campaign from the mailed flyer
Increased information-seeking and sharing	How often people sought out information about the health threat and shared it with others	Coordinate with hotline/call center on numbers and types/categories of calls Document numbers of calls, emails, and presentations with partner agencies	1,000 calls on vaccine availability, travel, and children's risk 5 emails to hospitals; 1 webinar; 16 calls from health care providers Social media shares
Reduced uncertainty + increased knowledge and understanding + alignment of risk perception with actual risk	A reduction in uncertainty about the health threat + an increase in knowledge about the health threat and reduction in psychological impacts of the health threat + people understood the actual risk to their health and not just their perceived risk of the health threat	Public opinion surveys Measurement of health intervention	Gather quantitative survey data through online and phone surveys Measure impact of pharmaceutical intervention by number of vaccines given
Maintained or increased source credibility	How the organization/agency responding to the emergency was perceived as credible by the audience	Public opinion surveys	Gather quantitative survey data through online and phone surveys

Table 10.4 (cont.)

Construct	Definition	Practical application	Example
Increased self-efficacy + behavior change	Increase in people who believed they could carry out a recommended public health action + long-term goal of emergency risk communication was to influence behavior among audiences to mitigate the health threat	Measurement of health intervention	Measure impact of pharmaceutical intervention by number of vaccines given

outreach event. Emergency risk communicators can also track information-sharing through the number of partner calls, emails, and presentations that were given to partners involved in the emergency response.

Reduced Uncertainty + Increased Knowledge and Understanding + Alignment of Risk Perception with Actual Risk

This grouping combines three risk communication outcomes: reduced uncertainty, increased knowledge and understanding, and alignment of risk perception with actual risk. These outcomes are more difficult to assess and attribute to one particular emergency risk communication message, but emergency risk communicators can gather data from public health interventions such as mass vaccination campaigns and the number of people who received a vaccine. At mass vaccination clinics, emergency risk communicators could survey people and ask them about their current knowledge of the health threat.

Maintained or Increased Source Credibility

Source credibility directly affects how likely audiences will be to take an action to protect their health.[43] Source credibility is made up of expertise and trustworthiness. Expertise is demonstrated through experience, organizational affiliation, and credentials. "Trustworthiness is situational and subjective and is grounded in shared values, history of interaction, reputation, and affiliation."[43]

Emergency risk communicators can measure source credibility in two ways:

1. Monitor the number of spokespeople that the agency is using. In previous emergencies, the employment of too many spokespeople leads to message inconsistency and conflicting information.[44]
2. Engage with local universities or polling companies to conduct public opinion surveys regarding the public's perception of the credibility of the organization.

Increased Self-Efficacy + Behavior Change

Self-efficacy and behavior change relate to the individual's belief that they can do something new and have the ability to carry out and maintain a new behavior.

Emergency risk communications can assess self-efficacy and behavior change through a health intervention's recommended actions. For example, at a mass vaccination clinic, emergency risk communications can track how many people received a vaccine.

Theory Callout: The Awareness, Desire, Knowledge, Ability, and Reinforcement Model

The awareness, desire, knowledge, ability, and reinforcement (ADKAR) model aims to assess, measure, and prepare the individual for change that accompanies large-scale changes within an organization. For example, the ADKAR model could support communications and organizational changes if a health agency undergoes a structural reorganization after a health emergency. The ADKAR model is a component of the Prosci change management framework, and it has become a common shorthand for addressing the change experience.[45] Large-scale, long-term change within organizations is successful when individuals are free from any barriers to sustaining change. The five key ADKAR principles to support an individual's empowerment to change are:

- *Awareness:* of the need for change
- *Desire:* to participate and support the change
- *Knowledge:* on how to change
- *Ability:* to implement required skills and behaviors
- *Reinforcement:* to sustain the change

During the COVID-19 response, the Texas Health Resources health care system used the ADKAR model to change internal processes of primary nursing (i.e., one nurse per patient) to team nursing (i.e., care coordinated and shared by a group).[46] The ADKAR model guided Texas Health Resources leaders to communicate, explain, and train care team members while implementing the process change. Using consistent messaging, listening to feedback, monitoring employee morale, and identifying barriers to change were key activities that the leaders engaged in while deploying the ADKAR model.

The EVALI Public Health Emergency and the Response by the Georgia Department of Public Health

Julie Mayo Lamberte, MSPH

Overview

The e-cigarette or vaping product use-associated lung injury (EVALI) public health emergency in the United States occurred between March 2019 and February 2020. According to CDC, EVALI arose when the users of e-cigarettes/vaping products reported suspicious respiratory, gastrointestinal, and nonspecific constitutional symptoms that a lung infection, such as pneumonia, would not cause. These e-cigarettes/vaping product users required hospitalization and respiratory support. It was reported that vitamin E acetate may have been responsible for the EVALI outbreak because it was discovered in patient lung fluid samples analyzed by CDC and in the e-cigarette or vaping product samples verified by the US Food and Drug Administration (FDA) and state labs. Vitamin E acetate was not present in lung fluid samples from people who did not have EVALI. In addition, there was not enough data to rule out the influence of other chemicals – such as THC (tetrahydrocannabinol, the main psychoactive compound in marijuana) or non-THC compounds – that were found in other reported EVALI cases. As of February 2020, there had been a total of 2,807 hospitalized cases in the United States, including the District of Columbia (DC) and two US territories (Puerto Rico and the US Virgin Islands). In addition, 68 EVALI-related deaths were verified in 29 states and DC.[47]

The Georgia Department of Public Health (DPH) headquarters are located in Atlanta, Georgia. Georgia DPH works in partnership with the 18 public health districts throughout the state of Georgia, serving the entire state. Each district incorporates one or more of 159 counties and their health departments.[48] On September 13, 2019, Georgia DPH confirmed three EVALI cases in the state of Georgia. Then, on September 25, 2019, the first EVALI-related death was reported.[48] This case study will focus on Georgia DPH's response to the EVALI public health emergency.

Timeline of Key Events
- March 2019: First hospitalization due to EVALI and the beginning of the EVALI public health emergency in the United States.[47]
- August 21, 2019: Georgia DPH published a Health Alert document about EVALI.[49]
- August 23, 2019: CDC reported the first death from EVALI in Illinois.[47]
- September 25, 2019: First death in Georgia reported by DPH.[48]
- October 9, 2019: Second death reported in Georgia. An updated Health Advisory was released to provide Georgia residents with more information about EVALI.[50]
- October 16, 2019: 21 cases identified in Georgia, including two deaths.[50]
- November 25, 2019: 42 cases and 6 deaths reported in Georgia.[51] Final update provided by DPH on their website and social media channels.
- February 2020: A total of 2,807 cases reported in the United States, including DC and two US territories (Puerto Rico and the US Virgin Islands). In addition, 68 EVALI-related deaths were verified in 29 states and DC.[47]

CERC Principles and Phase-Based Messaging
CERC includes an evidence-based structure designed by CDC. Described in the CERC introduction document,[52] the six CERC principles are Be First, Be Right, Be Credible, Express Empathy, Promote Action, and Show Respect.

In addition to the six CERC principles, phase-based messages should be considered when developing a disaster and emergency communication plan. The three phase-based message types after preparation for a disaster or emergency are initial, maintenance, and resolution/recovery.

- *Initial messages* should include all CERC principles. Also, initial messages should include the following key message components: uncertainty, commitment, self-efficacy, and empathy.
- *Maintenance messages* should include the CERC principles of Be Right, Be Credible, Promote Action, and Show Respect. The following are the key message components that should be included in maintenance messaging: deeper risk explanations, interventions, make a commitment to the community, and address misinformation and rumors.
- *Resolution/recovery messages* should include the CERC principles of Be Right, Be Credible, and Show Respect. Also, recovery messages should include the following key message components: focus on community health, health threat has been mitigated, and move toward a "new normal."

The goal of CERC is to provide the public with adequate communication so that crucial actions can occur during an emergency.[52]

CERC Analysis

During the EVALI public health emergency, Georgia DPH published a total of 11 media reports, which included five social media posts on Facebook and six publications on DPH's website. The following is an analysis of Georgia DPH's use of the CERC principles in six example messages.

Message 1

The first Georgia DPH message about EVALI was published on August 21, 2019 on DPH's website.[53] The following is an explanation of each CERC principle identified in this initial-phase message:

- *Be First:* August 21, 2019, was when this first message about the EVALI public health emergency was sent out in Georgia, before CDC reported on the first EVALI death in the United States.
- *Be Right:* Several sections in the Health Alert report stated what was currently known about EVALI, what was not known, and what DPH was doing to find out more information.
- *Be Credible:* Similarly to the Be Right CERC principle, this Health Alert document contained truthful information about EVALI.
- *Promote Action:* In this Health Alert document, there were many actions outlined for how health care providers could report EVALI.[53]

The CERC principles of Express Empathy and Show Respect were not present in this message.

Message 2

Another initial-phase message is the first Facebook post regarding the EVALI public health emergency.[49] The link provided in this post was to a news release published on Georgia DPH's website. Both the Facebook post and the link were posted on August 23, 2019. For this second example message, only the Facebook post was analyzed in terms of its use of the CERC principles.

- *Be First:* On August 23, 2019, this initial-phase message was published on Facebook regarding the EVALI public health emergency. This Facebook post appeared a few days following the initial-phase message on Georgia DPH's website (see Message 1).
- *Be Right:* The Facebook post stated that Georgia DPH "is investigating possible causes of respiratory illness related to vaping." This was an example of what DPH was doing to find out more information about EVALI. Also, the Facebook post detailed the symptoms of EVALI, representing examples of what was currently known about EVALI.
- *Be Credible:* Similarly to the Be Right CERC principle, the Facebook post detailed the typical symptoms of EVALI, which represented truthful information.
- *Promote Action:* The Facebook post stated at the end: "If you have a history of vaping and are experiencing breathing problems, seek medical care." Also, the post included a link to a news release for further information.[49]

The CERC principles not seen in the initial-phase Facebook message were Express Empathy and Show Respect.

Message 3

A news release from September 25, 2019, can be found on Georgia DPH's website regarding the first death in Georgia related to EVALI.[54] This is a maintenance-phase message because at that time period epidemiologists and other researchers were trying to determine what might have been causing EVALI and which populations were affected.

The following is an explanation of each CERC principle present in this maintenance-phase message:

- *Be Right:* The news release stated what was now known about EVALI, what was not known, and what DPH was doing to find out more information. The news release provided a specific affected population age range of 18–68 years old and stated that 78% of those affected by EVALI were male.
- *Be Credible:* Similarly to the Be Right CERC principle, this news release presented truthful information about EVALI.
- *Promote Action:* The last three paragraphs in the news release contained actionable items that the public could do to prevent EVALI and stated that people should seek medical care if they experienced these symptoms.
- *Show Respect:* The middle section of the news release gave somewhat respectful advice from the Georgia Governor and the DPH Commissioner to follow CDC recommendations and to stop using e-cigarettes or vaping devices until the specific cause of EVALI was found.[54]

The CERC principles not seen in this message were Be First and Express Empathy. These CERC principles are not typically seen in maintenance-phase messages.

Message 4

A maintenance-phase message on Facebook presenting a status update regarding EVALI was posted on October 10, 2019.[55] For this fourth example message, only the Facebook post was analyzed in terms of the CERC principles.

- *Be Right:* The Facebook post stated that Georgia DPH "is working with CDC and other state health department to investigate more than 1,000 cases." This is an example of what DPH was doing to find out more information about EVALI in the state of Georgia. Also, the Facebook post provided the latest information regarding that there was no specific e-cigarette or substance linked to the recent EVALI cases, which is an example of unknown information regarding EVALI. In addition, the updated list of EVALI symptoms represents an example of what was currently known about EVALI at that time.
- *Be Credible:* Similarly to the Be Right CERC principle, the Facebook post included updated symptoms of EVALI, which provided consistent information regarding the public health emergency.
- *Promote Action:* The Facebook post stated at the end: "People with a history of vaping who are experiencing breathing problems or any of these symptoms should seek medical care."[55]

The CERC principles not seen in this message were Be First, Express Empathy, and Show Respect. Be First and Express Empathy are not typically seen in maintenance-phase messages, however.

Message 5

Another maintenance-phase message gave a clinical alert report for EVALI.[50] The report was posted on Georgia DPH's website on October 16, 2019, regarding DPH's request for Georgia health care providers to report any possible cases of EVALI. This clinical alert report was a maintenance-phase message that contained the following CERC principles:

- *Be Right:* Two detailed pages of EVALI "Recommendations for Clinicians" provided actions that clinicians could undertake so that people who vape could limit their risk of EVALI and/or to allow patients to recover from EVALI.[50]

- *Be Credible:* Similarly to the Be Right CERC principle, the clinical alert report included an updated summary and background information regarding EVALI, providing reliable information regarding the EVALI public health emergency.
- *Promote Action:* Pages 2 and 3 of the clinical alert report provided thorough EVALI "Recommendations for Clinicians."

The CERC principles not seen in this clinical alert report were Be First and Express Empathy. These CERC principles are not typically seen in maintenance-phase messages.

Message 6

This message represents the final EVALI post on Georgia DPH's website.[51] There is no specific date on the post specifying when the page was last updated. However, the text "As of (11/25/2019)" is given on the post. This maintenance-phase message contained the following CERC principles:

- *Be Right:* Most of the post stated what was currently known about EVALI at that time in November 2019, what was not known, and what DPH was doing to find out more information.
- *Be Credible:* Similarly to the Be Right CERC principle, the post displayed reliable and up-to-date information about EVALI as of November 25, 2019.
- *Promote Action:* There were several parts of the post that contained actionable items that the public could do to prevent EVALI and advising the public to seek medical care if they experienced these symptoms. Also, medical professionals were directed to report EVALI cases using the Georgia Poison Center's hotline.

Be First and Express Empathy were not found in the post, as is usually the case for maintenance-phase messages. At the bottom of the web page helpful download links and websites for more information about the EVALI public health emergency were provided.

Implications

Overall, Georgia DPH did a pretty good job of covering the CERC principles in these six example messages. However, the CERC principle of Express Empathy was not demonstrated in any of the initial-phase messages. Also, DPH could have included the Show Respect CERC principle to a greater extent in the maintenance-phase messages.

Looking at Georgia DPH's website and Facebook channel, it can be concluded that its phase-based messaging was not complete and did not include recovery messaging. The public health emergency started in March 2019 and lasted through February 2020. Georgia DPH started posting information about EVALI in August 2019. There were no further posts about the EVALI public health emergency on DPH's website nor on its Facebook page after November 2019. DPH's other social media channels were also reviewed, and there was no EVALI messaging displayed on its Instagram or X feeds.

Interestingly, there were still documents and website postings regarding EVALI being updated by other public health departments, such as the Los Angeles County of Public Health, even past CDC's EVALI emergency response end date in February 2020. In March 2020, the County of Los Angeles published PDF document on their website entitled "Vaping Risks, Behaviors and Policy Responses: A View from Los Angeles County." This comprehensive guide described the history of EVALI, key definitions of vaping and e-cigarettes, current youth vaping trends in Los Angeles County, and EVALI recommendations.[56] In addition, the final document posted on the County of Los Angeles Public Health website was entitled "California Department of Public Health (CDPH) Health Alert: E-Cigarette, or Vaping, Product Use-Associated Lung Injury (EVALI) Cases during California's COVID-19 Response." This document was published on May 11, 2020. The Health Alert document described how there was still an ongoing threat of EVALI in California and that a few new cases of EVALI had been recently identified. The Health Alert provided up-to-date guidance for medical practitioners, local health departments, and Los Angeles County residents regarding EVALI in connection to COVID-19, and how both illnesses presented similar ongoing health risks.[57]

In conclusion, Georgia DPH could have done better with it EVALI public health emergency messaging. Other public health departments nationwide were still reporting on EVALI past CDC's public emergency end date in February 2020. Georgia DPH could have provided the public with at least one recovery/resolution message, such as announcing the ending of the EVALI public health emergency in February 2020, despite its overlap with the COVID-19 public health emergency.

End-of-Chapter Reflection Questions

1 How does your agency incorporate formative and process evaluation into health emergency responses?
2 How does your agency implement lessons learned based on communication activities? How could change management theory and the ADKAR model support sustained change in your organization?
3 Besides an AAR, how does your agency evaluate emergency risk communication? What would be a stretch goal for your agency regarding evaluating emergency risk communication activities?
4 How does your agency engage in disaster preparedness and public education after an emergency? What would be a stretch goal for your agency regarding public education after an emergency?

References

1 CDC. *Types of Evaluation*. National Center for HIV/AIDS, Viral Hepatitis, STD, and TB Prevention, editor. Atlanta, GA, CDC; n.d.

2 Roberti J, Jorro F, Rodríguez V, Belizán M, Arias P, Ratto ME, et al. Theory-Driven, Rapid Formative Research on Quality Improvement Intervention for Critical Care of Patients with COVID-19 in Argentina. *Glob Qual Nurs Res* 2021;**8**:23333936211015660.

3 McCann B, Hunter SC, McAloney-Kocaman K, McCarthy P, Smith J, Calveley E. Time for You: A Process Evaluation of the Rapid Implementation of a Multi-Level Mental Health Support Intervention for Frontline Workers during the COVID-19 Pandemic. *PLoS ONE* 2023;**18**(10):e0293393.

4 Mensah GA, Johnson LE, Zhang X, Stinson N, Jr., Carrington K, Malla G, et al. Community Engagement Alliance (CEAL): A National Institutes of Health Program to Advance Health Equity. *Am J Public Health* 2024;**114**(S1):S12–S17.

5 Types of Evaluation in Health Promotion and Disease Prevention Programs. *Rural Health Information Hub*. 2024. www.ruralhealthinfo.org/toolkits/health-promotion/5/types-of-evaluation (Accessed April 10, 2024).

6 What is the Kirkpatrick Model? *Kirkpatrick Partners*. 2024. www.kirkpatrickpartners.com/the-kirkpatrick-model (Accessed April 10, 2024).

7 *Study Guide for the Examination for Accreditation in Public Relations*. New York, Universal Accreditation Board/Public Relations Society of America, 2021.

8. CDC. *Crisis and Emergency Risk Communication October 2002*. Atlanta, GA, CDC, 2002.

9. CDC. *Crisis and Emergency Risk Communication October 2018*. Atlanta, GA, CDC, 2018.

10. Lohiniva AL, Sibenberg K, Austero S, Skogberg N. Social Listening to Enhance Access to Appropriate Pandemic Information among Culturally Diverse Populations: Case Study from Finland. *JMIR Infodemiol* 2022;2(2):e38343.

11. Mak S, Thomas A. Steps for Conducting a Scoping Review. *J Grad Med Educ* 2022;14(5):565–67.

12. FEMA. Glossary. n.d. https://training.fema.gov/programs/emischool/el361toolkit/glossary.htm (Accessed April 10, 2024).

13. Hotwash Guide. *Ohio School Safety Center*. n.d. https://dam.assets.ohio.gov/image/upload/ohioschoolsafetycenter.ohio.gov/Hotwash%20Guide.pdf (Accessed April 10, 2024).

14. FEMA. Hot Wash Form. n.d. https://training.fema.gov/is/flupan/references/02_course%20forms%20and%20templates/02_hot%20wash%20form-508.pdf (Accessed April 10, 2024).

15. Seeger M, Sellnow T, Ulmer R. *Communication and Organizational Crisis*. London, Bloomsbury Academic, 2003.

16. Tompkins PK. *Apollo, Challenger, Columbia: The Decline of the Space Program: A Study in Organizational Communication*. Oxford, Oxford University Press, 2004.

17. Moving Forward Summary Report. *CDC*. 2022. www.cdc.gov/about/organization/cdc-moving-forward-summary-report.html (Accessed April 10, 2024).

18. Weick K, Sutcliffe KM. *Managing the Unexpected: Assuring High Performance in an Age of Complexity*. San Francisco, CA, Jossey-Boss, 2001.

19. Liu LS, Ran GJ, Jia X. New Zealand Border Restrictions amidst COVID-19 and Their Impacts on Temporary Migrant Workers. *Asian Pac Migr J* 2022;31(3):312–23.

20. Parotto E, Lamberti-Castronuovo A, Censi V, Valente M, Atzori A, Ragazzoni L. Exploring Italian Healthcare Facilities Response to COVID-19 Pandemic: Lessons Learned from the Italian Response to COVID-19 Initiative. *Front Public Health* 2023;10:1016649.

21. Exercises. *FEMA*. 2023. www.fema.gov/emergency-managers/national-preparedness/exercises (Accessed May 25, 2024).

22. Koliou M, van de Lindt JW, McAllister TP, Ellingwood BR, Dillard M, Cutler H. State of the Research in Community Resilience: Progress and Challenges. *Sustain Resilient Infrastruct* 2018; doi: 10.1080/23789689.2017.1418547.

23. Holkup PA, Tripp-Reimer T, Salois EM, Weinert C. Community-Based Participatory Research: An Approach to Intervention Research with a Native American Community. *ANS Adv Nurs Sci* 2004;27:162–75.

24. Haboush-Deloye A, Marquez E, Dunne R, Pharr JR. The Importance of Community Voice: Using Community-Based Participatory Research to Understand the Experiences of African American, Native American, and Latinx People during a Pandemic. *Prev Chronic Dis* 2023; 20:E12.

25. Wojcik A. The Importance of Communication before and during a Public Health Emergency. *Dela J Public Health* 2019;5(4):20–30.

26. ASTHO. Evolving view of vaccination COVID-19, flu and RSV. 2023. www.astho.org/globalassets/pdf/covid/evolving-view-of-vaccination-covid-19-flu-rsv.pdf (Accessed April 10, 2024).

27. ASTHO. COVID-19 Public Health Communications Resource Hub. 2024. www.astho.org/topic/infectious-disease/covid-19/communications-resource (Accessed April 10, 2024).

28. DHS. National Preparedness Month. n.d. www.ready.gov/september (Accessed April 10, 2024).

29. CDC. Ready Wrigley. n.d. www.cdc.gov/orr/readywrigley/index.htm (Accessed April 10, 2024).

30. CDC. Campaigns: Zombie Preparedness. n.d. www.cdc.gov/orr/campaigns/index.htm (Accessed April 10, 2024).

31. Sovoia E, Lin L, Gamhewage G. A Conceptual Framework for the Emergency Risk Communications. *Am J Public Health* 2017;**107**(S2):S208–14.

32. Al Nashmi E, Bashir M. The Kuwaiti Government's Twitter Discourse during the COVID-19 Pandemic: Toward a Crisis Communication Model Using SCCT and CERC. *J Creat Commun* 2024;**18**:161–78.

33. Bernard NR, Basit A, Sofija E, Phung H, Lee JS, Rutherford S, et al. Analysis of Crisis Communication by the Prime Minister of Australia during the COVID-19 Pandemic. *Int J Disaster Risk Reduct* 2021;**62**:9.

34. Jin XL, Spence PR. Understanding Crisis Communication on Social Media with CERC: Topic Model Analysis of Tweets about Hurricane Maria. *J Risk Res* 2021;**24**(10):1266–87.

35. Kinsky ES, Chen L, Drumheller K. Crisis and Emergency Risk Communication: FEMA's Twitter Use during the 2017 Hurricane Season. *Public Relat Rev* 2021;**47**(4):10.

36. Lu JH. Themes and Evolution of Misinformation during the Early Phases of the COVID-19 Outbreak in China – An Application of the Crisis and Emergency Risk Communication Model. *Front Commun* 2020;**5**:7.

37. Lwin MO, Lu JH, Sheldenkar A, Schulz PJ. Strategic Uses of Facebook in Zika Outbreak Communication: Implications for the Crisis and Emergency Risk Communication Model. *Int J Environ Res Public Health* 2018;**15**(9):19.

38. Malik A, Khan ML, Quan-Haase A. Public Health Agencies Outreach through Instagram during the COVID-19 Pandemic: Crisis and Emergency Risk Communication Perspective. *Int J Disaster Risk Reduct* 2021;**61**:9.

39. Nour M, Alhajri M, Farag E, Al-Romaihi HE, Al-Thani M, Al-Marri S, et al. How Do the First Days Count? A Case Study of Qatar Experience in Emergency Risk Communication during the MERS-CoV Outbreak. *Int J Environ Res Public Health* 2017;**14**(12):16.

40. Ophir Y. Coverage of Epidemics in American Newspapers through the Lens of the Crisis and Emergency Risk Communication Framework. *Health Secur* 2018;**16**(3):147–57.

41. Troy CLC, Pinto J, Cui Z. Managing Complexity during Dual Crises: Social Media Messaging of Hurricane Preparedness during COVID-19. *J Risk Res* 2022;**25**(11–12):1458–75.

42. Dickmann P, McClelland A, Gamhewage GM, Portela de Souza P, Apfel F. Making Sense of Communication Interventions in Public Health Emergencies – An Evaluation Framework for Risk Communication. *J Commun Healthc* 2015;**8**(3):233–40.

43. Seeger M, Pechta L, Price S, Lubell KM, Rose D, Sapru S, et al. A Conceptual Model for Evaluating Emergency Risk Communication in Public Health. *Health Secur* 2018;**16**(3):193–203.

44. Scott BM. Spokespersons and Message Control: How the CDC Lost Credibility during the Anthrax Crisis. *Qual Res Rep Commun* 2005;**6**(1):59–68.

45. Hiatt J. The Prosci ADKAR Model. n.d. www.prosci.com/methodology/adkar (Accessed April 10, 2024).

46. Balluck J, Asturi E, Brockman V. Use of the ADKAR® and CLARC® Change Models to Navigate Staffing Model Changes during the COVID-19 Pandemic. *Nurse Lead* 2020;**18**(6):539–46.

47. CDC. Outbreak of Lung Injury Associated with the Use of E-Cigarette, or Vaping, Products. 2020. www.cdc.gov/tobacco/basic_information/e-cigarettes/severe-lung-disease.html (Accessed April 21, 2024).

48. Georgia Department of Public Health (DPH). About DPH. 2022. https://dph.georgia.gov/public-health-districts (Accessed April 21, 2024).

49. Georgia Department of Public Health (DPH). Georgia DPH Investigating Possible Vaping-related Illnesses. *Facebook*. 2019. www.facebook.com/GaDPH/posts/2371886426230292 (Accessed April 21, 2024).

50. Georgia Department of Public Health (DPH). Clinical Alert: Georgia Department of Public Health Urges Clinicians to Report Possible Cases of Vaping-Associated Lung Injury. 2019. https://dph.georgia.gov/document/document/dph-clinical-alert-oct-16-2019/download (Accessed April 21, 2024).

51. Georgia Department of Public Health (DPH). Severe Lung Disease among People Who Reported Vaping. 2019. https://dph.georgia.gov/vapinglunginjury (Accessed April 21, 2024).

52. CDC. CERC Introduction. 2018. https://emergency.cdc.gov/cerc/ppt/CERC_Introduction.pdf (Accessed April 21, 2024).

53. Georgia Department of Public Health (DPH). Health Alert: Severe Pulmonary Diseases among People Who Reported Vaping. 2019. http://dph.georgia.gov/document/document/dph-health-alert/download (Accessed April 21, 2024).

54. Georgia Department of Public Health (DPH). DPH Identifies First Death From Vaping-Associated Illness. 2019. https://dph.georgia.gov/press-releases/2019-09-25/dph-identifies-first-death-vaping-associated-illness#:~:text=DPH%20has%20identified%20nine%20cases,)%2C%2078%25%20are%20male. (Accessed May 25, 2024).

55. Georgia Department of Public Health (DPH). Severe Lung Disease among People Who Reported Vaping. *Facebook*. 2019. https://www.facebook.com/GaDPH/posts/2459466960805571 (Accessed April 21, 2024).

56. County of Los Angeles Public Health. Vaping Risks, Behaviors and Policy Responses: A View from Los Angeles County. 2020. https://publichealth.lacounty.gov/chie/reports/Vaping_CHIEBrief_March2020_Final.pdf (Accessed April 21, 2024).

57. County of Los Angeles Public Health. CDPH Health Alert: E-Cigarette, or Vaping, Product Use-Associated Lung Injury (EVALI) Cases during California's COVID-19 Response. 2020. http://publichealth.lacounty.gov/eprp/lahan/alerts/CDPHEVALI05112020.pdf (Accessed April 21, 2024).

Part IV Crisis Leadership

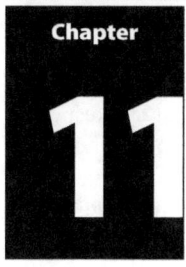

Chapter 11
Effective Communication during a Health Emergency
The Role of the Spokesperson and Working with the Media

Chapter Objectives
- List the four components of the spokesperson role.
- Describe why the spokesperson is critical to emergency response operations.
- Recall at least three ideal characteristics of a spokesperson.
- Describe common pitfalls facing spokespeople and how to avoid them.
- Explain three communication techniques when working with reporters.
- Recall agenda setting theory.

Prior to COVID-19, media briefings (also called press conferences) had a typical organizational format and room setup. For example, there would be a speaker with a podium or a panel of speakers sitting at a table with microphones, and on the other side of the room there would be a row of reporters with cameras and recording devices.[1] Everyone would be in the same physical place. COVID-19 drastically changed the structure of media briefings.[2] Today, sometimes everyone and everything is virtual, so there is one speaker and a lot of participants on a computer screen like in a Zoom online session. Or there could be a modified in-person media briefing, where there is a panel of speakers who are physically distanced from each other and a select number of reporters who are also physically distanced from each other.

Regardless of how the media briefing is set up, whether virtual or in-person, this chapter will focus on how to effectively communicate with the media under any circumstances. Three key topics are covered in this chapter. First is Spokesperson 101: What makes a good spokesperson and what are the common pitfalls facing a spokesperson? Second, how should spokespeople communicate with the media, including preparation, verbal and nonverbal communication, and key tips for handling questions from the media? And finally, how should we write a crisis message for the first 24 hours of a crisis?

Four Components of the Spokesperson Role
To deliver messages effectively as a spokesperson, it is vital to understand why the spokesperson role is so important during emergency responses. There are four key components of being a spokesperson.[3,4]

First, a spokesperson is the face of the issue or the emergency response that a health agency is responding to. This means that when members of the public, response partners, elected officials, and other stakeholders affected by an emergency want answers from a public health agency or are looking for information, the spokesperson is seen as the source of that information.

Second, a spokesperson publicly represents the health agency they work for. This means that anything that a spokesperson says or does – on social media or in real life, even when they think nobody's watching or listening – directly reflects on the health agency they are representing. When a person is designated as the official spokesperson for a public health agency, their actions are judged more critically than others who might be working on the response.

Third, it's crucial that a spokesperson stays on message. Staying on message means communicating the approved health agency messages, answering media questions in a way that brings the question back to the agency's message, and not deviating from approved messaging. The public health agency's media relations office, public health leadership team, and likely the legal and policy teams work hard to develop an appropriate communication strategy and key messages that adequately respond to a health crisis. Staying on message ensures that whatever the spokesperson says doesn't violate policy or create any sort of legal issues for the public health agency. As a spokesperson, it's critical to trust what your communications team has developed and deliver the content as fast as possible.

Fourth, and finally, being a spokesperson is not easy. This individual will face criticism, and in the modern world it is very easy to go online and be exposed to all kinds of comments and reactions that can be demoralizing for some professionals. Individuals who take on spokesperson roles must learn to take that criticism in their stride and to remember that such attacks or judgments are likely more about their agency's position than the spokesperson as a human individual. It is key that spokespeople remember that any health emergency and their position representing the health agency are both temporary. Any online criticism and attacks will eventually die down. It is important to maintain this mindset so as not to get distracted from the purpose of the role.

Importance of the Spokesperson Role during an Emergency Response

There are two key roles of a spokesperson that are critical to emergency risk communication during the health emergency: personalize the response agency and gain support for the health emergency response interventions.[3,4]

First, the spokesperson role takes the organization from being an "it" to a "we." As the face of the organization, a spokesperson must build trust and credibility for the public health agency leading the emergency response efforts. The spokesperson can remove psychological barriers that prevent audience members from taking protective actions through simple communication and messaging strategies. This means communicating effectively through verbal and nonverbal language to state that the health agency is committed to dealing with the crisis and mitigating the health threat. Through the spokesperson's words and actions, trust and credibility can be built with the community affected by the health emergency. Every time the health agency follows through on what the spokesperson said the health agency was going to do, more trust is built with the public. The role of a spokesperson changes the health agency from an impersonal, faceless organization into a personal group of people working to mitigate the health threat affecting the public.

The second reason the spokesperson is critical to the emergency response is they help gain support for the public health response operations. Health agencies use risk communication to reduce the incidence of illness, injury, and death during an emergency. The spokesperson is responsible for delivering those messages to various audiences. During COVID-19, various public health leaders around the world found themselves in local and national media spotlights. One of those public health leaders was Dr. Amy Acton, Director of the Ohio Department of Health, and she was one of the main spokespeople for the health department during the coronavirus response.[5] Representing Ohio state governor Mike DeWine, Dr. Acton was the spokesperson and subject matter expert who delivered key public health messages at statewide press conferences.[6] The messages she delivered focused on getting people on board with the public health interventions being implemented in Ohio. She became so well known for what she was doing that she developed a following not only in Ohio, but nationally. As time went on and public sentiment shifted regarding public health interventions, Dr. Acton encountered protestors at her home. Eventually, the pressure of being in this role lead her to resign after serving 1 year in the position. Because of her contributions, Dr. Acton was recognized in the special Women of the Year issue of *Time* magazine.[5] Dr. Acton is highlighted here as an exemplary spokesperson who used her role to garner public trust, credibility, and support for her health agency's emergency response operations and health interventions.

Characteristics of a Spokesperson

Spokespeople play a vital role during health emergencies in personalizing the health agency and gaining support for the health agency's emergency response operations. While media consultants advise spokespeople "to be natural" to successfully communicate with the media, this may not necessarily be the best advice. The Centers of Disease Control and Prevention (CDC) Crisis and Emergency Risk Communication (CERC) manual and recent research reveal the ideal and less-than-ideal characteristics of spokespeople.[7,8,9] Table 11.1 outlines the characteristics that contribute to a spokesperson's ability to successfully personalize a health agency and gain support for a health agency's response operations.

Ideal Characteristics of Spokespeople

- *Professional*: This characteristic is described as having relevant professional knowledge, technical expertise, and formal qualifications in a relevant field and appearing professional visually.[8]

Table 11.1 Characteristics of a spokesperson

Ideal characteristics	Less-than-ideal characteristics
Professional	Inappropriate demeanor
Experience working with the media	Lack of honesty/sincerity
Involved with health emergency decision-making	Poor emotional control
Trustworthy	Political bias
Charismatic	Lack of credibility
Clarity of speech (tone, rate, articulation)	
Relatable	

- *Experience working with the media:* This characteristic is described as understanding the media's needs, being a confident performer with the media, providing timely responses to the media, and being friendly with the media.[8]
- *Involved with health emergency decision-making:* This characteristic is described as being a person who actively participates in decision-making, being the head of the organization, or being a high-level manager or official within the agency.[8,10]
- *Trustworthy:* This characteristic is described as being trustworthy and having credibility.[8]
- *Charismatic:* This characteristic is described as being able to express oneself well, being calm and rational, being open and honest, having a healthy appearance, being moderate their temper, and being self-possessed.[8]
- *Clarity of speech (tone, rate, articulation):* This characteristic is described as having a stable tone and precise and consistent speech.[8]
- *Relatable:* This characteristic is described as being personable and authentic and appearing to be able to sympathize or understand what an affected community is experiencing.[8]

Less-than-Ideal Characteristics of Spokespeople

- *Inappropriate demeanor:* This characteristic is described as being equivocating, passive, vague, imprecise, verbose, or flattering to the media.[8]
- *Lack of honesty/sincerity:* This characteristic is described as concealing the truth or lying, not being honest, or not telling the truth for fear of losing one's job.[8]
- *Poor emotional control:* This characteristic is described as having a bad temper, being overly emotional, or threatening reporters.[8]
- *Political bias:* This characteristic is described as having an obvious political angle.[8]
- *Lack of credibility:* This characteristic is described as lacking credentials or being uninformed about the health emergency.
- *Unrelatable:* This characteristic is described as having a bureaucratic or haughty, overly official style.[8]

Mini-Case Study Application: Spokesperson Characteristics

Audience members, the public, and other stakeholders will judge spokespeople on these aforementioned characteristics. Therefore, this mini-case study application provides an opportunity to review and reflect on a relevant real-world situation.

In April 2010, an explosion on the Deepwater Horizon oil platform in the Gulf of Mexico, south of Louisiana, resulted in a massive industrial and environmental disaster as oil began leaking into the water. British Petroleum (BP) owned the oil rig and became responsible for the cleanup efforts. In May 2010, BP Chief Executive Officer (CEO) Tony Hayward said, "I want my life back" in response to the disaster.[11] This was an effort to personalize the situation, but for those small business owners, families, local elected officials, and individuals who lived in the area, the message fell flat and sparked public outrage.

In an effort to address the outrage, BP identified personnel who could support the response and attune culturally to the audience. Instead of a British CEO who appeared out of touch regarding the impacts of the disaster on locals, BP brought in Vice President Bob Fryar in June 2010 to help with on-the-ground response efforts. With a grounded presence and southern drawl, Bob delivered the following message to angry locals about the then-current cleanup operations.[12]

Statement by Vice President Bob Fryar

Good afternoon. This afternoon I've been out here on the Gulf Coast and Gulf Shores and I've been spending time with our cleanup crews. Before I'd like to share a little information about how that's going but, before I do that, I just want to talk a little bit about some of the other operations we have going on as you know from the beginning of this our goal has been very clear, we've had three areas we've been fighting: the subsea, offshore, and at the shoreline. Now this morning Admiral Allen shared with you exactly how the operation is going subsea, he talked about the cap that we put on onto the LMRP [lower marine riser package]. That operation has gone extremely well, over the last 24 hours we've been able to collect over 6,000 barrels of oil, so we're very pleased with that operation.

During this time, we're continuing to increase the flow of the pipe and to the drill ship. Tomorrow morning Admiral Allen will give you an update on exactly how much we've recovered. Over the 24-hour period again we're very pleased with how that operation is going very well in terms of the fight offshore. We have at this time over 2,500 vessels, which are now out doing various activities. They're out doing in situ burns, they're out skimming, and they're out doing surveillance for us. Just here in the Mobile area, we have over 1,000 vessels that are working. 900 of those are what we call our "vessel of opportunities," our VO program. And this program is a program that we have established that allows people to come and volunteer and bring their boats to get the basic training to come and operate in the operations. And they're doing a great job. They're out doing boom maintenance, they're doing surveillance, they're doing some skimming.

The bigger some of the shrimp boats, about skimming force, they've been very helpful. Some of the operations they've been doing also is they actually take boom, they've been dragging boom around and collecting the oil together in patches, and then the skimmers come in and they're able to skim up the oil from that boomed area, so the volunteers here have been a huge part of the cleanup, and we very much appreciate all the efforts they've done.

With respect to the shoreline again I've been here today up and down the beach working with the workers. Working with these local teams are folks that are from a local unemployment office, they've been a great help to us. They've come in and they've got here early this morning at 6:00. They've come in and they've very quickly and actively picked up the areas. The areas that we're finding up and down the beach, we're finding this very sporadic.

You know, it was great to see that the beaches were open today. There was a large number of people out on the beach and what we're finding is small patches of tar balls, small little splats of oil. The team is doing a great job cleaning this up. They're using rakes. They're using shovels.

We've brought in double the number of people that we need. Clearly, this is our top priority, and so is safety. So, what we're doing is we have doubled the number of people. We have people that are working 30-minute shifts and then taking breaks. We're getting them rested and rehydrated so we're just making sure that everything in this operation is done safely and that is our top priority in this operation.

The folks have done a good job that are out there actively cleaning this up. Again, most of the areas that I've been to today, they're able to get this cleaned up in 2 or 3 hours, and what we're finding out there, what we're seeing is that the crude oil is a very tarry substance. This oil has been out on the water for a long time volatile, the light ends of this have evaporated off. So, what you're seeing isa very tarry-type substance and so you know for the folks that are out on the beach, our advice to you is if you step on this, if you get this on you, simple soap and water will wipe it, you know, can clean this off. It's just like an asphalt road, it's a tarry substance that we're seeing out there.

So that's how our operations are going at the subsea offshore. The fight continues as well as the operations here. And I just want to end by just saying thanks to all the folks that are out here. At the sites that I was at there's one group of about 200, they had done a super job getting it cleaned up very quickly. Another group of about 100 just got into the area well. And what we've done is we've set up cells where we have people that are walking up and down the beach actively looking for this and as soon as they find it, they get on the phone and they call. And we've got a crew there very quickly. The teams have responded well and, you know, again, getting folks from the local unemployment office has been great, they're very appreciative and they're out there doing great work.[12]

Reflect upon and answer the following questions:
- Was Fryar professional and able demonstrate his knowledge of the emergency operations?
- Do you think he was credible? Why or why not?
- Do you trust him? Why or why not?
- Did he have charisma? Was he relatable?
- Did he demonstrate any of the less-than-ideal characteristics (e.g., inappropriate demeanor, lack of honesty/sincerity, poor emotional control, political bias, lack of credibility)?

Pitfalls of Spokespeople

There are four common pitfalls that can trip up a spokesperson: lying; using language that distances the spokesperson from their audience; aggressive behavior with reporters; and going off-message.[3] This section takes a look at these pitfalls and how they can negatively impact emergency risk messaging.

The first pitfall of a spokesperson is lying or clouding the truth. Always tell the truth and be as transparent as possible with the information that you have and the processes that you're using to find out what is causing the health threat. The truth will eventually come out – if it's not this year, it could be in 5 or 10 years. Lying damages organizational credibility and the spokesperson's personal reputation. An example of the truth coming out later is the Flint, Michigan, water crisis, in which government officials were criminally charged for their conduct during the health emergency for lying and professional misconduct.[13] Being open, transparent, and honest in organizational health emergency messages is critical to demonstrating the CERC principles of Be Right, Be Credible, and Show Respect.[14,15]

Another common pitfall for a spokespeople is using language that distances the spokesperson from the audience. This can typically occur among subject matter experts or technical experts who participate as spokespeople. Subject matter experts are knowledgeable in their field of study, which requires understanding subject-specific language and how to speak with other experts in the field. However, technical words that are common in a particular field may not be understood by a broad audience composed of individuals who don't have the same level of expertise as the speaker.[16] This might cause audiences to lose interest and so zone out. It's really important as a spokesperson that you use language that is relatable and easily conveys the key points of a complex topic in order to keep the attention of the audience. Making the message relatable and easy to understand ensures that the audience is able to take measures to protect their health, which is directly related to the CERC principle Promote Action.

Another common pitfall for spokespeople is becoming aggressive with reporters. Most spokespeople never intend to become aggressive or hostile with the media, but it is a common occurrence. Being aggressive with reporters can manifest through verbal and nonverbal actions. For example, interrupting or yelling at a reporter or rolling one's eyes or sighing are verbal and nonverbal actions that can be interpreted as aggression toward reporters. The key to avoiding this situation is engaging in self-management techniques, which empower the spokesperson to maintain personal homeostasis even in stressful situations. Self-management techniques include mindfulness, meditation, and physical activity.[17]

Since the role of the spokesperson during a health emergency is to humanize an agency and build trust and credibility with the audience, it is imperative for spokespeople to maintain professionalism and integrity during high-stress situations. If a spokesperson is unable to maintain their professional demeanor during a media briefing, their reaction may become the next news story instead of critical information about the health emergency. Being able to convey important health information during high-stress press briefings is necessary to demonstrating the CERC principles of Be Right, Be Credible, and Show Respect.

The final common pitfall for spokespeople is going "off-message." Often spokespeople think doing so is a great idea and that it will allow their message to resonate better with the audience than if they were to follow what their communication staff created and prepared for then. Unfortunately, this strategy can wreak havoc on the communications strategy that's in place, and it can have unforeseen impacts on stakeholder relationships. As an example, when CDC Director Dr. Rochelle Walensky had just come to work at CDC, she was feeling a little bit frustrated about the lack of concern people were showing regarding COVID-19. Her fear was that there was going to be another large wave of illnesses that was going to paralyze the US health care system, so she decided to go "off-message"[18,19,20] in the following statement:

> I would tell you the truth even if it was not the news you wanted to hear, now is one of those times when I have to share the truth and I have to hope and trust you will listen. I'm going to pause here. I'm going to lose the script and I'm going to reflect on the recurring feeling I have of impending doom. We have so much to look forward to, so much promise and potential of where we are, and so much reason for hope, but right now I'm scared.
> I know what it's like as a physician to stand in that patient room gowned, gloved, masked, shielded, and to be the last person to touch someone else's loved one because their loved one couldn't be there.
>
> I know what it's like when you're the physician, when you're the health care provider, and you're worried that you don't have the resources to take care of the patients in front of you. I know that feeling of nausea when you read the crisis standards of care and you wonder whether there are going to be enough ventilators to go around and who's going to make that choice. And I know what it's like to pull up to your hospital every day and see the extra morgue sitting outside.
>
> I didn't know at the time when it would stop. We didn't have the science to tell us. We were just scared. We have come such a long way. Three historic scientific breakthrough vaccines,

and we are rolling them out so very fast, so I'm speaking today not necessarily as your CDC Director and not only as your CDC Director but as a wife, as a mother, as a daughter, to ask you to just please hold on a little while longer.

I so badly want to be done. I know you all so badly want to be done. We are just almost there, but not quite that, and so I'm asking you to just hold on a little longer to get vaccinated when you can so that all of those people that we all love will still be here when this pandemic ends.[21]

Unverified reports indicate that the CDC Director's communication staff didn't know she was going say what she said, but news coverage did indicate it was unusual for an agency leader to experience a "emotional hiccup"[18] of this type during a media briefing. The important takeaway here is that when the spokesperson is also the director of an agency, there is explicit power and authority that comes with such a position. From a communications perspective, it is important to wield that power and authority carefully. Some media coverage of Walensky after this press briefing ranged from accusing her of crying wolf and that there was no such problem to criticism of her being too emotional.[18,22] Again, as mentioned earlier, it is important for spokespeople not to become the center of the story and instead to leverage the strategic communications that have been developed by the staff hired to do this specific type of communications work. Staying on-message, building a relationship with the audience, and maintaining agency credibility are critical activities for a spokesperson during a health emergency.

Working with Reporters

This section provides specific tips and techniques for working with reporters. Media relations is a vast field, so these tips and techniques only cover the basics of working with reporters.[23]

Practice and Preparation

Preparation really does pay off when engaging with the media. Risk communication researcher Vincent Covello analyzed thousands of media briefings and discovered that there are actually only 77 commonly asked questions by reporters during emergencies.[24] These questions include simple questions such as asking for the spokesperson's name and title to more complex questions about health risks, the cause of the emergency, the cost of emergency response operations, compensation for those affected by the emergency, and the long-term consequences of the emergency. Reviewing these commonly asked questions in preparation for a media interview gives a spokesperson the opportunity to prepare for potential questions that could arise during a media interview. Spokespeople ought to work with their communication staff to do practice run-throughs and mock interviews to prepare for what they might encounter during a media briefing or interview. The more a spokesperson can practice and deliver the key talking points, the more familiar the material becomes. Such familiarity enhances the credibility of the spokesperson when sharing these messages with reporters.

Nonverbal Communication

Effective nonverbal communication can enhance a spokesperson's interactions with reporters. For the purposes of this book, nonverbal communication includes physical appearance such as clothing and physical surroundings. For example, during a health emergency response in which a spokesperson is attending an on-site command post, it may not make sense to show up in a blazer or suit; wearing a fleece jacket with the agency's logo might be more appropriate. However, for a formal media briefing at the agency's headquarters, professional dress would be more appropriate.

When conducting virtual interviews, nonverbal communication consists of your surroundings, body language, camera position, and lighting. For example, the background and physical surroundings of the room impact message delivery. Communication staff might advocate for a simple background that conveys some of the individuality or personality of the spokesperson, or they might recommend using a virtual background that displays the logo of the health agency.

Regarding body language during media interviews, there are three areas to consider: eye contact, body posture, and facial expression. During a media interview, eye contact with the reporter creates a human connection. Lack of eye contact often is perceived as indicating that the interviewee does not know an answer, is lying, or is making things up, so it is recommended to maintain eye contact with the reporter. The second aspect of body language during media interviews relates to maintaining an open posture. For example, when standing at a podium or sitting at a table for a media briefing, make sure to adjust your body posture to avoid hunching forward or crossing your arms. These body postures can be perceived as closed postures, meaning they symbolize anger, aggression, or indifference. The best body posture to adopt is to place your hands on the podium or table or in your lap. Maintaining an open body posture demonstrates confidence and competence, which in turn builds trust and credibility for your organization and can help gain the public's support for the health department's interventions aimed at mitigating the health threat. Another area of body posture to be aware of as a spokesperson relates to unconscious movements or gestures one habitually engages in that can distract from the message being delivered. Often individuals will use their hands to gesture unnecessarily, tap their fingers out of nervousness, or swivel in their chair, and these unconscious actions can drive attention away from the speaker's message. However, it is possible to become aware of these unconscious movements and change them into more effective gestures. For example, college-level public speaking courses discuss how to use your hands and make gestures effectively to complement a point in a speech. Additionally, placing your hands on the podium or in your lap can anchor them and so reduce unconscious and unnecessary movements. Again, practice run-throughs and mock interviews with communication office staff and ask them for feedback on your nonverbal communication. Ask for assistance in identifying these unconscious movements and in breaking these habits. If the communication staff are not available, recording and reviewing yourself can be just as helpful. Reducing unconscious movements and gestures ensures a more professional delivery of emergency risk messages to the media.

The third aspect of body language relates to facial expressions. Faces can convey a lot of emotion. In the popular novel *Outlander*, the protagonist, Claire, unconsciously communicates through facial expressions: "Everything ye think shows on your face," her husband, Jamie, tells her.[25] For spokespeople representing a government agency, ensuring professionalism is important, especially when engaging with the media. Almost all interactions with the media – whether formal engagements such as media briefings or scheduled interviews or informal press gatherings such as at the site of an emergency or disaster – are recorded or documented. As a spokesperson for an agency, this means that every action in a public setting or on public social media accounts is publicly recorded and can be used by the media. In relation to nonverbal communications such as facial expressions, spokespeople ought to strive to convey confidence, power, calm, and personal warmth when engaging with the media and members of the public. Any frowns or expressions of disbelief that show up on your face during a press conference can become the focus of the story instead of the key messages about the health emergency and interventions to protect the public's health. As previously discussed regarding maintaining an open body posture, maintaining a positive, polite, and neutral expression throughout a media briefing conveys the sense of calm and confidence that is expected from a leader during a health emergency.

Verbal Communication

Verbal communication is defined as the use of words to deliver information.[26] For spokespeople, verbal communication includes tone, rate of speech, articulation, and other verbal sounds.

Tone of voice plays an important role when delivering a message and can convey emotion. Avoiding a monotone or a tone of voice that lacks inflection is important when delivering messages during health emergencies.

Tone of voice can also impact the rate or speed at which someone speaks. Speaking too fast can be perceived as being due to nervousness or a lack of confidence. Speaking too slowly can also impact how confident people feel in the speaker. When delivering a health emergency message, employ a conversational tone, meaning that you engage in delivering the message to the media in the same way as you might speak with a friend or colleague.

A third aspect of verbal communication is articulation, or the enunciation of words. When an individual is able to control their tone and rate of speech, they become able to clearly articulate their words, which flow naturally. Ensuring people hear and understand the words being spoken is another critical component of message delivery that spokespeople need to consider. If the audience is unable to correctly identify and understand the words being spoken, miscommunication and misunderstandings will occur.

A final aspect of verbal communication that spokespeople need to be aware of related to other verbal sounds, which can be playfully called "verbal garbage." These are the sounds and utterances that are used as pause fillers while the mind searches for the next word. Such sounds include "uh," "um," and "ah." When these verbal sounds are unconsciously deployed too often, much like the unconscious gestures discussed earlier, the audience can become distracted and lose interest in the overall message. Again, practicing the key messages and talking points will help spokespeople thoroughly learn these messages and so reduce the likelihood of engaging in verbal garbage.

Verbal communication is a critical skill that spokespeople need to master. Being aware of tone, rate, articulation, and verbal garbage will help spokespeople to become more effective and authentic communicators.

Addressing Public Speaking Anxiety

The comedian Jerry Seinfeld has a joke about the fear of public speaking: "According to most studies, people's number one fear is public speaking. Number two is death. Death is number two! Now, this means, to the average person, if you have to go to a funeral, you're better off in the casket than doing the eulogy."[27] Anxiety regarding public speaking can be so inhibiting that some people would rather not speak at all than have to deal with the fear and anxiety of speaking. To address this anxiety, engaging in mindfulness-based body movement practices can help. The following are three simple exercised to help reduce public speaking anxiety: shake it, twist it, and ground it.

1. *Shake it:* Stand with your feet placed shoulder width apart, with a neutral spine position and relaxed knees. Take a breath and exhale. Now begin to shake your body: Shake your hands, arms, legs, and whole body. Allow the anxiety to be recognized and shake it off. Do this for a minute. Pause. Check in and take note of what's present now.
2. *Twist it:* Stand with your feet placed shoulder width apart, with a neutral spine position and relaxed knees. Find balance and equal weight placement in your feet. Take a breath and exhale. Begin to twist your midsection or belly area gently to the right and allow your arms to swing with the movement, gently twisting and landing at the front and back of your body. Then twist to the left and allow the arms to swing with you. Allow the momentum of the movement and swing your arms to lead the movement. Do this for one minute. Pause and notice what's present now.
3. *Ground it:* If you are familiar with yoga, this action is called "mountain pose," or *tadasana*. *Tadasana* is called "mountain pose" as the essence or energy of the pose is to visualize a mountain – an unmovable, vast, large presence. To engage in the pose, stand with your feet placed shoulder width apart, with a neutral spine position and relaxed knees. Find balance and equal weight placement in your feet. Take a breath and exhale. Close your eyes. Begin to visualize a mountain. Take five long inhales and exhales. Open your eyes and notice what's present now.

Engaging in these simple practices can support internal self-management and help reduce anxiety. Even professional speakers engage in some form of centering or grounding practice before speaking. For example, vulnerability researcher Brené Brown repeats a mantra before going on stage to help calm her nerves.[28]

Mini-Case Study Application

Former New Zealand Prime Minister Jacinda Ardern was lauded as an exemplary crisis leader during COVID-19 for her confident, powerful, and practical way of communicating health information. The following is a transcript of a speech she gave on April 1, 2020.[29] In the transcript there is no verbal garbage, and the audio recording shows that she speaks with a level tone and uses inflection to highlight the importance of the message. She also engages in a conversational rate of speech and uses clear articulation.

> Good afternoon, everyone. I want to begin as I have done most days now and start by thanking New Zealanders for the ongoing work to make sure that they stay within their bubbles and stay at home during the period that we are at level 4 and the work that they are doing to break the chain of transmission. As you will have heard this morning there are 61 new cases today. While on the face of it that may seem a heartening number relative to some of the other figures that we've had now, I want to emphasize again that it is still too early to assess if our measures are successfully slowing transmission. Because COVID-19 takes a while to incubate we could still see increases in our numbers in the days to come – off the back of transmission in the community prior to the lockdown that may yet be rearing its head and visible symptoms.

If the virus is in the community in this way at present but not yet seen, then the worst thing we could do is be relaxed or too complacent and allow a silent spread. I think we only need to look at some of the *clusters of cases* [inflection emphasis by Ardern] that we have in our community to know just how quickly COVID-19 can spread if we weren't, for instance, currently at level 4 in the schooling community of Marist and Auckland the community of Meta Meta. If we weren't at level 4 we could see outbreaks that were far *far* [inflection emphasis by Ardern] worse down the track.

We also don't have a full picture of the extent of community transmission. That is why we have been so focused on increasing testing capacity, which over a period of time we've seen a 91% increase in that testing capacity. And we are working to continue to build that, it is why ultimately testing is so important to, obviously, our officials in the Ministry of Health as well. You'll have seen the Technical Advisory Group yesterday changing the definition for testing to encourage more testing to be undertaken.[29]

Effectively Working with Journalists during a Media Briefings and Interviews

There are three commonly known techniques to help you answer reporter questions: block and bridge; yes and; and acknowledging the feeling of the question. This section takes a look at each of these techniques, which can be easily applied during media briefings and interviews.

The first technique is called "block and bridge."[30] Basically, a successful block starts by acknowledging the question. A brief acknowledgment of the question lets the reporter know that the spokesperson has heard and understood what they're asking. This is then followed by an appropriate transition. The transition is the "bridge," and the bridge brings the spokesperson back to the talking points and the key messages that the health agency wants to communicate about the health emergency. The bridge would be something similar to, "What I think you're really asking is . . .." Or, "The overall issue is . . .." Or, "What's important to remember is . . .." Or, "It's not our policy to discuss this but what I can tell you is . . .."

These bridges are simply transitions to get the spokesperson back to the agency's talking points. The block and bridge is one of the most common techniques used when working with reporters. This technique is used when a question arises that the health agency is not ready to answer or the question is purposefully inflammatory. The spokesperson engages in respectful exchange with the reporter by acknowledging their question, but the spokesperson directs the focus back to the key health messages related to the health emergency response and to the health interventions aimed at mitigating the threat to the public's health.

A second common technique for answering reporter questions is "yes and."[31] This phrase might be familiar as it comes from comedic improvisation, but its application in media engagement is different. In the media context, when asked a question to which one has a negative answer, people typically respond with "yes but." Using this phrase can be perceived as a disclaimer or as negative news. Listeners tend to be more receptive if the speaker acknowledges their views with "yes and." For example, if asked about why vaccination is necessary when individuals have a right to choose their health actions, consider the following response: "Yes, we want to protect people's rights and we want them to stay alive to enjoy those rights." Using this technique acknowledges what was said and answers the question with a positive frame rather than a negative frame.

A third common technique for answering questions is to acknowledge the feeling behind the question.[31] This technique is often used during town hall meetings when there is potential for conflict and high emotion. When using this technique, spokespeople are avoiding the statement "I know how you feel," which may not be true and can infantilize the people asking the question. Instead, the spokesperson acknowledges what was said and legitimizes their situation. In response, a spokesperson can instead use "I statements," such as "I understand why you're angry," or "I understand your frustration, and anyone in this circumstance would likely feel the same way." Again, the spokesperson is acknowledging what was said and that the situation would be uncomfortable for anyone, and the spokesperson is also providing space for the individual to have their own feelings. This technique supports the CERC principle of Express Empathy by not negating the other's experience.

Mini-Application: Block and Bridge COVID-19 Media Briefing

The following mini-application comes from a March 26, 2021, media briefing hosted by the White House COVID-19 Response Team,[32] in which Dr. Anthony Fauci answered a question about the Wuhan lab leak theory and former CDC Director Robert Redfield's public comments about the lab leak theory.

> *Reporter question:* A colleague asked me to ask about Robert Redfield's comments this morning that he believes that the coronavirus escaped from the Wuhan Institute of Virology.
>
> *Dr. Anthony Fauci, Director of the National Institute of Allergy and Infectious Diseases and Chief Medical Advisor to the President of the United States:* OK, so when you think about the possibilities of how this virus appeared in the human population, obviously there are a number of theories. The issue that would have someone think it's possible to have escaped from a lab would mean that it essentially entered the outside human population already well adapted to humans – suggesting that it was adapted in the lab. However, the alternative explanation which most public health individuals go by is that this virus was actually circulating in China, likely in Wuhan, for a month or more, before they were clinically recognized at the end of December of 2019. If that were the case, the virus clearly could have adapted itself to a greater efficiency of transmissibility over that period of time – up to and at the time it was recognized. So Dr. Redfield was mentioning that he was giving an opinion as to a possibility, but again there are other alternatives that most people hold by.[32]

In this example, Dr. Fauci acknowledges the reporter's question and provides context for the lab leak theory and for Dr. Redfield's comment. He bridges back to his key message of "the alternative explanation which most public health individuals go by is that this virus was actually circulating in China ..." Dr. Fauci concludes there are multiple explanations for the origins of COVID-19, but his message is that most public health officials don't think it was due to a lab leak.

How to Work with the Media: One-on-One Interviews

This section provides key tips and techniques for conducting one-on-one media interviews. In the previous section, communication techniques for communicating at a media briefing were shared. This section looks at communicating with a single reporter.

Meeting with a single reporter in a one-on-one media interview is different than meeting with several reporters at once during a media briefing. As one-on-one media interviews take more time and are less efficient than media briefings in which several reporters receive the same information, it's important to understand why one-on-one interviews are important and how their structure is different.

One-on-one media interviews are important because they provide space for a more in-depth or investigative look at the health emergency. When agreeing to a one-on-one interview, it's important to understand the goal of the interview from the agency's perspective and from the reporter's perspective. A health agency might decide to do a one-on-one interview with a particular reporter or media outlet because the reporter has provided favorable coverage about the health emergency and is likely to provide an in-depth look at how the agency is handling the emergency. This type of interview benefits the agency and the reporter in that the reporter gets more detailed information about the health emergency operations and the health agency can bolster its credibility by providing more nuanced information about how it is working to stop the health threat and protect the community's health.

Most of the time, the media or press office will schedule interviews with reporters and will provide background information on the reporters and their recent published articles or video segments. The press office will typically organize the logistics of these interviews, including their time, location (physical or virtual), topic, and proposed date of publication. Location represents the biggest difference between a media briefing and a one-on-one interview. Media briefings are typically held in a press room or conference room with a podium and space for multiple reporters. One-on-one interviews are typically more intimate and can occur in an office, conference room, on the phone, on a video platform, or outside the agency's building. For in-person television interviews, the reporter will likely be bringing a cameraperson and will ensure the lighting and audio are of high quality. If the interview is being conducted virtually, ensure the background you use is professional or use a virtual filter that carries your agency's logo. For phone or radio interviews, the reporter will again work to ensure the best sound quality is obtained, but it's also key for the spokesperson to find a quiet location with good signal to limit any background noise.

When working one on one with reporters, there are three key tips to keep in mind: engage in on-message dialogue; use self-management techniques; and be mindful of verbal and nonverbal communication.

Due to the intimate setting of one-on-one media interviews, they can feel similar to informal conversations, and it is important for the spokesperson to be mindful of staying on-message. During a media briefing, a spokesperson can easily deliver remarks and then take questions. During a one-on-one interview, there is a back and forth between reporter and spokesperson. This dialogue can move dynamically into various areas depending on the topic, so spokespeople need to be prepared and able to use the block and bridge technique to draw the reporter back to the key messages that the health agency wants to share. Additionally, for one-on-one TV interviews, reporters like to use B-roll and multiple visual images during the interview. As such, be prepared to be asked to move around and respond to the same question a couple different times as the reporter and cameraperson look for the best visuals and to capture a solid answer to their questions. For example, they might want to have a visual image of the agency building in the background, and they might also want B-roll of the spokesperson and the reporter walking down a hallway together. Be prepared for some stops and starts throughout such an interview.

Some spokespeople thrive on media briefings and communicating with a large group of reporters; other spokespeople prefer one-on-one media interviews. Some might find one-on-one interviews stressful. As in media briefings, engage in self-management techniques to ground and center yourself before the interview and monitor internal reactions during the interview. Typically, a press officer will attend one-on-one interviews and can help stop the interview if the reporter's questions become hostile or veer into territory that was not agreed to when scheduling the interview.

Finally, be mindful of nonverbal and verbal communication activities. Regarding nonverbal communication, consider your physical appearance, body posture, body movements, eye contact, and facial expressions. Also consider the location and physical surroundings and what nonverbal messages the physical environment might be communicating. Regarding verbal communication, take note of your tone of voice, rate of speech, and articulation. It is important for the reporter to understand and hear what the spokesperson is saying.

Theory Callout: Agenda Setting Theory

Agenda setting theory looks at the relationship between the media and public opinion. In 1972, McCombs and Shaw studied how public awareness and the information shared by newspapers and broadcasters could shape perceptions of reality during a presidential campaign.[33] Those watching the news learned about particular issues, which influenced how much awareness they had of these issues. This type of relationship provides power to the media, allowing it to make editorial decisions about what information is shared, thus setting the agenda that will be discussed at the societal level.[33] Agenda setting theory explains the power of the media and how media outlets can influence public opinion through how they frame and report the information shared by a health agency. Agenda setting theory is still relevant today, as news media outlets and now social influencers have the power to set multiple agendas about what is being discussed in the news and on social media. It is important for emergency risk communicators to be aware of agenda setting theory because it provides understanding of other perspectives that may differ from the agency's perspective. While a health agency has a particular set of key messages that is wants to disseminate via the media, the media will receive the information, filter it through the media outlet's editorial agenda, reframe the information for the story, and then publish the story. Once the story is published, audience members – from the public to stakeholders to other agencies – will then read the story and will engage in their internal processing about the meaning of the story.

Maine Messaging during the Time of COVID-19: The Leadership Style of Dr. Nirav Shah
Lynn A. Walkiewicz, PhD, MSW

The COVID-19 Pandemic
On December 12, 2019, the first cluster of patients with an atypical disease were identified.[34] The disease didn't seem to respond to known treatments and dramatically affected the respiratory system. This was the beginning of major changes to the world. The strange

disease spread through China, into Thailand, through Japan and the Republic of Korea, and into Europe. On January 20, 2020, the first case was reported in the United States.[34] COVID-19 had come to the United States, although it did not have that name at the time. COVID-19 became the official name of the disease on February 11, 2020. The first official case was announced in Maine on March 12, 2020.[35]

Maine Governor Janet Mills took an assertive stance on tackling COVID-19. She had watched other states handle the pandemic, achieving mixed results regarding the safety of their people. Mills took a hard line, closing businesses and public spaces, mandating mask wearing, and mandating vaccination of health care workers when vaccines became available. Many citizens were upset with these actions, and they challenged her by keeping their businesses open, protesting in person, and other such actions. But Mills held her firm stance, greatly decreasing the number of deaths in Maine.

Governor Mills put Dr. Nirav Shah, head of Maine's CDC branch and Director of Public Health, in charge of the Maine response to COVID-19. Dr. Shah had only come to Maine in 2019 to rebuild a battered Maine CDC branch. He was a great choice as the head of Maine's CDC, but it was an interesting position in that Dr. Shah is obviously "from away." In Maine, if you haven't been born there, you are considered "from away." You could be an eighth-generation Mainer, but if you were born over the state line in New Hampshire you are "from away." People from away are not trusted as easily as natives.

According to the US Census, Maine has a white population of 90.8%.[36,37] According to other sources who slice the information differently, Maine is somewhere between the whitest state in the nation[38] and the fourth whitest.[39] As a state, Maine is behind the times in dealing with equity, be it from a race, gender, sexuality, or economic perspective. There is a large amount of racism and sexism in the state. Neo-Nazi extreme right-wing groups such as the Nationalist Social Club and the Proud Boys are active in Maine, and members of these groups in northern New England come to compounds in Maine for training.[40,41] Maine is 61.3% rural, with two of its 16 counties being 100% rural. It has the highest percentage of rural area in the nation,[36] and 90% of the state is undeveloped land.[42]

So, thinking that a man of obvious Indian descent would be able to reach the Maine population, when he was from away, hadn't been here long, and wasn't white, was quite a gamble on the part of Mills. The gamble paid off, however. Not only did Dr. Shah connect with the community during his presentations, but a Facebook "Friends of Dr. Shah" page was also created, and a local candy company created a Dr. Shah chocolate bar, with 10% of each sale going to a local food pantry.[43,44]

How did a brown-skinned man without a Maine accent gain such popularity? It was through his communication strategy. Shah doubled down on his presence in the public eye once COVID-19 started. He hadn't had much public exposure before then, but he became a daily presence after the onset of COVID-19. Dr. Shah gave a radio interview at 8:30 every weekday morning.[45] He also gave a television interview at noon every weekday.[46] His communication was forthright, honest, and truthful. He told stories, he wove in quotes from rock songs and movies, he integrated pop culture, and he drank Diet Coke on TV. He was empathetic, informative, and consistently available to the public. This case study provides specific examples of his communication and leadership through the lens of the CERC framework.

CERC Principles

CERC has six guiding communication principles[3]:

- Be First
- Be Right
- Be Credible

- Express Empathy
- Promote Action
- Show Respect

These six principles outline the components that should, if at all possible, be included in every public health emergency risk communication. The first three components deal with the information being presented. It's important to Be First to ensure that information is presented rapidly to clients. We have to Be Right – or at least as right as we can be – with the information that can be provided at the time because we want both to instruct the population to follow certain directives and not to be distributing incorrect information. We need people to trust the information we provide to them, which means that the people need to trust us. The only way that we can gain trust over time is through being truthful. When we get additional information or find that the information we have presented has changed, if we have been truthful, we can go back to the people and tell them the new information knowing that they will accept this news. The knowledge we have about a pandemic is fluid and needs to be continually updated. Be Credible, the third CERC principle, goes hand in hand with Be Right. What we express as the best information we have at the time needs to make sense and be logically explicable. If we have been truthful in presenting the data we have at the time, when we report that data have changes, it should be accepted because we have been credible.[3]

The last three CERC principles deal with how we have to treat the people receiving our messages. Express Empathy is incredibly important for making connections with people. It is these initial connections that we will be building on to create the trust that will allow us to Be Credible. Expressing empathy also lets people know that we are thinking about *them* and not just expressing vague ideals. We also want to Promote Action. People will need something to do in order to feel that they are responding, that they are doing something to fend off fear and engaging in actions than will make them safer. We need to tell them what actions are feasible and possible. They can choose whether to follow these actions or not, but providing them with these actions makes it easier to create initial movement toward a desired health behavior. Finally, we need to *Show Respect*. We are not telling people what to do because they are unintelligent or passive; we are providing actions because we respect people enough to know that they can accomplish them. Actions need to be personal and bite-sized; if an action is too large it might cause despair, preventing people from even beginning to engage in the action. But when we respect the *entire* person, regardless of their ability, functional needs, or intellectual status, we are more likely to build long-term relationships with them.[3]

CERC Stages of Messaging

In CERC, messaging follows four stages: precrisis, initial, maintenance, and resolution.[3] Each of the stages in this rhythm should contain the necessary information according to the CERC principles, but each stage is focused on different phases of the event being addressed, and so action messaging for each stage varies. Much of the precrisis stage takes place during what emergency managers call "blue sky" days. Blue sky days are days with no upcoming emergencies, during which we can build relationships, devise strategies, and make plans.

The precrisis stage includes drafting messages to different communities, ensuring that we can reach all communities using a variety of messaging paths, and creating partnerships with people who can help spread our messages. We should do as much preparation as we can and have those materials organized, particularly in terms of prescribed messaging, so that when an emergency arises, we can put out messages quickly by adding information that is specific to that emergency. Prescribed messages and message paths can be established and tested during blue sky times so that we can Be First and Be Credible.[3]

Initial messages are just that – they provide the initial information that we have to present to the public. In order to Be First, we have to have the components of the message and its presentation ready to go regarding the details of the event. We have to be able to calm any fears among the population and provide the necessary action steps for them to complete so that we can help each other as effectively as possible. We also need to promise to come back with updated information. This promise helps to establish credibility with the public, and it also allows us to update or change information regarding the event without losing the public's trust.[3]

Maintenance messages are those that come during the middle of an event. Empathy is needed to keep the populace coming back. Information needs to be updated, and action points need to be expressed and updated. Maintenance messages need to contain updated information in every session, so the populace has a reason to tune in to all of these messages. Whether it is updated statistics, new responses, or new actions for people to take to increase their own safety, we need to provide these details in the maintenance messages so that the populace remains aware of the dangers of the event.[3]

Finally, resolution messages come at the end of an event, thanking the populace for all they have done and informing the people that their assistance is no longer needed. They generally include a review of the event, responses to the event, and outcomes of the event. They may include notices of what went well, what didn't, and what changes will be made to be more effective when facing the next disaster event.[3]

Dr. Nirav Shah and the CERC Principles
Governor Mills put the leadership of the COVID-19 response in the hands of Dr. Nirav Shah. Dr. Shah consistently demonstrated the CERC principles in all of his messaging. His use of these principles generated a stalwart following among Maine people, thereby decreasing the amount of sickness and hospitalizations due to COVID-19 in the state: "The state has one of the lowest death rates and one of the highest vaccination rates."[47] Mills summarized his leadership succinctly in her goodbye statement to Dr. Shah:

> "Day after day, week after week, Dr. Shah spoke calmly and directly to the people of Maine, many of whom were scared and uncertain. He delivered to us the unvarnished truth, as best we knew it, and answered our questions with compassion, empathy, humor, and a clarity that gave us much-needed hope in our darkest of days," Gov. Janet Mills said in a statement last week. "I strongly believe that Maine's nation-leading success in confronting the pandemic is due in large part to Dr. Shah's leadership, and there is no doubt in my mind that he saved the lives of many Maine people. While I am saddened that we are losing Dr. Shah at the Maine CDC, I will be forever grateful for his work to protect and improve the health of Maine people."[47]

CERC Messaging Examples

Initial Messaging
The first COVID-19 case was diagnosed in Maine on March 20, 2020, Dr. Shah gave one of his press conferences on that day. He started with this statement: "I'd like to begin today's briefing by talking a bit about the ways in which some of the measures that we have recommended to everyone have affected people's lives."[46] That initial statement shows several of CERC's principles: Express Empathy, Promote Action, and Show Respect. He is recognizing that CDC instructions are causing changes in people's lives that may not be

welcome or comfortable, but he wants to reinforce that they are necessary actions to decrease exposure to COVID-19. He goes on to acknowledge the challenges faced and that many people have heeded the advice, and he says that masking and social distancing were acts "of good citizenship." After he pulls in the listener, he goes into the statistics – and tells the people what the statistics represent. He even admits that one of the numbers had changed because of a clerical error. Publicly acknowledging errors helps add to credibility.[46]

On December 16, 2020, Dr. Shah started his video update with a listing of lives lost. He offers compassion and sympathy to the families of those lost. He then talks about the demographics of those hospitalized, indicating that the majority of the hospitalized are unvaccinated. He continues to talk about the increase in testing volumes in Maine, and then he turns to discussing vaccines and vaccinations. He indicates that Mainers are vaccinating at a rate similar to 6 months prior and that the level of vaccinations shows that people are getting their boosters as requested. As he is speaking, the numbers of ill and vaccinated, among other statistics are shown near the bottom of the screen, alternating with the Community Vaccination Line phone number. This provides an additional method to connect people to resources. He continues to talk about the Omicron variation that was beginning to be seen at that time. He takes the time to explain the difference between how severe a variant is and how contagious it is; he uses this to discuss how concerning the contagiousness of the Omicron variant is and to update our information regarding COVID-19. He repeats statements that he thinks are very important. He asks questions such as, "So what does all of this mean to you, and what should you do today to be ready for Omicron?"[48] Putting the question so personally connects Shah to the person watching and sets them up for action items. Shah acknowledges, "Sometimes I feel like a thrower of wet blankets," but he goes on to say how these bad times can foster a cooperative spirit in residents.[46]

Maintenance Messaging
On September 30, 2021, Dr. Shah was a guest on WGAN News radio. It had been a couple of months since his last daily morning show during the worst of the pandemic – at this time he was just making occasional visits to the radio station. He and the host joke about how they had thought the pandemic was done and that they are so sorry he is back. This highlights how messaging changes. Dr. Shah and the host had truly expected the pandemic to be over by that time. They were preparing recovery messages. But the Delta variant had surged, numbers of hospitalizations and deaths were rising again, and Dr. Shah went back to writing maintenance messages. He says, "We are one of the most vaccinated states in the country. My hat goes off to Mainers for doing the hard work of getting vaccinated!"[45]

Dr. Shah indicates that the hospitalized are predominately unvaccinated; he states that 75% of the hospitalized are not vaccinated, and 100% of people in intensive care units are unvaccinated. He goes on to talk about how vaccination can prevent the worst of the ravages of the disease. Dr. Shah uses these figures not to scold the unvaccinated but to narrow down on a group of people – the unvaccinated – to encourage them to get vaccinated. His method was to encourage people to get vaccinated not as if they were resistant to vaccination but as if they simply hadn't had time to get vaccinated. Because this gentle encouragement was done without shaming, it shows his empathy. It also promoted action.[45]

On October 26, 2021, Dr. Shah published a series of tweets on the validity of the information he is offering. He takes on what he called the "gadflies," people "who do a little internet research, then play gotcha with the experts."[49] He writes, "Indeed, they prefer the role of a gadfly to spending years on knowledge acquisition. Why not? It's easier and you get to make waves. It's like having the only pin at a balloon party. It's a lot of fun for you, but pretty pesky for everyone else. But it's also low yield."[49] His analogies tie his arguments to individuals, not just a generic group. He goes on to engages a more academic mode: "But with one major difference: the debate that underlies a Kuhn-style paradigm shift is usually driven by a contrarian who *has* mastered the fundamentals of a field, and just sees them through a revolutionary lens."[49] He also speaks to how the attitude of the person influences the facts of a case. In this example, Dr. Shah is gently chastising the gadflies who argue against the veracity of his messages. His stressing of the scientific method undercuts the position of his opponents, making him seem more credible and supporting the truth of the statements that he is making.

Dr. Shah used his Twitter (now X) feed not only to communicate graphs, but also to share personal photos, such as those of his dogs in Halloween costumes.[49] Including these dog images in his Twitter feed made Dr. Shah personable, thereby making him more relatable. He managed to balance his scientific and personable image during COVID-19. He posted details of vaccination sites, CDC statistics, and pictures of his dogs.[49] His last post as Maine Public Health Director referred to all of the messages he had received during COVID-19 and how Mainers took care of each other, and he thanked everyone for what they had done.[49]

Recovery Messaging
Dr. Shah gave his final CDC regularly scheduled briefing on COVID-19 on June 30, 2021. He starts off by providing statistics: 69,033 total cases, 852 deaths, 2,077 hospitalized, 1,529,764 vaccinations given (90% of Mainers fully vaccinated), and 7.3 million pieces of personal protective equipment (PPE) delivered in the state.[50] Then he recounts the history of the pandemic, showing his empathy, starting by noting the changes to daily life and the sorrow and grief over those who had died. He notes that this is a declaration that ends the pandemic, but that COVID-19 continues, even though it will be considered an official pandemic in Maine. He uses this point to prompt the unvaccinated to get vaccinated. He says that COVID-19 vaccinations have fundamentally changed how we interact with the virus. Again, here he is softly chastising those that had not yet been vaccinated. He says that what we need to continue with is what saved Maine: "the spirit of community, understanding that we are all connected, and that none of us are an island."[50] He quotes one of his favorite proverbs: "If you want to walk fast, walk alone; if you want to walk far, walk together."[50]

This was not the first time Mainers heard this message from Dr. Shah, which he had repeated often while building his connections with the public and his credibility. He ends his message by thanking the interpreters, volunteers from across the state who stepped up to help at vaccine clinics and to take groceries to their neighbors, and his wife. He closes by offering heartfelt thanks to the people of Maine, saying that they should all be proud of the way they faced COVID-19, and thanking them for welcoming him and his family into their adopted home state. He is so grateful that "someone new to Maine, a guy from another state, could come to be viewed as someone to tune into."[50]

Dr. Shah posted a final message on YouTube on January 12, 2023.[51] The following quotations are from the YouTube message. He talks about how he wants to spread the great work that Mainers had done across the nation. "Maine walked far because we walked together." His self-deprecating humor is evident when he says that whether "it was in the volume of PPE delivered, the number of vaccines, or the cases of Diet Coke consumed, Maine led the nation." He says that he feels he is "letting us down, running around, and deserting us" by leaving the state. He calls Maine his home, and he says he is following in the footsteps of proud Mainers who answered the call to serve. "Be kind and take care of one another." I believe that being kind and taking care of each other are the ultimate stances that drive the CERC principles, and they also drove the behavior of Dr. Nirav Shah.[51]

Conclusion

Dr. Nirav Shah helped save Maine from the worst of the COVID-19 pandemic. As *Scientific American* says, his briefings "follow three principles: never shy away from the truth, answer questions directly, and acknowledge the statistics and numbers without overlooking the human element. Our national approach, he says, does not adhere to those principles."[52] He constantly utilized the CERC principles in his messaging. He has said, "... in a high-anxiety, low-trust situation like this, you have to empower people to act. Every five or six weeks, I take stock of where we are and come up with a couple of key asks of the people in Maine. For example, this week, I asked them to commit to get a flu shot. It's a concrete call to action, something everyone can do for themselves and their family. And it builds confidence and trust."[52]

All six of the CERC principles can be seen in the quotes given earlier. Be First: Dr. Shah was always the first to pass on news. Be Right: He acknowledged the statistics and numbers. Be Credible: He answered questions directly. Express Empathy: He acknowledged the high-anxiety, low-trust nature of this situation. Promote Action: He committed Mainers to get their flu vaccinations. Show Respect: He empowered people to act.

He did all this without pulling rank, without being a bully, and without scolding people. He did it with kindness, understanding, humor, and truth. Dr. Shah always took questions, always kept his cool, and spoke to the camera as if he were speaking to us individually. His communication skills helped to reduce the impacts of COVID-19 in Maine, which is all the more remarkable for it being a demographically old, rural, lower-education, lower-income populace overall. His consistency and humility should be standards for all people in Public Information Officer positions or for anyone who has to face the media.

End-of-Chapter Reflection Questions

1 Look back at previous chapters for which you've written initial, maintenance, and recovery messages. Choose one of them to read out loud and record yourself delivering your crisis messages. Have your coach or mentor provide feedback.

2 Reflect on a recent media interview you've given. Think about the three strategies for working with the media (block and bridge, etc.). Did you use any of them? If not, how could you have used one during the interview?

3 Take a personal inventory of the tips and techniques discussed in this chapter for self-management during high-stress situations. What are two techniques you could incorporate for your next high-stress situation?

4 Think of a leader you admire. Find a speech or media interview they've recently given. What do you notice about their verbal and nonverbal communication skills and styles? How does this leader vary their tone of voice, rate of speech, and inflection to make key points? What do you notice about their body language?

5 Imagine you are working in a call center. Members of the public are calling with questions regarding an infectious disease outbreak. How can you use the messages you've developed to answer these questions?

6 Review your agency's policies regarding call centers during health emergencies. What gaps need to be addressed? What are the strong points of the current policies and plans?

References

1. Olariu I, Bogdan N. A Conceptual Approach on Press Conference. *Stud Sci Res Econ* 2015;**21**:317.

2. Schuman N. How to Conduct a Successful Virtual Press Conference. *PR News*. 2020. www.prnewsonline.com/virtual-press-conference (Accessed April 2, 2024).

3. CDC. *Crisis and Emergency Risk Communication October 2018*. Atlanta, GA, CDC, 2018.

4. Abu-Akel A, Spitz A, West R. The Effect of Spokesperson Attribution on Public Health Message Sharing during the COVID-19 Pandemic. *PLoS ONE* 2021;**16**(2):e0245100.

5. Filby M. Two years after COVID-19 pandemic began, Dr. Amy Acton reflects on her place in history. *The Columbus Dispatch*. 2022. www.dispatch.com/in-depth/opinion/2022/03/13/amy-acton-ohio-usa-today-women-of-the-year/6844804001/ (Accessed March 1, 2024).

6. The Columbus Dispatch. Governor DeWine, Dr Amy Acton news conference. 2020. www.youtube.com/watch?v=7v4WmwZl_8g (Accessed April 2, 2024).

7. CDC. *Crisis and Emergency Risk Communication October 2002*. Atlanta, GA, CDC, 2002.

8. Lyu SY, Chen RY, Wang SF, Weng YL, Peng EY, Lee MB. Perception of Spokespersons' Performance and Characteristics in Crisis Communication: Experience of the 2003 Severe Acute Respiratory Syndrome Outbreak in Taiwan. *J Formos Med Assoc* 2013;**112**(10):600–607.

9. Demeshko A, Buckley L, Morphett K, Adams J, Meany R, Cullerton K. Characterising Trusted Spokespeople in Noncommunicable Disease Prevention: A Systematic Scoping Review. *Prev Med Rep* 2022;**29**:101934.

10. Buckley L, Morphett K, Rychetnik L, Land M-A, Cullerton K. Spokespeople in Public Health: Important Characteristics from the Perspective of Australian Public Health Professionals. *Health Promot J Austr* 2024;**35**(3):829–34.

11. CNN. Hayward – Life Back. *YouTube*. 2010. www.youtube.com/watch?v=EZraCNZZ7U8 (Accessed April 2, 2024).

12. Fryar B. Oil Spill – BP News Conference Orange Beach Alabama Pt1. *YouTube*. 2010. www.youtube.com/watch?v=RjJ7zId3bM8 (Accessed April 2, 2024).

13. Booker B. Ex-Michigan Gov. Rick Snyder and 8 Others Criminally Charged in Flint Water Crisis. *NPR*. 2021. www.npr.org/2021/01/14/956924155/ex-michigan-gov-rick-snyder-and-8-others-criminally-charged-in-flint-water-crisis (Accessed April 10, 2024).

14. Noar SM, Austin L. (Mis)communicating about COVID-19: Insights from Health and Crisis Communication. *Health Commun* 2020;**35**(14):1735–39.

15. Seeger M. Best Practices in Crisis Communication: An Expert Panel Process. *J Appl Commun Res* 2006;**34**(3):232–44.

16. Plain Language Materials and Resources. *Centers for Disease Control and Prevention*. 2023. www.cdc.gov/healthliteracy/developmaterials/plainlanguage.html (Accessed April 2, 2024).

17. Strategies for controlling your anger: Keeping anger in check. *American Psychological Association.* 2011. www.apa.org/topics/anger/strategies-controlling. (Accessed April 2, 2024).
18. Elliott P. In a Break with Washington's Usual Posture, the CDC Director Makes an Emotional Plea. *Time.* 2021, March 30.
19. Quinn M. CDC director Rochelle Walensky warns of "impending doom" amid COVID-19 spikes. *CBS News.* 2021, March 30.
20. Pettypiece S. CDC director warns of "impending doom" as Covid cases rise. *NBC News.* 2021, March 29.
21. *Press Briefing by White House COVID-19 Response Team and Public Health Officials.* Washington, DC, The White House, 2021.
22. Yuldoshboev S. CDC Director Who Weeped on TV about "Impending Doom" Says Data Suggests "Vaccinated People Do Not Carry the Virus, Don't Get Sick". *Daily Caller.* 2021, March 30.
23. Johnson RRJ, Fraser MR. *A Communications Playbook for Public Officials.* Arlington, VA, ASTHO, 2022.
24. Covello VT. Risk Communication. In: Frumkin H, editor. *Environmental Health: From Local to Global.* New York, Jossey Bass/John Wiley and Sons, Inc., 2005; 988–1009.
25. Gabaldon D. *Outlander.* New York, Bantam Doubleday Dell Publishing Group, 1992.
26. Vleugels C. *Human Communication Coursebook for Speech Class.* Stillwater, OK, Oklahoma State University, n.d.
27. Jerry Seinfeld. *IMDb.* n.d. www.imdb.com/title/tt0697754/characters/nm0000632 (Accessed April 2, 2024).
28. Curtin M. Even Brené Brown Gets Nervous at Public Speaking Engagements. Here Are Her 3 Tricks for Calming Nerves. *Inc.* 2019. www.inc.com/melanie-curtin/even-brene-brown-gets-nervous-at-public-speaking-engagements-here-are-her-3-tricks-for-calming-nerves.html (Accessed April 2, 2024).
29. Prime Minister Jacinda Ardern's Covid-19 news conference – 1 April 2020. *YouTube.* 2020. www.youtube.com/watch?v=E319CIMzI3k (Accessed April 2, 2024).
30. IEEE. *Media Training 101: How to Interact with the Press.* Piscataway, NJ, Institute of Electrical and Electronics Engineers, n.d.
31. CDC. *Crisis and Emergency Risk Communication October 2014.* Atlanta, GA, CDC, 2014.
32. White House COVID-19 Response Team. Media Briefing. *YouTube.* 2021. www.youtube.com/watch?v=LmCHGHrwSVQ (Accessed April 1, 2024).
33. Public Affairs and Agenda Setting: Passive On-Lookers or Active Participants? *University of Oklahoma.* n.d. www.ou.edu/deptcomm/dodjcc/groups/00C3/Literature%20review.html (Accessed April 2, 2024).
34. CDC Museum COVID-19 Timeline. *Centers for Disease Control and Prevention.* 2023. www.cdc.gov/museum/timeline/covid19.html (Accessed April 2, 2024).
35. Response Timeline. *State of Maine.* 2023. www.maine.gov/covid19/timeline (Accessed March 1, 2023).
36. Census: Maine most rural state. *MaineBiz.* 2012. www.mainebiz.biz/article/census-maine-most-rural-state (Accessed March 1, 2023).
37. Maine: 2020 Census. *United States Census Bureau.* 2020. www.census.gov/library/stories/state-by-state/maine-population-change-between-census-decade.html (Accessed March 1, 2023).
38. Singh N. What Are the Whitest States in the US? *International Centre for Education and Training.* 2022. https://icetonline.com/what-are-the-whitest-states-in-the-us/?utm_source=rss&utm_medium=rss&utm_campaign=what-are-the-whitest-states-in-the-us (Accessed March 1, 2023).
39. Whitest States 2023. *World Population Review.* 2023. https://worldpopulation

review.com/state-rankings/whitest-states (Accessed March 1, 2023).

40. Makuch B. Neo-Nazi "Building White Ethnostate Now Working with Local Extremist Group." *Vice News*. 2022. www.vice.com/en/article/maine-neo-nazi-christopher-polhaus-white-ethnostate/ (Accessed March 1, 2023).

41. In 2021, 4 Hate Groups were Tracked in Maine. *Southern Poverty Law Center (SPLC)*. 2021. www.splcenter.org/states/maine (Accessed March 1, 2023).

42. Maine: Forestry in the Pine Tree State. *Northeast–Midwest State Foresters Alliance*. 2023. www.northeasternforests.org/content/maine (Accessed March 1, 2023).

43. Fans of Dr. Nirav Shah [Maine]. *Facebook*. 2023. www.facebook.com/groups/fansofdrshah (Accessed March 1, 2023).

44. Shah Bars. *Wilbur's of Maine Chocolate Confections*. 2023. www.wilburs.com/product/shah-bars-2 (Accessed March 1, 2023).

45. WGAN News Radio. Dr. Nirav Shah. 2021. https://soundcloud.com/newsradio-wgan/dr-nirav-shah-193896607?utm_source=wgan.com&utm_campaign=wtshare&utm_medium=widget&utm_content=https%253A%252F%252Fsoundcloud.com%252Fnewsradio-wgan%252Fdr-nirav-shah-193896607 (Accessed March 1, 2023).

46. News Center Maine. Maine Coronavirus COVID-19 Briefing. 2020. *YouTube*. www.youtube.com/watch?v=Uyj97QNvP60 (Accessed March 1, 2023).

47. Nirav Shah guided Maine through COVID's Uncertainty. *Bangor Daily News*. 2023. www.bangordailynews.com/2023/01/18/opinion/editorials/shah-covid-uncertainty (Accessed March 1, 2023).

48. Maine Public Radio. CDC Briefing December 15. 2021. *YouTube*. www.youtube.com/watch?v=AMtWWVwAbz4 (Accessed March 1, 2023).

49. Shah N. Twitter. *Twitter/X*. 2023. https://twitter.com/nirav_uscdc (Accessed March 1, 2023).

50. Maine Public. Maine CDC Briefing June 30. 2021. *YouTube*. www.youtube.com/watch?v=EC8DYYOZyiM (Accessed March 1, 2023).

51. Shah N. Maine CDC Leadership Announcement. *YouTube*. www.youtube.com/watch?v=PzhMD2c7G8Y2023 (Accessed March 1, 2023).

52. Shell E. How Straight Talk Helped One State Control COVID. *Scientific American*. 2020. www.scientificamerican.com/article/how-straight-talk-helped-one-state-control-covid/ (Accessed March 1, 2023).

Part IV Crisis Leadership

Chapter 12

Crisis Leadership
Staying Steady on Unsteady Ground

Chapter Objectives
- Describe the challenges of public health leadership since the COVID-19 pandemic.
- Identify at least two personal assessments to support self-reflection.
- List at least three factors that lead to burnout.
- Describe the "window of tolerance" and its importance in self-regulation.
- Describe at least six leadership qualities.
- Write your own leadership origin story.
- Recall transformational leadership theory.

Many people in leadership positions – positions with legitimate authority and responsibility to manage people and oversee projects – speak of a desire to be the leader, manager, or supervisor they never had. This chapter explores various qualities that leaders can utilize to provide and receive support when faced with stressors and challenges in both their work and personal lives. The COVID-19 pandemic presented a unique and unprecedented set of stressors for public health leaders: the Centers for Disease Control and Prevention (CDC) decisions overruled by the White House; shortages of personal protective equipment (PPE) for health care workers; the lack of medical countermeasures at the beginning of the outbreak; faulty COVID-19 tests and the lack of a national testing strategy; and the politicization of masks and vaccines later in the outbreak response. Public health leaders faced many kinds of harassment, including death threats at work, doxing (publishing of confidential information to facilitate harassment), protesters at their homes, and kidnapping threats.[1,2,3]

Public health leaders often pursue careers in public health based on mission-driven ideologies such as serving their community or nation by helping people access health services, protecting people from communicable diseases, or furthering research on public health threats. Essentially, these people are looking to serve a greater good, and working on population-level health aligns with their natural inclination to serve. Many public health practitioners were not prepared for the lack of civility in American society that led to such backlash regarding public health policies: "The general decline in civility in political discourse in the US has made ad hominem attacks commonplace and hollowed out traditional ways of grappling with value conflicts."[2]

Many public health practitioners found themselves sidelined and unable to effect any real change due to the politics that overtook the pandemic response. Even at the federal government level, CDC found itself caught in political battles with both Republican and Democratic White House administrations. CDC is an independent agency that conducts research and provides guidance to state governments, physicians, researchers, and government officials.[4] CDC medical professionals are guided by the standards of their profession rather than the political whims of the Capital Beltway.[4] CDC, being based in Atlanta, GA, is generally insulated against political interference based on its geographic distance from Washington, DC. In addition, it only has six political appointees on staff, and most of the work it conducts is carried by its 11,000 staff scientists and medical professionals – not political appointees.[4]

Many people who pointed fingers at the Trump administration for interfering with CDC during the pandemic turned a blind eye when the Biden administration did the same thing.[4] While the Trump administration often downplayed the severity of the COVID-19 pandemic and ignored guidance from CDC officials, the Biden administration shared a similar mindset when it came into office. For example, in May 2021, the White House announced that wearing masks was no longer necessary.[5] This message was regarded as premature by CDC and caught the entire public health system off guard. Neither CDC nor local health departments were provided with sufficient time to properly prepare to operationalize guidance for those still at risk of contracting the virus. Later, in September 2021, the Biden administration again pressured CDC to move faster to provide science-based guidance regarding the need for booster shots.[6] Although the Biden administration wanted to change the political narrative surrounding the pandemic, rushing CDC to make decisions when the evidence was not yet available is another example of political interference.

So how do public health leaders rise above the politics that are now so intertwined with public health? How do public health leaders combat burnout, underfunded budgets, a shrinking workforce, lack of trust from the public, incivility, and political interference? This chapter explores different qualities that leaders can learn and master to help them navigate the inevitable difficulties of their professional lives. These qualities also support leaders when facing stressors such as difficulties and challenges both at work and in one's personal life.

Knowing Thyself

Etched above the entrance to a temple of Apollo at Delphi, Greece, are the words "know thyself." Echoed by Socrates and Plato in the phrase "the unexamined life is not worth living," and further alluded to by Aristotle, who wrote "to know thyself is the beginning of wisdom,"[7] the human drive to understand one's inner workings and how to maximize one's potential in the world are paramount to our human experience. Self-reflection, self-awareness, and understanding one's strengths and weaknesses are necessary for those stepping into leadership roles that will test their steadfastness, commitment, and true inner wisdom.

Modern society faces great challenges, including environmental issues, increasing economic divides in terms of socioeconomic status, the degradation of university education, the speed of technological advancement, potential job losses due to artificial intelligence, increased partisanship and incivility, and a lack of willingness to compromise to find solutions that will serve the whole of humanity.

To address these challenges, leaders need to be fully available without inner conflicts or predetermined agendas to listen to all voices, to see all proposals, and with true discernment to be able to facilitate action that serves the greater whole and not the loudest faction. Knowing thyself represents the ability to know one's personality or ego, what drives it, and what soothes it, and to be able to recognize when one's ego is running the show instead one's most mature and autonomous self.

In his book *Conscious Leadership*, John Mackey, Whole Foods CEO, recounts a time when his ego was running the show, and he engaged in a heated debate with an activist about animal rights.[8] Mackey, a vegetarian but not a vegan, believed Whole Foods had stringent standards regarding animal welfare. After the debate he engaged in self-reflection and was able to see that the activist was correct and there was a misalignment in the company's practices regarding animal welfare. To address this misalignment, Mackey led an initiative to develop a more robust set of animal welfare standards and encouraged agriculture partners to update their animal welfare practices too.[8] By acknowledging that his ego was running the show, Mackey was able to correct course and offer a solution that was more in alignment with the company's values regarding animal welfare.

There are ample examples of Donald J. Trump often acting based on egoistic narcissism during his presidential term.[1,2] A recent study examined the impacts of grandiose and vulnerable narcissism on mask wearing and vaccination during the COVID-19 pandemic.[9] *Grandiose narcissism* is described as having a strong self-focus, being less responsive to criticism, tending to ignore the needs of others, being willing to exploit others for personal gain, and desiring to elevate one's social status regardless of the costs to relationships. *Vulnerable narcissism* is described as having fragile self-esteem, unsure attachment, and emotional instability and being inauthentic. The study revealed that those with grandiose narcissism were less likely to wear a mask and less likely to get a vaccine. In contrast, those with vulnerable narcissism were more likely to wear a mask and get vaccinated as they are more sensitive to judgment and more likely to adhere to social norms. One caveat for grandiose narcissists is as follows:

> However, if those higher in grandiose narcissism do wear a mask, then they are more likely to tell others to wear one as well. This may appear contradictory but makes sense once unpacking the subdimensions of grandiose narcissism: demand for mask-wearing for mask-wearers is a function of authority-seeking and exhibitionism. In this way, narcissism's influence depends on the individual and conditions; telling others to wear a mask fulfills authority-seeking demands, if one is a mask-wearer, and this demand appears to eclipse other narcissistic influences.[9]

Had Trump pivoted his narcissism into the action of wearing a mask with "MAGA" printed on the front, perhaps the outcome of the 2020 presidential election would have been different. His inability to get past his frustration at having to do something he didn't like to do – wear a mask – altered the mask policy in the United States. This example is important to highlight because, as leaders have legitimate authority to make decisions, those decisions can have positive and negative consequences on thousands or millions of people's lives. Being a leader requires the assumption of great responsibility to make decisions that will affect people's lives, meaning leaders will be held accountable for those actions. It behooves leaders to know when they are acting from a place of true inner wisdom or making decisions based upon egoistic maneuvering stemming from unresolved inner conflicts.

Personality Assessment Tools

There are ample tools and tests available to guide leaders in their self-exploration of their personality or ego. This section will highlight four different such personality tests.

Myers–Briggs Type Indicator

The Myers–Briggs Type Indicator is an extremely popular personality assessment. It was developed based on the work of Carl Jung, a psychoanalyst and psychiatrist who created Jungian psychology, also known as analytical theory.[10] It divides the psyche into three parts: personal unconscious, collective unconscious, and ego. In alignment with Plato, Socrates, and Aristotle, Jung deeply explored his own conscious and subconscious mind to truly "know thyself." Inspired by Jung's work, nurse Isabel Myers developed the Myers–Briggs Type Indicator during the World War II to facilitate better working relationships between health care professionals, particularly nurses. Using Jung's theory that fundamental individual differences in mental and emotional functioning were based upon individual preferences, she developed a questionnaire to identify these preferences.[10]

There are four main categories of the Myers–Briggs Type Indicator assessment: energy, perceiving, judging, and orientation.

- *Energy* has to do with one's propensity toward extraversion or introversion. Extraverts gain energy from those around them, engaging their attention and focus on external experiences. In contrast, introverts gain energy in solitude and focus their energy internally on inner thoughts or solo activities.
- *Perceiving* looks at how one processes information through the senses or through intuition. Sensing types prefer to gather information using the five senses of sight, sound, taste, touch, and smell. They want to gather data and make sense of this information before making decisions. In contrast, intuitive types rely upon instincts, identifying the big picture and patterns before gathering concrete facts.
- *Judging* identifies individual preferences regarding decision-making based on thinking or feeling. Thinkers rely on logic and facts, while feelers rely on seeking harmony when resolving an issue.[10]
- *Orientation* applies to one's preferred lifestyle. Judging types prefer an ordered, predictable, and settled lifestyle; in contrast, perceiver types prefer a flexible and unpredictable lifestyle.

DISC Assessments

The DISC behavioral instrument is based on the work of psychologist William Moulton Marston. The DISC instrument classifies behaviors into four personality types: Dominant, Influencer, Steady, and Conscientious. It also provides methods that leaders can use to work with each personality type.[11]

- *Dominant* types are straightforward communicators who make quick decisions and are results-oriented. They are likely to take the initiative on projects and have a lot of energy to devote to projects.
- *Influencer* types are outgoing, persuasive, and charismatic. Influencers excel when the organizational environment supports personal success. Influencers are often good delegators and spread enthusiasm across their team.
- *Steady* types are consistent, dependable, and easygoing. They are often good at carrying out tasks or teaching others how to do work activities or learn new skills. Steady types appreciate established work patterns and routines.
- *Conscientious* types are thorough, attentive perfectionists who can think ahead and prevent problems.[11] They prefer detail-oriented jobs that require an elevated level of

quality and accuracy. They prefer to define their own personal authority and often work alone but can work within a team to carry out a work task.

Gallup Strengths Finder

The Gallup Strengths Finder was created to focus on the strengths that individuals bring to their jobs rather than their individual weaknesses. Gallup research indicates that people who are able to focus on their strengths every day at work "are six times as likely to be engaged in their jobs and more than three times as likely to report having an excellent quality of life in general."[12] The Gallup Strengths Finder identifies 34 themes that represent a common language of strengths (see Table 12.1). To find a person's strengths, purchase the Clifton Strengths online assessment and answer each question quickly with the first thought or idea that comes to mind. The results of the assessment will provide your top five strengths.

Table 12.1 The 34 themes of the Gallup Strengths Finder

achiever	command	deliberative	harmony	learner	self-assurance
activator	communication	developer	ideation	maximizer	significance
adaptability	competition	discipline	includer	positivity	strategic
analytical	connectedness	empathy	individuation	relator	woo
arranger	consistency	focus	input	responsibility	
belief	context	futuristic	intellection	restorative	

The Enneagram

The Enneagram is an ancient wisdom teaching that was infused with modern psychological knowledge by Dr. Claudio Naranjo in the 1970s. The name "Enneagram" comes from the Greek word *ennea* meaning nine, as the teaching focused on nine personality types. "Each of nine types is associated with a particular set of emotional, cognitive and behavioral inclinations or compulsions that together form a basic worldview and *modus operandi*."[13] Since the 1970s, the Enneagram has been studied, researched, and adapted by counselors, psychologist, spiritual seekers, and business consultants to provide a framework for individuals to investigate and explore the deeper ego mechanisms that drive a person's decision-making and lifestyle choices.

The nine personality types are described as follows[14]:

- *Type 1: The Perfectionist* – view the world against a preset ideal of how the world should be.
- *Type 2: The Helper* – often have trouble communicating needs, they tend to over-help others to meet their unspoken needs.
- *Type 3: The Performer* – their worldview is focused on success and getting things done in the world.
- *Type 4: The Artist* – value emotions and authenticity and often focus their attention on their own inner world.
- *Type 5: The Observer* – often introverted, being more focused on intellectual pursuits than social interaction.

- *Type 6: The Devil's Advocate* – worldview is often focused on safety and security, and they often have issues with authority figures; tend to be loyal, but can become paralyzed by indecision.
- *Type 7: The Adventurer* – extroverted, outgoing individuals focused on having fun and adventures.
- *Type 8: The Boss* – worldview is focused on strength and power and they are often more comfortable moving toward conflict in a way to gather clarity about a situation.
- *Type 9: The Mediator* – easygoing individuals who see all sides of a situation; often have a challenging time saying "no" or taking a stance of their own.

As leaders begin to understand their inner ego mechanisms, it is necessary for them to cultivate practices to help identify those mechanisms and return to their true center. The following sections outline those practices that support leaders as they develop inner resilience when faced with difficulties and challenges.

Stressors

Stress is inevitable in modern life. Whether a person faces good stress (e.g., pressure to help achieve a goal or level up a skillset) or bad stress (e.g., work anxiety that leads to constant fear), the ability to allow stress to move through the body without repressing it is key. When bad stress becomes chronic, burnout can occur. Burnout is defined as becoming exhausted due to excessive demands on one's energy, strength, or resources in the workplace.[15] Due to the novel nature of the COVID-19 pandemic and the unforeseen strain it inflicted on an already stretched health care system, burnout was a major consequence of the pandemic.

The 2021 Public Health Workforce Interests and Needs Survey discovered that many were leaving the public health work force, and the pandemic was cited as a cause:

> Nearly one-third of state and local public health employees (32%) said they are considering leaving their organization in the next year – 5% to retire and 27% for another reason. Among those who said they're considering leaving, 39% said the pandemic has made them more likely to leave. Looking out further, 44% said they are considering leaving within the next five years.[16]

One study found that 48% of physicians and 63% of nurses reported burnout.[17] Health care workers identified occupation stressors as fear of exposure or getting sick, job-related anxiety or depression, and work overload. Many of these health care workers intended to reduce their hours or leave their positions because of these stressors.

Additional environmental factors that can contribute to burnout include[18]:

- Increased work hours
- Bureaucratic/administrative work
- Electronic health records (increased screentime)
- Failure to achieve work–life integration
- Increased focus on productivity
- Lack of leadership support
- Lack of meaningful work
- Lack of collegiality at work
- Lack of individual and organizational value alignment
- Lack of flexibility/work control

In addition to environmental factors that contribute to burnout, when an individual faces too much stress without adequate time and space to self-reflect and allow the body to process its reaction to such stress, burnout occurs. Dr. Dan Siegel, a professor of psychiatry, developed a framework called the "window of tolerance." He suggested that when people work within this window of tolerance they can function and thrive in everyday life.[19] However, due to work and life stressors, people tend to move out of the window of tolerance and into either a state of either hyper- or hypo-arousal. When a person is hyper-aroused, they experience anxiety, anger, fight-or-flight reactions, or a sense of being overwhelmed. When a person is hypo-aroused, they feel numb, shut down, withdrawn, frozen, passive, or shameful. The goal is to be able to move from a hyper-aroused or hypo-aroused state back into the window of tolerance where one finds one's optimal functioning state.

To move from these states when faced with daily stressors, a person needs to be able to identify when they are faced with a stressor, to recognize when they've moved out of the window of tolerance, and to engage in practices that return them to the window of tolerance.

Identifying Stressors

When engaging in work that is high stress, such as responding to a novel virus during a global pandemic that has drastically altered one's daily life, it is important to recognize the activities or situations that cause stress. By identifying the stressor and labeling it as a stressor, the mind can become aware of the external condition that is causing such inner struggle or conflict. When a person can identify a stressor, they can develop techniques to cope with the stress.

Recognizing States of Hyper- or Hypo-Arousal

Sometimes individuals are not able to recognize stressors until they are actively experiencing a body sensation such as anger, frustration, or numbness. It is important to be aware of feelings, thoughts, or body sensations that align with hyper-arousal (anger, irritability, frustration) or hypo-arousal (withdrawn, numb, overwhelmed).[19] By identifying these emotions, one can become aware that the mind has become dysregulated and has moved out of the window of tolerance. A person can begin to engage in techniques that will help them to regulate their nervous system and move them back into the window of tolerance.

Practices to Return to the Window of Tolerance

There are many practices and techniques that can help a person regulate their nervous system when they have become dysregulated. These practices include:
- Deep breathing
- Meditation
- Taking a walk
- Yoga
- Visualizations
- Eye movement desensitization and reprocessing (EMDR) paddles
- Lying under a weighted blanket

Deep breathing, meditation, yoga, and mindfulness practices continue to be studied by researchers to understand their impacts on the body and one's overall health and well-being.[20] When leaders take account of their personalities, recognize when they are engaging in activities that could lead to burnout, and take steps to self-regulate their nervous systems for optimal functioning, they can begin to cultivate deeper leadership qualities to support their optimal functioning in the world.

Leadership Qualities

Numerous leadership studies focus on understanding what makes a good leader (i.e., authenticity, conscientiousness, extroversion, agreeableness, openness, steadfastness) and what contributes to being a bad leader (i.e., narcissism, need for achievement, risky behavior).[21,22,23] Leaders have turned to Buddhism, Zen wisdom, or the Yoga Sutras of Patanjali to cultivate mindfulness and self-awareness within their leadership styles.[21,24] Management consultants and business researchers have focused on an individual's psychological traits to understand how they impacts one's leadership style.[22,25] In June 2010, vulnerability and shame researcher Brené Brown gave a talk at TEDxHouston about her research. Her talk is one of the most viewed on TED.com, with more than 5 million hits, and it is available in 38 different languages.[26] Brené Brown has cultivated her own leadership training focusing on how vulnerability and courage are necessary for modern leaders.

The following subsections focus on leadership qualities derived from crisis and emergency risk communication (CERC) research, modern psychological studies, leadership development, and ancient wisdom teachings. Developing these leadership qualities can help public health leaders remain grounded and focused during health emergencies.

Courage

Courage isn't the absence of fear. Courage is the conviction to speak up when it is needed regardless of politics or organizational agendas.[24] Courage is the boldness to move forward and face the reality of a situation. The following quote from Greek historian Thucydides is an example of courage: "The bravest are surely those who have the clearest vision of what is before them, glory and danger alike, and yet notwithstanding, go out to meet it."

Compassionate Empathy

Compassionate empathy involves not only understanding a person's predicament and feeling with them, but also being spontaneously moved to help, if needed.[27] Leaders can cultivate compassionate empathy through words and actions during crisis responses. Authentically communicating compassionate empathy as the Governor of North Dakota did during the COVID-19 response can build trust and demonstrate authenticity (see Chapter 6).

Steadfastness and Consistency

Steadfastness and consistency are qualities that help leaders stay the course even when the situation becomes more challenging or complex over time. Being able to face continued struggles and move forward despite the obstacles represent true steadfastness.[23]

Calm Stillness

Calm stillness flows out of mindfulness – the ability to observe without judgment or reaction and communicate one's understanding of a situation without being impacted by inner conflict.[21] The quality of calm stillness can be demonstrated through a sense of inner groundedness. Imagine a tree rooted into the earth; despite high winds moving its branches around, the tree itself stays grounded, unmoving. Another example of calm stillness can be exemplified through the yoga pose of *tadasana*, or mountain pose. The intention of this yoga pose is to become as immense, solid, and steady as a mountain.

Joy

The feeling of joy and excitement is needed in leaders to celebrate wins and milestone achievements. The quality of joy does not need to be forced or mechanically felt each day, but rather expressed when true joy and excitement are occurring. When leaders celebrate wins with employees, trust deepens among the staff and throughout the organization.

Curiosity

Curiosity is a fuel that sustains kinetic energy and ensures things continue to move forward. Being curious about your employees and about the work they are doing can help to develop relationships and deepen trust throughout the organization.

Humility

Leaders are often in positions of power and authority. The flipside of humility is narcissism – a focus on one's own importance. It is important for leaders to maintain a sense of humility and cultivate a personal understanding that organizational work is ultimately completed by teams of people. The following quote from the Apple founder Steve Jobs is an example of humility: "Great things in business are never done by one person; they're done by a team of people."

Generosity

Generosity comes from an inner contentment and a lack of a desire for wanting more.[25] At its core, generosity is about giving to others with a feeling of true openness and abundance and without need for reciprocation. Generosity doesn't necessarily relate to material goods and resources. Giving people access to you through office hours and mentoring sessions are also acts of generosity.

Integrity

Integrity is a commitment to acting morally and ethically, following a consistent set of behaviors, beliefs, and values.[28] Leaders demonstrate integrity when they "walk the walk and talk the talk." The following quote from civil rights activist Reverand Martin Luther King Jr. is an example of integrity: "On some positions, cowardice asks the question, 'Is it safe?' Expediency asks the question, 'Is it politic?' And vanity comes along and asks the question, 'Is it popular?' But conscience asks the question, 'Is it right?' And there comes a time when one must take a position that is neither safe, nor political, nor popular but he must do it because conscience tells him it is right."

Accountability

Accountability is taking responsibility for one's actions and the consequences of those actions. Instead of dodging a situation, a leader must be willing to do what it takes to ensure the job is completed.[25] If something happens that negatively impacts the situation, be accountable for what happened. Being accountable and taking responsibility can build relationships and develop trust with others.

Discernment

Discernment is the ability to separate similar objects, ideas, thoughts, and activities with precision. It is the ability to clearly delineate between an apple and an orange. Discernment involves using a combination of intellect and intuition to make decisions.[25]

Vulnerability

Brené Brown defines vulnerability as daring to show up and let ourselves being seen.[26] Being vulnerable in modern society is becoming increasingly challenging as the public sphere and media environment become more uncivilized.[29] Leaders showing up as their full selves is needed more than ever.

Self-Awareness and Boundaries

Any leader needs to use self-awareness to establish boundaries in order to ensure a healthy and balanced life. There are only so many hours in a day and there is only so much energy an individual can expend. Being aware of when that energy is depleting and establishing health boundaries to ensure one's ability to recharge are necessary for leaders, especially during long emergency responses. Yoga practitioners who study the Yoga Sutras of Patanjali are familiar with the concept of *svadhyaya*, or the study of the self. By taking time to self-reflect, a person can learn more about their wants, desires, fears, and hopes. As one continues to "know thyself," one is also cultivating more self-awareness. Modeling self-awareness and healthy boundaries empowers your employees to do the same.

Active Listening

Active listening is a critical action of professional discourse, and it requires deliberate practice to develop a mastery of it.[30] There are four parts to active listening:

- Receive the information
- Understand/process
- Evaluate
- Respond (or follow up later)

By actively listening to others and engaging in thoughtful dialogue one can develop trusting relationships. Employees appreciate being seen and heard by their leaders, which fosters a better work environment, especially during high-stress situations such as health emergency responses.

Beginner's Mind

Leaders often arrive in their leadership role because of their vast expertise and professional experience. The quality of beginner's mind comes from Zen Buddhism wisdom teachings and asks students to engage in openness toward whatever activity they are engaging in, regardless of their proficiency or knowledge. Cultivating beginner's mind allows leaders to view their organization through fresh eyes and provides spaces for a free exchange of ideas and possibilities to carry out work activities without relying on rigid and preconceived ideas.

Love and Respect

The qualities of love and respect come from a place of honoring all of humanity. In this regard love is defined as "when we allow our most vulnerable and powerful selves to be deeply seen and known, and when we honor the spiritual connection that grows from offering that with trust, respect, kindness, and affection."[26] This definition is not limited to romantic love but extends to love and respect for each person that may cross our paths either at work or in our personal lives.

Acceptance

Leaders provide guidance, vision, and support within organizations to carry out organization missions, increase profits, or serve a community. Through strategic planning, a specific set of goals and objectives are outlined to achieve milestones; however, as many leaders know, especially those who have experienced and managed a crisis, "the best laid plans of mice and men often go awry." The leadership quality of acceptance is the ability of a leader to accept and allow that things are not and may not go forward as planned. Accepting the situation and facing reality can provide space for new ideas and solutions to emerge.

Mini-Application: Leadership Origin Story

Part of "knowing thyself" is reflecting on who we are and how we appear in the world. Through storytelling and personal narratives, people can share how they came to be who they are today.[31] A study of top-level managers in the United States revealed that leadership origin stories fall into four general categories: being, engaging, performing, and accepting[31,32]:

- *Being* is defined as having personal attributes that inspire.
- *Engaging* is defined as facilitating collective actions.
- *Performing* is defined as carrying out positional duties.
- *Accepting* is defined being recognized by others as having the capacity to serve.

For this practical application, answer the following questions to develop your leadership origin story[31,32]:

1. When and how did you become a leader?
2. What is your definition of leadership?
3. How do you see yourself as a leader?
4. How do you engage in leadership duties in your current position?

Theory Callout: Transformational Leadership Theory

"Transformational leadership identifies and examines leadership behaviors that strengthen employees' awareness of the importance and values of task outcomes by articulating a vision for the future, providing a realistic action plan to reach necessary goals, and giving individualized support to employees."[33,34] Transformation leadership is made up of four dimensions[33,34]:

- *Idealized influence:* Employees align with leaders' values, beliefs, and ethical or moral orientations.
- *Inspirational motivation:* Leaders articulate their vision to inspire and motivate their staff.
- *Intellectual stimulation:* Leaders support curiosity to find innovative solutions and challenge status-quo perspectives.
- *Individual consideration:* Leaders engage with employees personally rather than engaging with an impersonal group of people.

Government agencies are known for their bureaucratic red tape, dysfunctional and inefficient processes, and slow results and outcomes. Leveraging transformational leadership theory within a government agency can empower employees to move beyond the stereotypes of government and engage fully in their work to make a meaningful difference in serving the community through public health activities.

Analyzing Prime Minister of New Zealand Jacinda Ardern's COVID-19 Communication Using the CERC Framework

Kishla Askins, MPH

The human tragedy of COVID-19 has impacted the lives of the global community in a multitude of ways. Many lessons are to be learned from the pandemic that inform future responses. This case study will compare the former Prime Minister (PM) of New Zealand (NZ) Jacinda Ardern's communication during the COVID-19 pandemic to the CDC CERC guiding principles.

Overview of the COVID-19 Pandemic

The coronavirus pandemic originated in Wuhan City, China, as reported by the World Health Organization (WHO) on December 31, 2019, as a pneumonia of unknown cause that infected 44 patients in 4 days. New Zealanders (NZers) first heard about this "mystery virus" on January 6, 2020.[35] By the third week of January, the first cases were being reported in Thailand, Japan, Korea, the United States, France, Canada, and Malaysia. At the same time, China's first known death due to the virus was made public.[36,37] On January 30, 2020, WHO Director General Tedros Adhanom Ghebreyesus declared a Public Health Emergency of International Concern (PHEIC), which alerted countries to take specific measures associated with surveillance and disease reporting.

As the coronavirus expanded its footprint into Africa, Europe, South America, the Middle East, and other parts of Asia, the first case was transmitted to NZ. By this point, WHO named the disease COVID-19, and the virus severe acute respiratory syndrome coronavirus 2 (SARS-CoV-2). Deaths outside of China (e.g., in the United States) were reported, while new threats to cruise ships emerged. Consequently, travel, global supply, the economy, health care networks and facilities, and international events were all impacted because of the pandemic. Although not well publicized, the WHO–China Joint Mission, including Canada, Germany, Japan, Nigeria, Korea, Russia, Singapore, and the United States, traveled to Beijing and Wuhan for an on-the-ground discussion regarding the outbreak.[36,37]

WHO, recognizing worldwide impact and the spread of the coronavirus, declared COVID-19 a pandemic on March 11, 2020. While many countries were experiencing significant increases in COVID-19 cases, NZ remained stable until March 17, 2020. At that point, NZ's cases jumped from 8 to 20, with no recorded deaths. In comparison, Italy had 3,500 cases with almost 350 deaths, China reported 72,000 cases with 1,800 deaths, the United States had 6,300 cases with 1,700 deaths, and next door in Australia there were 455 cases and 5 deaths.[38] In April 2020, COVID-19 had a global reach of 2.5 million cases and had resulted in almost 170,000 deaths.[38] NZ focused on flattening its COVID-19 curve.

Background

NZ was led by PM Jacinda Ardern under the crown of England's Queen Elizabeth. In 2017, at the age of 37, Ardern was the world's youngest female elected head of government, and she was only the second world leader to give birth while in office. Despite these impressive credentials, this young world leader was no stranger to crisis. In fact, she had been recognized for her consistent management of three significant tragedies that took place in her first term. These events included: a terrorist attack on the Christchurch Mosque, killing 50 people; the Whakaari/White Island volcanic eruption, resulting in 21 dead and 26 severely injured; and the COVID-19 pandemic. From a communications standpoint, she was well prepared, as she earned a Bachelor of Communication Studies in politics and public relations from the University of Waikato; this might have informed her expert messaging and use of the CERC principles during these crises.[39] The PM was staffed with a Ministry of Health and National Emergency Management Agency to handle crises such as COVID-19, natural disasters, and interruptions of daily essential needs (e.g., water, power, and food).[40]

Before a discussion on PM Ardern's crisis communication can take place, it is important to understand potential elements that influence the way a communicator crafts their messages. NZ is a significantly smaller country than the United States, with a population of 4.8 million people (about twice the population of Mississippi) that is growing by 1% each year. Sitting southeast of Australia, in the Pacific Ocean, NZ is approximately 103,000 square miles in area, with a population density of 46 people per square mile. It has two large cities, in which almost 40% of the population resides. The population is composed predominantly of European descent; however, about 15% are Māori (aborigine people of NZ) and 12% are of Asian ethnicity. The religious status of NZ is around 50% Christian, while the other 50% either does not identify, is unstated, or includes Hindu, Buddhist, or Islamic. Most significant is NZ's geographic location and trade of imports and exports; China is NZ's top trade partner, at almost 30% of its exports.[41]

CERC Principles, Phases, and Analysis

Barbara Reynolds says, "The right message at the right time from the right person can saves lives."[42] PM Ardern is a credible spokesperson who led with empathy and respect and expended her political will to incorporate decisive action when necessary. It is difficult to talk about communication without considering her additional role as the leader of NZ. Although leadership is not a specific part of the CERC principles, it has a clear relationship with trust, respect, and success in managing a crisis. Paraphrasing Winston Churchill, "cometh the hour, cometh the man" is meant to imply that the "right leaders will come to the fore during times of crisis."[43] PM Ardern's leadership could inspire a different rhetoric: "cometh the crisis, cometh the woman." She skillfully influenced "what we say, when we say it, and how we say it."[42]

The six principles of CERC – Be First, Be Right, Be Credible, Express Empathy, Promote Action, and Show Respect – are guideposts for managing messaging during a crisis.

Because PM Ardern had already been confronted with significant crises, she was primed to incorporate these key principles at the appropriate phases of the CERC rhythm. These phases provide the framework for engaging with the community, empowering decision-making, and evaluating the situation. NZ has moved through the preparation, initial, and some parts of the maintenance phases of the CERC rhythm; however, lessons from other countries reveal that this progression could include periods of regression as well, requiring a communication strategy that addresses movement back and forth within the phases from initial to resolution.[42]

Be First
The COVID-19 pandemic was well on its way to impacting the entire world when the first cases were reported in NZ. Unlike an isolated crisis that involves a start and stop timeline, a localized geography, and a clear retrospective picture of the incident, being first in this pandemic is difficult to ascertain when much of the world was already impacted by the time NZ and the PM were confronted with it. The expectation of the Be First principle is that time is the enemy. This concept of Be First must also balance the importance of time-sensitive information with accuracy. The dissemination of information to the public should be from the most credible source (e.g., public health department or appropriate organization) known to stakeholders and their constituencies.[42]

NZ initiated communication on January 24, 2020, via a news release by the Ministry of Health, the expected source for a public health emergency. The message conveyed elements of the precrisis phase: public understanding, public preparation, risk of imminent threat, and incorporation of expertise.[44] It communicated a commitment to deliver information promptly and accurately as to present information as it became available. It reassured the public that there was an established expert advisory group in place, and it prepared health professionals for their first cases of COVID-19. Additionally, the message confirmed that NZ had a plan that was specific for pandemics, and that NZ was currently at the "readiness stage." This release signaled the importance of the issue while presenting a calming message that the government was well positioned in its current state.[45] It also answered the expected risk questions: When do I seek medical treatment? What can I do to prevent this? What should I expect in terms of symptoms? Do I have to take special precautions regarding contact? And what are the special travel restrictions?[42] The initial message released to the citizens of NZ was as follows:

> This novel coronavirus causes pneumonia. Symptoms are similar to the regular flu and include coughs, fever and breathing difficulties. People who have died from the virus are understood to have been adults already in poor health. All travelers to NZ who become sick within a month of their arrival are encouraged to seek medical advice and contact Healthline or a doctor and share their travel history. It is important to mention recent travel from Wuhan and any known contact with someone with severe acute respiratory illness who has been in Wuhan.
>
> People can take steps to reduce their risk of infection. This includes regularly washing hands, covering your mouth & nose when you sneeze, staying home if you are sick and avoiding close contact with anyone with cold or flu-like symptoms.[45]

Be Credible
Normally, a spokesperson must establish credibility with the media and/or public; however, PM Ardern was a proven and credible spokesperson in crises after her successful management of the Christchurch terrorist act in early 2019. She received global recognition for her cultural sensitivity, empathy, decisive action on gun control, and respect of all

residents of NZ. She did not need to establish credibility, only maintain her reputation by managing this crisis just as she had handled the others – with empathy and competency. As the pandemic progressed, Ardern took the helm of the daily press conferences from the Minister of Health, signaling her expanded engagement. She did this in concert with experts, maintaining their importance and collegial communication. By taking the lead spokesperson position, she provided the "it" to "we" human connection by reintroducing a familiar and established face leading the efforts of the response. She encompassed the key points of "what makes a good spokesperson" with her competence, communication, empathy, honesty, and deference to expertise while others around the world were fumbling.[46] As an example of her honesty during the crisis, she prepared NZ for more restrictions of their movements with the following address:

> The worst-case scenario is simply intolerable. It would represent the greatest loss of New Zealanders' lives in our history, and I will not take that chance. I am not willing to put the lives of our citizens in danger. The government will do all it can to protect you. Now I'm asking you to do everything you can to protect all of us. Kiwis – go home. We currently have 102 cases, but so did Italy once, now the virus has overwhelmed their health system, and hundreds of people are dying every day.[47]

In an article entitled "Arise Saint Jacinda, a Leader for Our Troubled Times," it was argued that Ardern's mastery of minutiae and frank admission of the problems NZ was facing added to her credibility as a communicator and leader. While responding to the COVID-19 pandemic, she recognized the complexity of delivering education equipment (e.g., laptops) to children for homeschooling as delays plagued her government, remarking, "I know this is a complex project that is being undertaken at a pace so we know it will take time to get it right." In the interim, she set up dedicated educational TV channels as "not the solution but an offering of [her] recognition that there is a problem."[48]

Spokesperson

Part of being an effective spokesperson is understanding one's audience while transitioning through the phases of CERC. This understanding helps inform the careful crafting of communication products so that they will be received and understood. Factors such as accessibility, cultural considerations, and age influence communicating with NZers: "Effective emergency communication requires an understanding of target audiences with differing needs, perceptions and characteristics."[42] Appreciating the difficulties children may be experiencing during the pandemic, PM Ardern held a special press conference for children. Her ability to leverage something so personal as being a parent and understanding of the unique needs of children speak to her level of skill gained through personal experience and professional training. Although a communication major herself, she convened this press conference with a communication specialist for children, demonstrating humility and deference to expertise. The following message from March 18, 2020, won the hearts of parents and children alike:

> Kids asked a lot of questions most of the time, and right now they understandably have plenty about Covid-19. They asked questions about the virus, how they are transmitted, how to keep their grandparents safe, and how soap works. Children seem to be less severely impacted by the virus than older people, with their symptoms more mild and of shorter duration. We want to try to explain what is happening in a way that is easy [for children] to understand. We try to avoid worrying them and remind them that you are being very safe to protect them and other New Zealanders.[49]

Another remarkable example of her special attention to reaching out to children during the crisis was her ability to recognize the importance of Easter and how COVID-19 might impact this celebration. In doing so, she managed to shift the focus from a potentially negative outcome to a positive alternative for celebrating Easter in the following message:

> You'll be pleased to know that we do consider both the tooth fairy and the Easter Bunny to be essential workers. So, I say to the children of NZ, if the Easter Bunny doesn't make it to your household, then we have to understand that it's a bit difficult at the moment for the bunny to perhaps get everywhere. Maybe you draw an Easter egg and pop it into your front window and help children in your neighborhood with their own Easter egg hunt, because the Easter Bunny might not get everywhere this year.[50]

Express Empathy

Reynolds and Quinn stated that an open and empathetic style of communication most effectively engenders public trust, uniting a population.[51] As noted in the CERC Manual, it is important to consistently convey empathy in the initial phase of an emergency response. Consistent with her genuine and honest communication style, Ardern stated:

> For those of you who are parents or caregivers, you will have questions about schools and education facilities. At Alert Level Two, schools will be closed if there is a case that affects a school, as we have been doing to date. Sending children home at this stage though, doesn't necessarily reduce transmission in the community, but I can assure you we are constantly monitoring these settings to keep children safe. As a mum, I can assure you that is my key consideration.

> Till then, I know this current situation is causing huge disruption and uncertainty. And right now, I cannot tell you when that will end. This alert system is designed to help us through that – so please do stay tuned as we share daily updates – especially as alert levels can move from one level to the next in a short space of time, as we have seen elsewhere in the world.[52]

Promote Action

Ardern's ability to promote action was as consistent as her empathy. Just as she instituted gun control measures swiftly after the Christchurch terrorist act, she continued this decisive leadership in her response to COVID-19. On March 21, 2020, PM Ardern addressed NZers in a rare unscheduled press conference to announce a national lockdown and alert system to provide clear direction for NZ's next steps in its fight against COVID-19. Her four-tiered alert system was designed to impact the entire country or individual towns as needed and ranged from Alert Level One to Alert Level Four. This COVID-19 response system established a common language for NZers to understand what moving from one alert level to another meant and the actions they had to take to contain and stop the transmission of the coronavirus. Promoting action was certainly one element of her communication, but sprinkled throughout her messages were words of empathy, relatability, respect, honesty, and unity.

Incorporating a clear understanding of the psychology of crisis should inform communication. Ardern empowered NZers to take action that would reduce the threat of COVID-19. She did this by acknowledging the anxiety and uncertainty that are byproducts of crises and are best solved by providing stakeholders with actionable items to help relieve such feelings of hopelessness. As NZ moved through the initial challenges of the pandemic and embarked on the maintenance phase of the CERC rhythm, she appropriately engaged with NZers' feelings of fear, helplessness, and uncertainty.[53] Presenting a steadfast and calm demeanor, she would communicate hard truths but also provide proactive steps that people could take to protect their health in an effort to reduce the public's anxiety over the unfolding pandemic. Consistent with her unique style, Ardern delivered a sobering and calming outlook for NZers while giving them clear and concise direction in the following message:

> I'm speaking directly to all New Zealanders today to give you as much certainty and clarity as we can as we fight COVID-19. Over the past few weeks, the world has changed. And it has changed very quickly. In February it would have seemed unimaginable to close NZ's borders to the world, and now it has been an obvious step as we fight COVID-19. This is because we are experiencing an unprecedented event – a global pandemic that is now in NZ, we have moved to fight by going hard, and going early. That's why we have to focus on one simple goal – to slow down COVID-19.
>
> And finally, we are asking that you limit your movement around the country. This will help us track and contain any spread of COVID-19. That means cutting non-essential domestic travel. Every unnecessary movement gives COVID-19 a chance to spread.
>
> For now, I ask that NZ does what we do so well. We are a country that is creative, practical, and community minded. We may not have experienced anything like this in our lifetimes, but we know how to rally, and we know how to look after one another, and right now what could be more important than that? So, thank you for all that you are about to do. Please be strong, be kind, and unite against COVID-19.[52,54]

On April 9, PM Ardern addressed the nation again, halfway through the national lockdown and implementation of the alert system. Understanding the difficulties endured thus far, she called upon NZers for additional action and patience. A particularly good example of giving people more "things to do," she did this with full transparency by highlighting the sacrifices of the many and shortcomings of the few. While creating an umbrella of sacrifice and action by NZers, she empowered them to do more for the sake of their country and fellow NZers. A call for sustained action is sometimes difficult, but Ardern framed this message with empathy, stern leadership, and inspiration:

> We are turning a corner, and your commitment means our plan is working. But to succeed, we need it to keep working. Success does not mean we change course. Removing restrictions now would allow the virus to spread rapidly once again and we would be back to the starting line within two weeks. While most people are doing the right thing, some are not. We cannot let the selfish actions of a few set us back. And we won't. Especially after all that everyone has sacrificed to get us here. I have read messages from those who have lost loved ones they couldn't come together to grieve for, brand new parents whose most joyful time has been made so difficult because of separation. Help us get ready as a nation for the marathon we must all run together. I know we can do this. And I know that, because we are already. So, as we head into Easter I say thank you to you and your bubble. You have stayed calm, you've been strong, you've saved lives, and now we need to keep going.[55]

Show Respect
COVID-19 illustrated the variance in the pandemic's timeline of impact; NZ's initial phase was not the same as China's or the United States'. While the rhetoric of other world leaders destroyed relationships, shifted the blame, or put Chinese citizens at risk, PM Ardern took a different course of action. Out of respect for the Chinese, she recognized the loss that

China has suffered due to COVID-19 during a February Chinese New Year celebration in NZ. While in the company of the Chinese Ambassador, diplomatic corps, and parliamentary and numerous other Chinese organizations, she guided global society toward unity and kindness with the following message:

> I want to start by acknowledging the backdrop of the Coronavirus outbreak on these New Year celebrations. I especially wish to pay my respects to those who have died from the virus, those who are sick, and their families and loved ones. The strength of the bilateral relationship means that while there has been much that has been affected in recent week, there is also a sound footing for us to restore, normalize and indeed advance our relationship once the current outbreak is over.[56]

Leadership

There are many articles focused on PM Ardern's leadership during crises. She received a great deal of support not only from her people but also from global leaders and citizens. She was as effective on gun control, climate change, and child poverty as she was in her messaging and responses during the COVID-19 crisis. Some might argue that leadership is not an essential part of communication. However, it can also be argued that implementing the appropriate tone, temperament, respect, and empathy starts with leadership. In the book *You're It: Crisis, Change, and How to Lead When It Matters Most*, Marcus et al. discuss meta-leadership during crises. Meta-leaders "wield influence well beyond their formal authority," and people will follow them and their messages.[57]

The CERC traits interwoven throughout Ardern's leadership provided individuals with purpose of action, engaging them in unity and in the fight against the virus instead of allowing fear and denial. She framed NZ's response to the coronavirus pandemic in the "Unite Against COVID-19" campaign. This campaign message was regularly displayed as a backdrop during press conferences and on Facebook, Twitter, Instagram, LinkedIn, and the NZ government website. Unity as a consistent and successful theme used during response efforts to the emergency reminded NZers of their strength and resilience. Ardern expressed that "all New Zealanders are impacted by crises and together, they will be successful for all Kiwis."[58]

In alliance with NZers, and recognizing the economic struggles they were facing due to COVID-19, Ardern announced that the collective government (including herself) was taking a pay cut for the next 6 months. Again, this was an act to illustrate her understanding of her people and their needs, as well as being a potential economic forecast for the next 6 months. This speech is just one example of Ardern knowing what to say and when to say it. The empathy, tone, and action expressed demonstrated her connection to the problem and to her people. This show of solidarity was unifying as these economic challenges highlighted the income inequality issue that was further exacerbated by the pandemic. On April 15, 2020, Ardern made the following significant announcement:

> Today I can confirm that myself, government ministers and public service chief executives will take a 20% pay cut for the next six months as we acknowledge New Zealanders who are reliant on wage subsidies, taking pay cuts and losing their jobs as a result of COVID-19's global pandemic. We feel acutely the struggle that many New Zealanders are facing. And so, too, do the people that I work with on a daily basis. It is about leadership and showing solidarity in NZ's time of need. If there were ever a time to close the gap between groups of people across NZ in different positions, it is now. I am responsible for the Executive branch. Myself and Ministers is where we can take action and that is why we have.[59]

The *Atlantic* article entitled "New Zealand's Prime Minister May Be the Most Effective Leader on the Planet" addressed Ardern's leadership style, focusing on her empathy and how it resonated with her people. PM Ardern said in many speeches, "Know us by our deeds." She has stated that "it is important for NZ that the only kind of leadership that we can offer globally is moral. When you have individuals, who can harness the moral voice with authenticity and sincerity, that becomes an immensely powerful moment."[54]

In offering moral leadership, Ardern recognized the need for change in this brave new world as it embarked on life after COVID-19. NZ may not have had a lot to offer regarding national security, pandemic research, or solutions for future outbreaks, but Ardern offered a powerfully unifying crisis leadership style that was successful while being genuinely focused on people and the good in the world. This style of leadership could rewrite the crisis communication playbook, or at least reinforce the benefits of using the CERC principles to influence international leadership when it comes to crises. Ardern provided lessons on empathetic leadership, respectful rhetoric, embracing multiculturality, global unity, and decisive action for people instead of for politics.

"When we think of wartime presidents, we think of Franklin D. Roosevelt or Abraham Lincoln."[60] This was not a time of war as these figures would have known it, but it was a global pandemic of a scale not seen in the modern era. Global leadership and crisis communication during a pandemic will be informed and molded by those who changed the course of history. Ardern is not Roosevelt or Lincoln, but she was a worthy PM of NZ: "Cometh the crisis, cometh PM Ardern."

End-of-Chapter Reflection Questions

1 Reflect on your personal self-management and self-regulation activities. On a scale of 1–10 (10 being the highest), how would you rate yourself? What could be improved? What would be a stretch goal to improve your self-management and self-regulation activities?

2 Burnout and mental health issues have gained more attention since the COVID-19 pandemic. Reflect on what you know about burnout. Have you personally experienced burnout? Have your coworkers? How did you or others address burnout? What resources did (or does) your employer offer to address burnout?

3 Imagine you wanted to implement a new strategic initiative with your health agency. How could you use transformational leadership theory to share your vision and empower your employees regarding this new initiative?

4 Challenge yourself to a 21-day reset to support your nervous system. Consider trying meditation, yoga, or breathing exercises for 21 days. Journal about your experience. How did this 21-day reset impact your leadership style?

5 Take a personal inventory of yourself and the leadership qualities listed in this chapter. How many do you exhibit? What qualities do you want to cultivate?

6 Reflect upon leaders you admire. Why do you admire them? What qualities do they possess? How do they inspire you to be a better leader?

References

1. Abutaleb Y, Paletta D. *Nightmare Scenario: Inside the Trump Administration's Response to the Pandemic that Changed History*. New York, HarperCollins Publisher, 2021.
2. Mello MM, Greene JA, Sharfstein JM. Attacks on Public Health Officials During COVID-19. *JAMA* 2020;**324**(8):741–42.
3. Cappelletti J. Whitmer kidnapping plot co-leader sentenced to 19 years in prison. *PBS*. 2022. www.pbs.org/newshour/politics/whitmer-kidnapping-plot-co-leader-sentenced-to-19-years-in-prison (Accessed May 23, 2024).
4. Schiff E, Mallinson DJ. Trumping the Centers for Disease Control: A Case Comparison of the CDC's Response to COVID-19, H1N1, and Ebola. *Adm Soc* 2023;**55**(1):158–83.
5. Linskey A, Abutaleb Y, Sun LH, Pager T. Biden vowed to "follow the science" but left many out with sudden mask guidance. *The Washington Post*. 2021. www.washingtonpost.com/politics/biden-masks-cdc/2021/05/20/6467e66e-b974-11eb-a5fe-bb49dc89a248_story.html (Accessed May 23, 2024).
6. Banco E, Owermohle S, Cancryn A. Tensions mount between CDC and Biden health team over boosters. *Politico*. 2021. www.politico.com/news/2021/09/13/cdc-biden-health-team-vaccine-boosters-511529 (Accessed May 23, 2024).
7. LeDoux J, Brown R, Pine D, Hofmann S. Know Thyself: Well-Being and Subjective Experience. *Cerebrum* 2018;**2018**:cer-01-18.
8. Mackey J, McIntosh S, Phipps C. *Conscious Leadership: Elevating Humanity through Business*. New York, Penguin, 2020.
9. Hatemi PK, Fazekas Z. The Role of Grandiose and Vulnerable Narcissism on Mask Wearing and Vaccination during the COVID-19 Pandemic. *Curr Psychol* 2022;**42**:19185–95.
10. Woods RA, Hill PB. Myers–Briggs Type Indicator. *StatPearls*. 2022. https://pubmed.ncbi.nlm.nih.gov/32119483/ (Accessed May 23, 2024).
11. Slowikowski MK. Using the DISC Behavioral Instrument to Guide Leadership and Communication. *AORN J* 2005;**82**(5):835–43.
12. Rath T. *Strengths Finder 2.0*. New York, Gallup Press, 2007.
13. Seekers after truth: A program for growth through the exploration of the personality. *The Naranjo Institute*. 2011. www.naranjoinstitute.org.uk/enneagram.html (Accessed May 13, 2024).
14. Chesnut B. Beatrice Chestnut. n.d. www.beatricechestnut.com (Accessed May 13, 2024).
15. Freudenberger HJ. Staff Burn-Out. *J Social Issues* 1974;**30**(1):159–65.
16. de Beaumont. Findings 2021. 2021. https://debeaumont.org/phwins/2021-findings (Accessed May 13, 2024).
17. Sinsky CA, Brown RL, Stillman MJ, Linzer M. COVID-Related Stress and Work Intentions in a Sample of US Health Care Workers. *Mayo Clin Proc Innov Qual Outcomes* 2021;**5**(6):1165–73.
18. Singh R, Volner KDM. Provider Burnout. *StatPearls*. 2023. https://pubmed.ncbi.nlm.nih.gov/30855914/ (Accessed May 24, 2024).
19. Siegel DJ. *The Developing Mind: How Relationships and the Brain Interact to Shape Who We Are*, 2nd edition. New York, Guilford Publications, 2012.
20. NIH. Meditation and Mindfulness: What You Need to Know. 2024. www.nccih.nih.gov/health/meditation-and-mindfulness-what-you-need-to-know (Accessed May 15, 2024).
21. Doornich JB, Lynch HM. The Mindful Leader: A Review of Leadership Qualities Derived from Mindfulness Meditation. *Front Psychol* 2024;**15**:1322507.
22. Judge TA, Piccolo RF, Kosalka T. The Bright and Dark Sides of Leader Traits: A Review and Theoretical Extension of the Leader Trait Paradigm. *The Leadership Quarterly* 2009;**20**(6):855–75.

23. Wilson S, Newstead T. The Virtues of Effective Crisis Leadership: What Managers Can Learn from How Women Heads of State Led in the First Wave of COVID-19. *Organ Dyn* 2022;**51**(2):100910.
24. Compassion Institute. Compassion Institute homepage. 2024. www.compassioninstitute.com (Accessed May 15, 2024).
25. Maxwell JC. *The 21 Indispensable Qualities of a Leader.* Nashville, TN, Thomas Nelson, Inc., 1999.
26. Brown B. *Daring Greatly.* New York, Avery, 2012.
27. Goleman D. *Emotional Intelligence.* New York, Bantam Book, 1995.
28. Karthikeyan C. A Meta Analytical Study on Leadership Integrity: A Leadership Ethics Perspective. *Int J Manage IT Eng* 2017;**7**(4):240–63.
29. Bybee KJ. *How Civility Works.* Stanford, CA, Stanford University Press, 2016.
30. Tennant K, Long A, Toney-Butler TJ. Active Listening. *StatPearls.* 2023. https://pubmed.ncbi.nlm.nih.gov/28723044/ (Accessed May 18, 2024).
31. Zheng W, Meister A, Caza BB. The Stories That Make Us: Leaders' Origin Stories and Temporal Identity Work. *Human Relations* 2021;**74**(8):1178–210.
32. Meister A, Zheng W, Barker CB. What's your leadership origin story. *Harvard Business Review.* 2020. https://hbr.org/2020/08/whats-your-leadership-origin-story (Accessed May 18, 2024).
33. Lindert L, Zeike S, Choi KA, Pfaff H. Transformational Leadership and Employees' Psychological Wellbeing: A Longitudinal Study. *Int J Environ Res Public Health* 2022;**20**(1):676.
34. Lai F-Y, Tang H-C, Lu S-C, Lee Y-C, Lin C-C. Transformational Leadership and Job Performance: The Mediating Role of Work Engagement. *Sage Open* 2020;**10**(1):2158244019899085.
35. Kronast H, Sadler R. Coronavirus: Timeline of New Zealand's response to COVID-19. *Newshub.* 2020. www.newshub.co.nz/home/new-zealand/2020/04/coronavirus-timeline-of-new-zealands-response-to-covid-19.html (Accessed April 1, 2020).
36. World Health Organization. Situation report – 1. 2020. www.who.int/docs/default-source/coronaviruse/situation-reports/20200121-sitrep-1-2019-ncov.pdf?sfvrsn=20a99c10_4 (Accessed April 1, 2020).
37. World Health Organization. WHO timeline: COVID-19. 2020. www.who.int/news-room/detail/08-04-2020-who-timeline—covid-19 (Accessed April 1, 2020).
38. World Meters. COVID-19 coronavirus pandemic. 2020. www.worldometers.info/coronavirus (Accessed April 1, 2020).
39. Wikipedia. Jacinda Ardern. 2020. https://en.wikipedia.org/wiki/Jacinda_Ardern (Accessed April 1, 2020).
40. National Emergency Management Agency. National Crisis Management Center. 2020. www.civildefence.govt.nz/about/national-crisis-management-centre (Accessed April 1, 2020).
41. World Population Review. New Zealand population 2020. 2020. https://worldpopulationreview.com/countries/new-zealand-population (Accessed April 1, 2020).
42. Centers for Disease Control and Prevention. CERC introduction. 2018. https://stacks.cdc.gov/view/cdc/120677 (Accessed April 1, 2020).
43. Robson D. What makes a good leader during a crisis? *BBC.* 2020. www.bbc.com/worklife/article/20200326-covid-19-what-makes-a-good-leader-during-a-crisis (Accessed April 1, 2020).
44. Reynolds B, Seeger M. Crisis and Emergency Risk Communication as an Integrative Model. *J Health Commun* 2005;**10**(1):43–53.
45. Ministry of Health. Novel coronavirus update – 24th January 2020. 2020. www.health.govt.nz/news-media/news-items/novel-coronavirus-update-24th-january-2020 (Accessed April 1, 2020).

46. Centers for Disease Control and Prevention. CERC spokesperson. 2014. https://emergency.cdc.gov/cerc/ppt/CERC_Spokesperson.pdf (Accessed April 1, 2020).

47. Ainge-Roy E. Kiwis go home: New Zealand to go into month-long lockdown to fight coronavirus. *The Guardian*. 2020. www.theguardian.com/world/2020/mar/23/kiwis-go-home-new-zealand-to-go-into-month-long-lockdown-to-fight-coronavirus (Accessed April 1, 2020).

48. Clark P. Arise Saint Jacinda, a leader for our troubled times. *Financial Times*. 2020. www.ft.com/content/d26564b4-80ba-11ea-82f6-150830b3b99a (Accessed April 1, 2020).

49. Roy E. Jacinda Ardern holds special coronavirus press conference for children. *The Guardian*. 2020. www.theguardian.com/world/2020/mar/19/jacinda-ardern-holds-special-coronavirus-press-conference-for-children (Accessed April 1, 2020).

50. Chappell B. The Easter Bunny is an essential worker. *National Public Radio*. 2020. www.npr.org/sections/coronavirus-live-updates/2020/04/07/828839205/the-easter-bunny-is-an-essential-worker-new-zealands-ardern-says (Accessed April 1, 2020).

51. Reynolds B, Quinn S. Effective Communication during an Influenza Pandemic. The Value of Using a Crisis and Emergency Risk Communication Framework. *Health Promot Pract* 2008;**9**(4):13S–17S.

52. Ardern J. COVID-19 update. *Beehive.govt.nz*. 2020. www.beehive.govt.nz/speech/pm-address-covid-19-update (Accessed April 1, 2020).

53. Centers for Disease Control and Prevention. CERC psychology of a crisis. 2019. https://emergency.cdc.gov/cerc/ppt/CERC_Psychology_of_a_Crisis.pdf (Accessed April 1, 2020).

54. Friedman U. New Zealand's prime minister may be the most effective leader on the planet. *The Atlantic*. 2020. www.theatlantic.com/politics/archive/2020/04/jacinda-ardern-new-zealand-leadership-coronavirus/610237 (Accessed April 1, 2020).

55. Ardern J. Prime Minister's remarks halfway through alert level 4 lockdown. Beehive.gov.nz. 2020. www.beehive.govt.nz/speech/prime-minister's-remarks-halfway-through-alert-level-4-lockdown (Accessed April 1, 2020).

56. Ardern J. PM speech at parliamentary new year celebration 2020. Beehive.govt.nz. 2020. www.beehive.govt.nz/speech/pm-speech-parliamentary-chinese-new-year-celebration-2020 (Accessed April 1, 2020).

57. Marcus L, McNulty E, Henderson J, Dorn B. *You're It: Crisis, Change, and How to Lead When It Matters Most*. New York, Public Affairs, 2019.

58. New Zealand Government. Unite against COVID-19. *Twitter*. 2020. https://twitter.com/covid19nz?ref_src=twsrc%5Egoogle%7Ctwcamp%5Eserp%7Ctwgr%5Eauthor (Accessed April 1, 2020).

59. New Zealand's Jacinda Ardern takes 20% pay cut during coronavirus pandemic. 2020. *YouTube*. www.youtube.com/watch?v=vmep4N0MBr8 (Accessed April 1, 2020).

60. Elving R. Trump tries on the mantle of "wartime president." *National Public Radio*. 2020. www.npr.org/2020/03/22/819672681/trump-tries-on-the-mantle-of-wartime-president (Accessed April 1, 2020).

Index

Abrysvo, 167
acceptance, 206, 210, 215, 315
accessibility, 66, 86, 115, 119, 122, 124, 126
ACIP (Advisory Committee on Immunization Practices), 92–93, 171
active listening, 62, 152, 237, 314
Acton, Amy, 17, 19, 20, 283
ADKAR model, 257, 272
after-action review (AARs), 3, 11, 26, 191, 261, 262–63
agenda setting theory, 262, 295
alerting systems, 108
anaphylaxis, 6, 92–93, 94
anthrax, 7, 177
anxiety, 9–10, 69, 114–15, 248, 252, 291, 320–21
Ardern, Jacinda, 291–92, 317–19, 320, 321–23
ASPR (Administration for Strategic Preparedness and Readiness), 87
audiences, 51, 52–54, 140–43, 145–47, 178–80, 237–39, 286–88
  accessibility, 66, 86, 115, 119, 122, 124, 126
  appropriate language, 66
  emotional communication, 134
  external, 51, 53, 60, 115
  focused action, 145, 179, 218, 237
  health literacy, 62
  identification, 3, 27, 51, 60, 146, 150
  internal, 51, 52, 60, 244
  information needs, 60
  key, 3, 10, 141, 145, 178, 237
  limited English proficiency (LEP), 33, 66
  multiple, 58
  relationships or network affiliation, 51
  segmentation, 53–57, 146, 149–51, 179–80, 184, 238
  application, 55–60, 63–64, 86
  foodborne illness outbreak, 184
  information needs, 51
  medical audiences, 86
  medical communities as segment, 87–89, 91–92, 96
  MMR immunization, 238, 242
  origins, 54
  process, 54
  risk explanations, 131
  segment identification, 51
  stakeholder vs. partner, 60
  We Can Do This campaign, 218
  tailoring communication to, 203

Be Credible principle, 8–9, 18, 70, 71, 131, 249, 274–75
Be First principle, 8–22, 69–70, 154–56, 249, 274–76, 296–97
Be Right principle, 8, 69–70, 154, 156–57, 274–76, 296–97
beginner's mind, 314–15
behavior change, 202–3, 205, 207, 215, 268, 271–72
Berkley Media Studies Group, 231
Besser, Richard, 144
Beyfortus, 167
Biden, Joseph, Jr., 235
Biomedical Research Alliance, 211
block and bridge technique, 292
body language, 114, 132, 289, 301

boomerang effect, 208–9
Boston Congress of Public Health (BCPH), 127, 128–29, 132–34
boundaries, 314
British Petroleum (BP), 284
Brown, Brené, 312, 314
Bryan, Albert, 170
Buddhism, 312, 314
Burgum, Doug, 143–44
burnout, 114, 208, 236, 305, 306, 310–12, 323
Buser, Genevieve, 89
Butte County, CA, 127–29, 134
Buttigieg, Pete, 40, 41, 43, 44, 46

Cacioppo, John, 97
California, 63, 128–29, 133, 144, 171, 234, 277
California Camp Fire, 127–29, 131–35
call centers, 33, 121, 152, 186–87, 220–21, 244–45, 261
calm stillness, 313
campaign implementation, 204
case studies, 3, 8, 16, 21, 35–36, 55, 56, 67
  audience segmentation for outbreaks, 55–56
  California Camp Fire, 127–33
  CDC COCA Call COVID-19 Vaccines, 92–94
  DHHS digital campaign and vaccine uptake, 209–17
  East Palestine Train Derailment, 39, 46
  Ebola epidemic, 96–103
  EVALI, 272–77
  Flint Water Crisis, 153–59
  Georgia COVID-19 response, 246–51
  H1N1 initial crisis message, 144–45
  Jackson Water Crisis, 67–69

327

case studies (cont.)
  Louisiana Mpox outbreak, 189–95
  Mount Carmel Legionnaires' disease outbreak, 16–21
  New Zealand COVID-19 response, 316–23
  Odwalla Juice Outbreak, 63
  Oregon Health Authority COVID-19 resilience plan, 232–33
  spokesperson characteristics, 284–85
  Triangle Lake pesticide use, 7
  University of Oregon meningitis outbreak, 171–72
censorship, 177
Centers for Disease Control (CDC), 81–83, 84, 85, 93, 94, 100, 101, 103, 191–94, 257–73, 306
  anthrax bioterrorism response, 8
  Clinician Outreach and Community Activity call, 91
  cooperative agreement funding, 25
  COVID-19 response, 226, 305–6
    data graphics, 85
    faulty tests, 1, 85, 236
    vaccine information, 93
  Ebola response, 82–103, 229
  Health Alert Network, 109
  hurricane response Katrina, 11, 140
  meningitis vaccination recommendations, 171
  monkeypox information, 189, 192
  Mount Carmel Legionnaires' disease outbreak, 18
  pandemic preparation, 249
  recommendations childhood vaccination, 6
  SARS response, 31
  scientific guidance, 88
  smallpox information, 109
  structural reconsideration, 257–63
  Zika virus information, 79, 81–83, 84
  Zombie Preparedness campaign, 265
CERC communication phases, 8, 10–12, 130, 131, 139, 140, 248
  evaluation, 10, 11, 18, 69, 190–91
  initial, 167, see initial communication phase
  maintenance, 11, see maintenance phase
  recovery, 11, 43, 44, 225–26, 237–45, 250–51
  resolution, 11, 18, 40, 70, 71, 132, 159
CERC principles, 8–9, 17, 18, 101, 102, 130, 131, 133, 155–59, 249, 250, 251, 273–76, 297–98
  case studies
    California Camp Fire, 127, 130, 131–33, 134, 275
    Dallas Ebola outbreak, 100–2
    EVALI, 272–77
    Flint Water Crisis, 154–59
    Georgia COVID-19 response, 246–51
    Georgia public health crisis, 249–50, 252, 276
    Jackson Mississippi messaging, 70–72
    Louisiana Mpox outbreak, 191–92
    Maine COVID-19 response, 296, 298–301
    New Zealand COVID-19 response, 317–19
    train derailment, Ohio, 39, 46
    We Can Do This campaign, 204, 210, 216, 218–20
  CERC phases and, 10, 17–21, 44, 275–76
  individual principles
    Be Credible, 8–9, 18, 70, 71, 131, 249, 274–75
    Be First, 8–22, 69–70, 154–56, 249, 274–76, 296–97
    Be Right, 8, 69–70, 154, 156–57, 274–76, 296–97
    Express Empathy, 8–9, 40, 45–46, 133, 147–49, 225–26, 273–74
    Promote Action, 18, 70, 72, 154–55, 158, 160, 273–76
    Show Respect, 8–10, 18, 154–55, 159, 160, 273, 275–76
  messaging stages and, 297–98
  middle management and, 95
  origin, 9
  self-efficacy messaging and, 78
  spokesman selection and, 45, 69
CERC principles, case studies Legionella, Ohio, 16–21
CERC principles, case studies, Maine COVID-19 messaging and, 298–301
CERC Rhythm, 18, 160, 318, 320
chatbots, 121, 127
chlamydia, 189, 191
Chokwe Antar Lumumba, 68
chronic disease, 10, 12, 233
chronic obstructive pulmonary disease (COPD), 16
Churchill, Winston, 317, 323
Cieslak, Paul, 174–75
Circle of Comfort strategy, 237
Clark, Tom, 92
clearance procedures, 16, 28, 38, 100, 126
Clinician Outreach and Community Activity (COCA), 91–92
commitment statements, 43, 142, 225, 228
communication audits, 25–26, 259, 260–61
communication channels, 33–34, 84, 107, 108, 110–12, 150–51, 184–86, 241–44
  external, 58, 107, 115, 121
  internal, 52, 107, 108, 112–13, 236, 245

Index

business collaboration channels, 111–12
hospital information-sharing, 111
Microsoft Teams, 112–13
project management tools, 112
secure alerting systems, 108–11
webinars and conference calls, 113–15
communication objectives, 145, 147, 174, 179, 181, 218, 240
communication products, 91–92, 107–21, 151, 174, 179–85, 220, 243
by communication channel, 151, 185
chatbots, 127
prepared responses, 121
social media, 125
community analysis, 202
community-based participatory research (CBPR), 7, 203, 264
Community Engagement Alliance (CEAL), 258
community grief, 234, 236
community memorials, 11, 225, 234–35, 253
community preparedness, 27, 52–53
community resilience, 225, 233, 241, 257, 264
community right to know, 64, 65, 160
community-based organizations, 7, 47, 51, 73, 216, 222, 264
complaint reviews, 259, 261
conference calls, 91, 113–14, 146–51, 184, 238–43
consensus recommendations, 36–37, 47, 260
consent, 65, 211
consent language, 211
consistency, 46, 109, 155, 266, 301, 312
content analysis, 259, 260
contraceptive services, 79
Covello, Vincent, 288
COVID Collaborative, 202

COVID-19, 2–3, 126, 201–2, 226–28, 232–33, 234, 235
behavior prediction, 221
challenges for healthcare professionals, 95
data dashboards, 86, 116
economic disruption, 227
emerging media forms, 126
empathy during, 143
Georgia, 246, 247–48, 249, 251, 253, 258
identification, 246
incubation, 291
long COVID, 219
Maine, 296, 298, 300
media briefings, 281
memorials, 234–35
misinformation, 227
New Zealand, 317, 318, 319–22
physical distancing, 112
staff impacts, 236
testing, 167
vaccines, 92, 93, 170–71, 210, 213, 214–15
hesitancy, 210
success, 210
website messaging, 121, 124, 169
COVID-19 pandemic, 11, 12, 175–76, 210, 233, 245–47, 305–6
credibility, 140, 251, 282–84
acknowledgment of error, 299
commitment statements, 142, 228, 250, 252
correct information-building, 69, 101, 169
high-level officials, 73
lack of, 101
loss of, 101, 102–3, 116, 157, 159–60
Mount Carmel Health System, 19
nuanced information, 294
spokespeople, 288, 318–19
Crisis and Emergency Risk Communication framework, 9–10, 25–47, 209
Crisis and Emergency Risk Communication Toolkit, 35

crisis communication team, 28–29, 76, 111, 152
crisis communication teams sustainable, 29
crisis communications, 5, 7–8, 36, 39, 127, 131–33, 134
crisis leadership, 3–4
culpability, 208–9
curiosity, 313

Daschle, Tom, 7
data dashboards, 86, 111, 121–22, 195, 250
data graphics, 84–85
data reporting, 88, 91–92
data, patient-identifiable, 111
Deepwater Horizon disaster, 284
defamation, 64
Department of Health and Human Services (HHS), 84–85, 109, 154, 157–59, 189–90, 209–10
Department of Homeland Security (DHS), 110, 178, 265
Department of Public Health (DPH), 246–48, 272–76
desensitization, 208–9
design, 203–4
DeWine, Mike, 40–46, 283
Diana, Princess of Wales, 235
diffusion of innovation theory, 205–6
DISC assessments, 308
discernment, 306, 314
disinformation., 175, 227, *see also* misinformation; rumor
dissonance, 208–9
diversity, equity, and inclusion, 30
DMA (designated market areas), 210–11, 212, 213–15, 216
Douglas Complex Fire, 35
Duchesne, Juan, 89

Earlier, Faster, Smoother, Smarter, 267–68
Ebola, 1, 14, 97–103, 177, 229, 230
Eccles, Jacquelynne, 207

e-cigarette or vaping product use-associated lung injury (EVALI) emergency, 272–77
e-cigarettes, 272–76
education entertainment, 5, 207
Ekman, Paul, 143, 228
elaboration likelihood model, 76, 96
email newsletters, 34, 269
Emergency Operations Coordination, 27, 52–53
Emergency Public Information and Warning, 27, 52–53, 121
emergency response plans, 2, 10, 73, 103, 172
Emergency Support Function, 10, 32, 59, 61
empathy
  cognitive, 143
  compassionate, 143, 312
  crediblity and, 318–19
  emotional, 143
  expression, 297
  maintenance messaging, 298
  recovery messaging, 300
  statements omitting, 43–44
EMResource, 111
Enneagram, 309–10
Environmental Protection Agency (EPA), 40–45, 70–71, 110, 154
epidemic of apprehension, 208–9
epidemiology, 29–30, 73, 76–77, 80, 84–86, 103, 110–11
Epi-X, 91, 108, 110–11
ERC conceptual model, 268–72
evaluation
  impact, 259
  process, 204, 258, 277
  program, 231, 257–58, 259
evaluation phase, 10, 11, 18, 69, 190–91
expectancy-value theory, 208
Express Empathy principle, 8–9, 40, 45–46, 133, 147–49, 225–26, 273–74

extended parallel process model (EPPM), 206–7
external audiences, 51, 53, 60
Eyster, Mike, 172

Facebook, 119, 125, 129, 132, 269–70, 274–76
Fauci, Anthony, 2, 293
FCC (Federal Communications Commission), 117
FCPH (Franklin County Public Health), 18–19
FDA (Food and Drug Administration), 93–94, 110, 170–92, 212
Federal Emergency Management Agency (FEMA), 110, 117, 225, 263, 265
Flint, Michigan, 15, 153–60, 286
flu, 26, see influenza
focus groups, 37–38, 203, 258, 259–60, 266–67
foodborne illness, 145–50, 179–84, 240, 242–43
formative evaluation, 258
Frieden, Tom, 97, 100, 101
Fryar, Bob, 284–85

Gallup Strengths Finder, 309
generosity, 313
Genesee County Community Action Resource Department, 155
Genesee County Health Department (GCHD), 154, 157–58
Georgia, 57, 246–48, 249, 273, 274
Georgia Department of Public Health, 246, 249, 250, 252, 272–77
Glendale, 35
gonorrhea, 189
Google, 122, 123
Google Translate, 122
GovDelivery, 118–19
government censorship, 177
Grey's Anatomy, 208
grief, 234, 236, 248, 300
Grunig, James E., 54
guidance, scientific for medical professionals, 88, 91–92
Gupta, Sanjay, 126

Hanna-Attisha, Mona, 154, 156
Harris, Kamala, 235
Hart, Ariel, 246
Health Alert Network (HAN), 87, 91, 108–9, 146–51, 180–85, 238–43
  sample message, 109–10
Health belief model (HBM), 3, 201, 206–21
Health Care Coalitions (HCC), 53, 87–91
health communication, 5
health communication campaigns, 201, 202, 204, 205, 207–9, 218–21, 225, 229, 262
  design, 203
  differences from emergency risk communication, 204–5
  emergency risk communication and, 204–6
  examples
    We Can Do This, 218–20
  implementation, 203–4
  infrequency of discussion in emergency context, 201
  maintenance, 204
  overview, 202
  reasons for use, 201–2
  results dissemination, 204
  stages
    community analysis, 202–3
    design and initiate, 203, 204
  student vaccinations, 174
  system activation, 208
  unintended consequences, 208–9
Health Insurance Portability and Accountability Act (1996), 65
health literacy, 54, 62
health promotion, 5, 10
health records, 65, 127
healthcare emergency readiness coalitions (HERC), 111
healthcare providers, 5–6, 87–90, 92–94, 146–50, 179–80, 238
HIV, 167, 189, 194, 245

hospitals, 56, 57, 65, 147
  admission of e-cigarette users to, 272–73
  as audience segment, 57
  ASPR Hospital Preparedness Program, 87
  COVID-19 pandemic, 208, 247, 258, 298, 299
  Lane County measles outbreak, 56
  McLaren Flint, 156
  Mount Carmel Grove City, 16–21
hotlines, 115, 117, 121, 127
hotwashes, 237, 245, 263
humility, 301, 313, 319
Hurley, Katrina, 96
hurricanes, 140
  Katrina, 11–12, 140, 264
  Rita, 12
Husel, William, 19
hyper-arousal, 311
hypo-arousal, 311

impact evaluation, 259
Incident Command System (ICS), 52, 53, 59, 61, 113, 115, 186
Indiana, 45, 111
influenza, 26, 176, 183, 261
  avian, 149, 183, 238, 241
infodemic, 175–76, 177, 195
information needs, 52–53, 59, 60, 61, 63, 76, 86, 88–91, 107–8
  audience segmentation and, 63–64, 86, 179, 218
  changing, 139
  during health emergencies, 60–63
  internal public health audiences, 60
  media, 61
  medical community, 87–88, 91, 92, 94
  partners, 59
  partners and stakeholders, 67, 73
information-sharing, 27, 52–53, 59, 108
initial phase, 10, 42, 97–98, 101–2, 139–40, 190–91, 249, 250
  case studies
    East Palestine Train Derailment, 41–42

duration, 11, 40, 140
information accuracy, 10
messaging, 140, 146, 218, 249
press conferences, 41
Instagram, 72, 85, 123, 125, 191, 269, 276
integrity, 313
internal audiences, 51, 52, 60, 244
internal communications, 52, 107, 108, 112–13, 236, 245
interventions
  nonpharmaceutical, 27, 52–53, 81–82, 90, 167, 173
  pharmaceutical, 11, 164, 167, 174, 176, 201
interviews, 55, 126, 288–89, 292, 293–95, 296, 301
  epidemiological, 261
  in-depth, 259, 260–61
  intercept, 259–60
  one-on-one, 294–95
  semistructured, 37, 258

Jackson Water Crisis, 67–68, 70–73
Joint Information Center, 8, 25, 27, 28, 29–31, 258, 261
Jones, Lauren, 172, 173
joy, 313
Jung, Carl, 308

Kabat-Zinn, Jon, 245
Kanter, Joseph, 192
Kegeles, Stephen, 221
Kemp, Brian, 246–48
key audiences, 3, 10, 141, 145, 178, 237
Khan, Ibad, 92
Kitsap County, 118

Lane County Health and Human Services (LCHHS), 56, 171, 172
leadership, 17, 26, 296, 298, 315, 317, 322–23
leadership qualities, 305, 312, 315, 323
  acceptance, 315
  accountability, 4, 102, 117, 157, 160, 257, 314
  active listening, 62, 152, 237, 314

beginner's mind, 314–15
calm stillness, 313
compassionate empathy, 312
courage, 312
curiosity, 313
discernment, 306, 314
generosity, 313
humility, 313
integrity, 313
joy, 313
love and respect, 315
self-awareness, 306, 312, 314
steadfastness and consistency, 312
vulnerability, 4, 70, 132, 207, 312, 314
legal authority, 4, 66
Legionella, 16, 20, 158–59
Legionnaires' disease, 16–20, 21, 156–57, 158, 160, 177
Leventhal, Howard, 221
Lewin, Kurt, 264
libel, 64
literature reviews, 88, 259, 262
long COVID, 219
long-term, 59, 176–77, 201–2, 205–6, 220–21, 264–65, 268–69
long-term health emergencies, 201–2, 205–6, 220–21, 229
long-term health emergencies, 229
Los Molinos, 206
Louisiana, 189–94, 284
love and respect, 315
Luedtke, Patrick, 172, 174

Mackey, John, 307
Maine, 296, 298–301
maintenance phase, 11, 41, 42, 43, 45, 131, 165, 178–81, 274–76
  audience segmentation, 179–80, 190
  case studies
    California Camp Fire, 132
    East Palestine Train Derailment, 40–44, 45, 46
    Ohio Ebola outbreak, 101
  communications planning, 237–38
  duration, 40

maintenance phase (cont.)
  Georgia vaping crisis, 275–76
  media management, 19
  messaging during, 41–45, 80, 164, 165, 298, 299
  misinformation pushback, 18
  Oregon meningitis outbreak, 173
  overview, 11
  public communication, 20
  rumor management, 164–65, 169
  transition to recovery phase, 225–26
  trust and credibility, 176
  uncertainty and, 176
Markey, Ed, 235
Marston, Wiliam Moulton, 308
Mask Policy, 247, 307
masks, 56, 132, 133, 143–44, 167, 305–6, 307
McCluhan, Marshall, 114
McKibben, Sean, 20
measles, 56–57, 89, 148, 182, 238, 240
  messaging examples, 145–47, 151, 179, 238, 240, 241, 243
media briefings, 32–33, 60, 115–17, 119, 120, 169, 287–89, 293, 295
  body language, 289
  contingency plans, 116
  debriefs, 116
  information concerning, 59, 60–61, 116, 294
  journalist Q&As, 292–93
  location, 115, 294
  media notification, 116
  messaging during, 116, 141, 169, 294
  pre-COVID-19, 281
  sign language interpretation, 30
  social media embeds, 126
  spokeperson identification, 116
  support personnel, 115
  townhalls and, 119
  virtual, 281
media inquiries, 33, 258
media interviews, 30, *see* interviews

media monitoring, 29, 177, 259–62
media naturalness theory, 114
media relations, 4, 29–30, 150–51, 174, 180–85, 242–43, 288
media richness theory, 107–8
memorandum of understanding (MOU), 16
memorials, 11, 225, 234–35, 253
men who have sex with men (MSM), 189
meningitis, 171, 173, 175
MERS, 38
message testing, 16, 25, 26, 36–38, 203, 205
Messonnier, Nancy, 2
Michigan, 15, 117, 153–54, 155, 156–57, 159–60, 286
microcephaly, 77, 81, 84
Microsoft Office, 112
Microsoft Teams, 112, 113
Middle Eastern respiratory syndrome (MERS), 38
Miller, Katherine, 236
Mills, Janet, 296, 298
mindfulness, 3, 143, 245, 287, 291, 312–13
misinformation, 42–43, 127, 164–65, 170–83, 195
Mississippi Emergency Management Agency, 72
monkeypox, 3, 165–67, 189–94
Mount Carmel Health System, 16–19, 20, 21
Move Your Way campaign, 5
Mpox, 3, *see* monkeypox
MSW, 295, 301
multiyear emergencies, 201
Murthy v. Missouri, 178
Myers–Briggs Type Indicator (MBTI), 308

Naranjo, Claudio, 309
narcissism
  grandiose, 307
  vulnerable, 307
National Assessment of Adult Literacy, 62
National COVID-19 Memorial Wall, 235

National Emergency Management Agency (New Zealand), 317
National Incident Management System (NIMS), 8, 30
National Opinion Research Center (NORC), 211
National Research Council, 6
National Transportation Safety Board (NTSB), 43–44
Nationalist Social Club, 296
neomycin, 6
network manipulation, 187–88
new normal, 11, 40, 225–26, 230, 232–33, 234, 240
New Orleans, 189–90, 194
New York City Health Department, 167
New Zealand, 264, 316–22, 323
Nilsen, Thomas, 6
nirsevimab, 167–68
nonpharmaceutical interventions (NPIs), 27, 52–53, 81–82, 90, 167, 173
nonverbal communication, 116, 281, 288–90, 294–95
North Dakota, 143–44, 312

Obama, Barack, 78–80, 83, 154
Obama, Michele, 204
obfuscation, 208–9
ODH (Ohio Department of Health), 17, 18–19, 20, 283
Odwalla Juice Outbreak, 63–64
Ohio Emergency Management Agency, 41, 42
opportunity cost, 208–9
Oregon, 65, 66, 89, 111, 171–74, 230, 232–33
Oregon Department of Forestry, 7, 35
Oregon Health Authority (OHA), 7, 88, 171, 173, 174, 230, 232–33
outcome evaluation, 258–59, 262

outrage factors, 14–15
Oxitec, 83

palivizumab, 168
parasocial interaction, 207
partner agencies, 10, 31, 36–37, 120, 126, 152, 186
Pence, Michael, 168
Personality Assessment Tools, 307
pharmaceutical interventions, 11, 164, 167, 174, 176, 201
phase-based messaging, 8, see CERC communication phases
podcasts, 121, 126
police powers, 66
PPE (personal protective equipment), 2, 89, 90, 91–92, 247, 300, 305
precrisis planning, 3, 8, 10, 35–36, 51, 69, 265
prepared response (PR), 121, 152, 186
preparedness activities, 4, 10, 25, 36, 38, 249
press conferences, 40–44, 46, 99, 100, 129, 132, 133
Privacy Act (1974), 64–65
process evaluation, 204, 258, 277
program evaluation, 231, 257–58, 259
project management tools, 112, 152
Promote Action principle, 8–9, 18, 38–39, 154–55, 158, 190, 273–76
Proud Boys, 296
public education, 92, 209–10, 211, 216–17, 229–30, 264–65, 277
public education campaigns, 210, 211, 216–17, 229–30, 264–65
public health emergency preparedness (PHEP), 4, 25, 26, 52–74, 87, 231
  PHEP capabilities, 28, 52
public health law, 8, 64, 66
Public Health Workforce Interests and Needs Survey, 2

public information officers, 2, 12, 16, 28–30, 32, 132, 152
public inquiries, 117, 259, 260–61
public speaking anxiety, 290–91
Puerto Rico, 83, 273

quality improvement, 4

rapid response, 4
recovery messages, 77, 80, 145, 225, 226, 229, 234
recovery phase, 11, 43, 44, 225–26, 237–45, 250–51
  messaging, 44
  policy changes during, 11
Redfield, Robert, 293
Rehabilitation Act (1973), 66
reorganization, 263, 272
resilience, 225, 232–34, 241, 247, 257, 264, 310
resolution phase, 11, 18, 40, 70, 71, 132, 159
respiratory syncytial virus (RSV), 165–67, 265
response timeliness, 21
retrospective sensemaking, 263
Reynolds, Barbara, 317, 320
RICE framework, 266
right to know, 64, 65, 160
RISE program, 233
risk
  dread, 13
  explanation, 42–43, 80–81, 131, 158–59, 165, 173, 181
  perception, 3, 12, 13, 15, 268–70, 271
risk communication, 5–7, 15, 17, 40, 43, 46, 266–67
ritualized actions, 234
Rogers, Everett, 206
Rosenstock, Irwin M., 221
rumors, 32–33, 83, 169–83, 187, 188
  algorithmic manipulation, 188
  California Camp Fire, 132
  diminished trust, 188
  maintenance phase, 169, 249
  measles outbreak, 181–82, 183
  misinformation and, 175
  social network position, 188
  Spiro–Starbird virality framework, 187–88
  spokespeople addressing, 169–70
  uncertainty, 188
  viral, 188
  websites addressing, 169
  Zika virus, 81, 83

Sandman, Peter, 14
Sandy Hook Elementary, 237
Santa Barbara, 171
scientific guidance, 88, 91–92
search engine optimization (SEO), 121, 123–24
Seeger, Matthew W., 268–69
Seinfeld, Jerry, 290
self-awareness, 306, 312, 314
severe acute respiratory syndrome (SARS), 31, 176
Shady Cove, 35
Shah, Nirav, 295–96, 298–301
SharePoint, 112
Shimabukuro, Tom, 92
Show Respect principle, 8–10, 18, 154–55, 159, 160, 273, 275–76
showing respect, 251, 273–74, 286, 287
slander, 64
Slovic, Paul, 13
Slow the Spread campaign, 210
smallpox, 109, 189
smoke inhalation, 35–36
social media management, 29, 30, 84
social media, 96, 125, 177, 210–11, 250–51, 266–67, 269, see also Facebook; Instagram; Twitter
social networks, 187–88
social norming, 208–9
social reproduction, 208–9
social resilience, 234
source credibility, 41, 44, 71, 139, 268, 270, 271
Southern Decadence, 189–90, 194
spokespeople, 28, 30, 115, 116, 117, 119, 120, 281–84, 286, 287, 288, 289, 290, 294

Index

spokespeople (cont.)
  addressing rumors, 169, 244
  body language, 289
  CDC, 8
  characteristics, 283–84
  components of role, 281
    dealing with criticism, 282
    face of issue, 281
    message consistency, 282, 283, 287
    representative of health agency, 282
  coordination with others, 46, 116, 119, 152, 244
  credibility, 318
  designation, 28, 45
  empathy, 62, 143, 228
  identification, 28, 116
  information currency, 220
  key tips for, 139, 152, 164, 186, 220, 244
  language used, 286, 290, 293
  location, 115–16, 289, 294
  nonverbal communication, 290
  officials as, 29, 174, 288
  one-on-one interviews, 295
  pitfalls, 286–87
  politicians as, 42, 43, 45, 73, 319
  preparation, 116, 288
  professionalism, 287
  quantity, 8, 271
  recovery phase, 244
  response techniques, 292–93
  responsibilities, 30
  scientists as, 29
  talking points, 117
  townhalls, 119
  Trinity Health, 19
  truthfulness, 286
stakeholder management theory, 57, 67
stakeholder type, 58–59
Starbird, Kate, 176, 187
steadfastness, 240, 306, 312
Stiles, Kattaryna, 88
STIs (sexually transmitted infections), 167, 189–94
Streck, Richard, 20
stress, 69, 96, 103, 114–15, 236, 245, 310–11

structural reconsideration, 263
subject matter experts (SMEs), 25, 26–30, 36, 76, 141, 286
Superstorm Sandy, 264
surveys, 3, 37, 211–12, 259–60, 310
Synder, Rick, 154
system activation, 208–9
Szent-Gyorgi, Albert, 13

talking points, 60–61, 116–17, 125, 151–52, 179–85, 243, 292
This Is Our Shot campaign, 170–71
TikTok, 121, 126
Time For You program, 258
tone of voice, 116–30, 290, 295–301
tools
  online meeting, 252
  project management, 112
  videoconferencing, 114, 115
Toomley, Kathleen, 252
townhall meetings, 60, 107, 119–21, 177, 259, 262
training, 29, 264
transformation leadership theory, 315
translators, 30
transparency, 21, 140, 141, 159, 250, 251, 252
Triangle Lake, 7
Trinity Health, 19, 20
Trump, Donald J., 40, 41, 43–44, 45, 129, 306, 307
trust
  development, 177, 190, 248–49
  in government, 176
  loss of, 187–88, 250
Twin Arches memorial, 235
Twitter, 70, 72, 118–25, 155, 156, 300

Uganda, 77, 229–30
uncertainty reduction theory, 152–53
unintended consequences of health communication campaigns, 208
University of Oregon, 171–74
US Ad Council, 202

Vaccine Adverse Event Reporting System, 93
vaccines, 6, 92–94, 166, 167, 170, 171, 194, 209–17
  confidence, 213–14
  cost, 172
  COVID-19, 92, 93, 170–71, 210, 213, 214–15
  Pfizer–BioNTech, 93
  hesitancy, 1, 202, 210
  influenza, 183
  mandates, 15, 174
  measles, 182
  meningitis, 173
  misinformation, 181
  MMRV, 6
  monkeypox, 192–94
  novelty, 14
  respiratory syncytial virus, 168
  safety, 93, 210, 219
  schedules, 148
  smallpox, 109
  uptake rates, 202
  Zika virus, 79, 81
Vacunateya, 170–71
value-based messaging, 232
verbal communication, 153, 288, 290, 295
vicarious learnings, 263–64
Virgin Islands, 83, 170, 273

Walensky, Rochelle, 229, 287–88
Warren, Elizabeth, 235
Washington State Health Department, 230
We Can Do This campaign, 204, 210, 216, 218–20
WEA (wireless emergency alerts), 117–18
Weaver, Karen, 154
webinars, 91–92, 94, 113, 115, 119, 186, 220
websites, 107, 109, 116–17, 120, 121–25, 210, 275–76
  anchor text, 123–24
  content, 122
  inbound and outbound links, 125
  keywords, 69, 123–24
  managers, 30, 84
  page titles, 123–24

Whole Foods, 307
wildfires, 12, 26, 35–36, 140, 226, 233
window of tolerance theory, 311
Wireless Emergency Alert system, 117–18
workforce, 2–3, 4, 29, 231–32, 233, 236, 244–45
World Health Organization, 77, 78–79, 125, 127, 175, 227–28, 316–17
Wuhan, 246, 293, 316, 318

X, 70, *see* Twitter

'yes and . . .' technique, 292
Young, Ashley, 79
YouTube, 72, 119, 125, 156, 158, 191, 300

Zika virus, 77–84, 110
Zoom, 114–15, 119
  fatigue, 113–15

For EU product safety concerns, contact us at Calle de José Abascal, 56–1°, 28003 Madrid, Spain or eugpsr@cambridge.org.

www.ingramcontent.com/pod-product-compliance
Lightning Source LLC
LaVergne TN
LVHW021942060526
838200LV00042B/1892